SMALL
ANIMAL
CARDIOLOGY
SECRETS

SMALL ANIMAL CARDIOLOGY SECRETS

JONATHAN A. ABBOTT, DVM, Dip ACVIM (Cardiology)
Associate Professor
Department of Small Animal Clinical Sciences
Virginia-Maryland Regional College of Veterinary Medicine
Virginia Polytechnic Institute and State University
Blacksburg, Virginia

HANLEY & BELFUS, INC.
An Affiliate of Elsevier

HANLEY & BELFUS
An Affiliate of Elsevier

The Curtis Center
Independence Square West
Philadelphia, Pennsylvania 19106

Note to the reader: Although the information in this book has been carefully reviewed for correctness of dosage and indications, neither the authors nor the editor nor the publisher can accept any legal responsibility for any errors or omissions that may be made. Neither the publisher nor the editor makes any warranty, expressed or implied, with respect to the material contained herein. Before prescribing any drug, the reader must review the manufacturer's current product information (package inserts) for accepted indications, absolute dosage recommendations, and other information pertinent to the safe and effective use of the product described.

Library of Congress Cataloging-in-Publication Data

Small Animal Cardiology Secrets / edited by Jonathan Abbott.
     p. ; cm.—(The Secrets Series®)
     Includes bibliographical references and index.
     ISBN 1-56053-352-8 (alk. paper)
        1. Dogs—Diseases—Examinations, questions, etc. 2. Cats—Diseases—
Examinations, questions, etc. 3. Veterinary cardiology—Examinations, questions,
etc. I. Abbott, Jonathan, 1965– II. Series.
     [DNLM: 1. Cardiovascular Diseases—veterinary—Examination Questions.
2. Diseases—therapy—Examination Questions. 3. Cat Diseases—therapy—
Examination Questions. 5. Veterinary Medicine—methods—Examination Questions.]
SF992.C37 S62 2000
636.7'089612—dc21

                                  00-023234

SMALL ANIMAL CARDIOLOGY SECRETS   ISBN 1-56053-352-8

Permissions may be sought directly from Elsevier's Health Sciences Rights Department in Philadelphia, USA: phone: (+1)215-238-7869, fax: (+1)215-238-2239, email: healthpermissions@elsevier.com. You may also complete your request on-line via the Elsevier Science homepage (http://www.elsevier.com), by selecting 'Customer Support' and then 'Obtaining Permissions'.

Last digit is the print number: 9 8 7 6 5 4 3

CONTENTS

CONTRIBUTORS

Jonathan A. Abbott, D.V.M., Dip ACVIM (Cardiology)
Associate Professor, Department of Small Animal Clinical Sciences, Virginia-Maryland Regional College of Veterinary Medicine, Virginia Polytechnic Institute and State University, Blacksburg, Virginia

Julie Armstrong, D.V.M.
Department of Veterinary Internal Medicine, Western College of Veterinary Medicine, University of Saskatchewan, Saskatoon, Saskatchewan, Canada

Clarke E. Atkins, D.V.M., Dip ACVIM (Internal Medicine and Cardiology)
Professor of Medicine and Cardiology, Department of Clinical Sciences, College of Veterinary Medicine, North Carolina State University, Raleigh, North Carolina

Catherine J. Baty, D.V.M., Ph.D.
Hitchings-Elion Fellow, Burroughs Wellcome Fund, University of North Carolina-Chapel Hill, Chapel Hill, North Carolina

Andrew W. Beardow, B.V.M.&S., MRCVS, Dip ACVIM (Cardiology)
Vice-President, Cardiopet, Veterinary Referral Centre, Little Falls, New Jersey

Darlene R. Blischok, D.V.M.
Cardiology Resident, Veterinary Referral Centre, Little Falls, New Jersey

John D. Bonagura, D.V.M., M.S., Dip ACVIM (Cardiology)
Professor, Department of Veterinary Medicine and Surgery, University of Missouri-Columbia, Columbia, Missouri

Betsy R. Bond, D.V.M.
Staff Cardiologist, Department of Medicine, The Animal Medical Center, New York, New York

Davin J. Borde, D.V.M.
Cardiology Resident, Veterinary Heart Institute, Gainesville, Florida

Maribeth J. Bossbaly, V.M.D., Dip ACVIM (Cardiology)
Veterinary Cardiologist, Heartsound Consultants, Veterinary Specialty and Emergency Center, Langhorne, Pennsylvania

Janice McIntosh Bright, B.S.N., M.S., D.V.M.
Associate Professor of Cardiology, Department of Clinical Sciences, College of Veterinary Medicine and Biomedical Sciences, Colorado State University; Cardiologist, Veterinary Teaching Hospital, Fort Collins, Colorado

William A. Brown, D.V.M., Dip ACVIM (Cardiology)
Veterinary Cardiology Consultants, Birmingham, Michigan

Dana A. Buoscio, D.V.M., Dip ACVIM (Cardiology)
Chicagoland Veterinary Cardiology, Willowbrook, Illinois

Clay A. Calvert, D.V.M.
Professor, Department of Small Animal Medicine, College of Veterinary Medicine, University of Georgia, Athens, Georgia

Nigel A. Caulkett, D.V.M., M.V.Sc., Dip ACVA
Associate Professor, Department of Veterinary Anesthesiology, Radiology and Surgery, Western College of Veterinary Medicine, University of Saskatchewan, Saskatoon, Saskatchewan, Canada

Teresa C. DeFrancesco, D.V.M., Dip ACVIM (Cardiology)
Clinical Assistant Professor, Department of Clinical Sciences, College of Veterinary Medicine, North Carolina State University, Raleigh, North Carolina

Marilyn Dunn, D.M.V., M.V.Sc., Dip ACVIM (Internal Medicine)
Staff Internist, Department of Small Animal Medicine, Centre Vétérinaire DMV, Ville St-Laurent, Quebec, Canada

Charles S. Farrow, B.Sc., D.V.M., Dip ACVR
Professor of Medical Imaging, Consultant in Veterinary Instructional Development, Western College of Veterinary Medicine, University of Saskatchewan, Saskatoon, Saskatchewan, Canada

Virginia Luis Fuentes, M.A., Vet.M.B., D.V.C., MRCVS
Assistant Professor, Department of Veterinary Medicine and Surgery, University of Missouri-Columbia, Columbia, Missouri

Rebecca E. Gomph, D.V.M., M.S., Dip ACVIM (Cardiology)
Associate Professor of Cardiology, Department of Small Animal Clinical Sciences, The University of Tennessee College of Veterinary Medicine, Knoxville, Tennessee

John-Karl Goodwin, D.V.M., Dip ACVIM (Cardiology)
Adjunct Assistant Professor, Division of Cardiology, University of Florida College of Veterinary Medicine, Director and Staff Cardiologist, Veterinary Heart Institute, Gainesville, Florida

Robert L. Hamlin, D.V.M., Ph.D., Dip ACVIM (Internal Medicine and Cardiology)
Professor of Veterinary Physiology and Pharmacology, Department of Veterinary Biosciences, College of Veterinary Medicine, Ohio State University, Columbus, Ohio

David H. Knight, D.V.M., M.Med.Sc.
Professor of Cardiology, Department of Clinical Studies, School of Veterinary Medicine, and Chief, Section of Cardiology, Veterinary Hospital, University of Pennsylvania, Philadelphia, Pennsylvania

Nancy J. Laste, D.V.M., Dip ACVIM (Cardiology)
Staff Cardiologist, Angell Memorial Animal Hospital, Boston, Massachusetts

Michael B. Lesser, D.V.M., Dip ACVIM (Cardiology)
Head of Medicine, Advanced Veterinary Care Center, Lawndale, California

Carroll Loyer, D.V.M., Dip ACVIM (Cardiology)
Veterinary Cardiologist, Englewood, Colorado

Steven L. Marks, B.V.Sc., M.S., MRCVS, Dip ACVIM (Cardiology)
Assistant Professor of Internal Medicine, Department of Veterinary Clinical Sciences, Louisiana State University School of Veterinary Medicine, Baton Rouge, Louisiana

Matthew S. Mellema, D.V.M.
Veterinary Medical Teaching Hospital, School of Veterinary Medicine, University of California-Davis, Davis, California

Paolo Porzio, D.V.M., M.Vet.Sci., Dip ACVIM (Internal Medicine)
Assistant Professor, Department of Clinical Studies, Ontario Veterinary College, University of Guelph, Guelph, Ontario, Canada

Carl D. Sammarco, B.V.Sc., MRCVS, Dip ACVIM (Cardiology)
Cardiopet Inc., Veterinary Referral Centre, Little Falls, New Jersey

Donald P. Schrope, D.V.M.
Staff Cardiologist, Veterinary Referral Centre, Little Falls, New Jersey

Margaret M. Sleeper, V.M.D.
Section of Cardiology, Veterinary Hospital, University of Pennsylvania, Philadelphia, Pennsylvania

Francis W. K. Smith, Jr., D.V.M.
Clinical Assistant Professor, Department of Medicine, Tufts University School of Veterinary Medicine, North Grafton, Massachusetts

Patti S. Snyder, D.V.M., M.S., Dip ACVIM
Associate Professor, Department of Small Animal Clinical Sciences,, University of Florida College of Veterinary Medicine, Gainesville, Florida

Mark E. Stamoulis, D.V.M., Dip ACVIM (Cardiology)
Clinical Assistant Professor, Department of Medicine, Tufts University School of Veterinary Medicine, North Grafton, Massachusetts

Rebecca L. Stepien, D.V.M., M.S., Dip ACVIM (Cardiology)
Clinical Assistant Professor, Department of Medical Sciences, University of Wisconsin School of Veterinary Medicine, and Clinical Cardiologist, University of Wisconsin Veterinary Medical Teaching Hospital, Madison, Wisconsin

Wendy A. Ware, D.V.M., M.S.
Associate Professor, Department of Veterinary Clinical Sciences and Biomedical Sciences, Iowa State University College of Veterinary Medicine, Staff Cardiologist, Veterinary Teaching Hospital, Ames, Iowa

Kathy N. Wright, D.V.M.
Assistant Professor, Division of Cardiology, Department of Pediatrics, The University of Cincinnati/Children's Hospital Medical Center, Cincinnati, Ohio

PREFACE

In recent years, the discipline of veterinary cardiology has evolved to a remarkable extent; diagnostic capabilities have improved considerably, which has led to changes in therapeutic approach. The catalog of cardiac medications that are available to the practicing veterinarian is ever expanding and new interventional techniques have been added to the management of congenital heart disease.

This volume is not intended to take the place of traditional textbooks; rather, it conforms to a format that has been successful when adapted to other medical and veterinary disciplines. Each chapter consists of a series of questions that relate to specific areas of veterinary cardiology; each followed by an answer. The depth and detail of the answers vary considerably; in some instances the question spurs a discussion of pathophysiologic mechanisms or the efficacy of a therapeutic approach, while in others the answer is simply a statement of fact. The value of this format lies in its similarity to the teaching method that is used by most clinical veterinary educators; questions are used to test knowledge, to stimulate discussion, and to prompt the student to assimilate facts. It is my hope that this book is of value to those for whom it was written: students, house officers, and practitioners with an interest in the fascinating discipline of veterinary cardiology. Finally, I wish to thank the contributing authors who took the time to share their expertise and knowledge.

Jonathan A. Abbott, D.V.M., Dip ACVIM (Cardiology)

Dedication

This book is dedicated to
our patients,
and also to ARA and MHA.

Jonathan A. Abbott

I. Cardiovascular Function and Dysfunction

1. CARDIOVASCULAR PHYSIOLOGY

Robert L. Hamlin, D.V.M., Ph.D.

1. What is cardiac performance?

The cardiovascular system serves to deliver oxygen and nutrients to body tissues and to remove the waste products of metabolism. In order to accomplish this, the heart must generate force in order to propel blood through the vascular system and it must do so while maintaining a blood pressure that is adequate to perfuse vital tissues. Cardiac performance is a general term that refers to pumping ability; it depends not only on the strength, or contractility, of the myocardium but also on cardiac filling and the physiologic state of the blood vessels. Clinically important factors that determine cardiac performance include the following: (1) heart rate; (2) force of contraction; (3) interference to flow of blood; (4) the amount of oxygen present in the myocardium; and (5) the stiffness of the myocardium.

2. What determines heart rate? How does heart rate relate to cardiac performance?

Heart rate (HR) is expressed as the number of times the heart beats each minute. For dogs it varies from 35 (during sleep) to over 240 during maximal exertion and/or excitement. The normal values for these states are not known; but what is known is that heart rates, contrary to common belief, are no different between large dogs and small dogs.

HR is determined by how frequently a wave of stimulation (also called a wave of depolarization) travels through the heart and shocks it into contraction. This wave of depolarization begins normally in the sinoatrial node (SAN) located at the juncture of the right atrium and cranial vena cava. The SAN has an intrinsic rate of discharge of approximately 100 times per minute, but the rate of discharge may be accelerated by heating (e.g., fever) or slowed by cooling (e.g., hypothermia). More importantly, the rate of discharge of the SAN is accelerated when norepinephrine—produced by sympathetic efferent traffic—binds to B1-receptors on the SAN, or it is slowed when acetylcholine—produced by parasympathetic or vagal efferent traffic—binds to the cholinergic receptors.

HR can be measured by listening with a stethoscope, by feeling the heart thump against the thoracic wall (i.e., the apex beat), by feeling femoral arterial pulsations, or from an electrocardiogram. (Actually, the electrocardiogram only tells you whether the heart was electrically stimulated to beat, not whether or not it beat!)

The relationship between heart rate and cardiac output is direct except at heart rates that are so rapid that ventricular filling is impaired. If other factors that affect cardiac performance remain unchanged, increases in HR result in increases in cardiac output. However, when HR is very high, ventricular filling is impaired and cardiac performance declines; this phenomenon is particularly pronounced in large, diseased hearts. Because of this and because heart rate is an important determinant of myocardial oxygen consumption, diseased hearts tend to tolerate tachycardia poorly.

3. What is "sinus arrhythmia"? What is its physiologic basis?

For dogs—but much less so for cats—heart rate speeds during inspiration and slows during expiration. This is known as a respiratory sinus arrhythmia (RSA), and the RSA is caused by decreasing (during inspiration) and increasing (during expiration) vagal efferent traffic to the SAN.

1

Those changes in vagal tone result from irradiations to the vagal centers in the medulla from juxtaposed ventilatory center discharge and the intactness of the parasympathetic nervous system.

4. In a very approximate way, heart rate is inversely related to systemic blood pressure. What is the explanation for this relationship?

HR varies inversely with systemic arterial blood pressure (BP) and, therefore, BP may be somewhat monitored by HR. The higher the BP, the lower the HR, and vice versa. This relationship to sustain BP normal occurs because of the baroreceptor reflex in the following way:

1. BP falls.
2. High-pressure baroreceptors in the aortic arch and carotid sinus detect less stretch.
3. The receptors send fewer afferent volleys along the vagus and glossopharyngeal nerves to the brain.
4. The medulla oblongata perceives fewer volleys and, after "discussions" with the hypothalamus, decides to take remedial action, which is speeding of the HR by decreasing vagal efferent traffic to the SAN.
5. Because HR is increased, which caused the amount of blood pumped by the heart to increase, the BP returns toward normal. (Of course, concurrent sympathetically mediated vasoconstriction also helps in the return of pressure toward normal.)

Should BP increase instead of having decreased, the HR will decrease, because the baroreceptors will "tell" the medulla that the BP is too high, and the medulla will slow HR and dilate systemic arterioles, thus restoring normal BP.

5. What determines the force of ventricular contraction?

The force generated by the left ventricle (the ventricle usually of greatest importance for the clinician) is determined by 3 factors:

1. The volume of blood within it just before it contracts (termed the preload).
2. The rate of cross-bridge cycling (termed myocardial contractility or the inotropic state) of the contractile machinery (actually the heavy meromyosin heads that are tiny cross-bridges extending between two other proteins) of the myocardium.
3. The interference the left ventricles perceive to ejecting blood (termed the afterload).

6. How and why does preload affect the force of contraction?

Preload (PL) is a prime determinant of the force of contraction because it determines the number of contractile units (heavy meromyosin heads) that are cycling and the amount of calcium available to permit the cycling. This relationship determines the Frank-Starling law of the heart that states that, all else being constant, the force of ventricular contraction is determined by the degree of stretch on the myocardial fibers just before they contract. In other words, the heart pumps out whatever returns to it; or yet another way, the heart cannot pump out what it does not receive.

7. What factors determine the preload?

The PL is determined by the end-diastolic pressure (EDP) (i.e., the pressure within the ventricle just before it begins to contract) minus the pleural pressure (i.e., the pressure on the outside of the heart), all divided by the stiffness (i.e., elasticity modulus) of the ventricular wall. (The same is true for how big a balloon gets when you blow it up. The size is determined by the pressure inside minus the pressure outside all divided by how stiff the balloon is.)

The EDP is determined by the pressure of blood in the lungs, since it is that pressure, upstream from the left ventricle, which pushes blood into the ventricle. The pressure of blood within the lungs is determined by how much blood is in the lungs, which is determined by two factors: how much blood is somewhere else, and how thoroughly the left ventricle removes blood from the lungs and pumps it into and through the arteries.

How much blood is somewhere else (i.e., not in the lungs) is determined by the degree of constriction or relaxation of the smooth muscle in the systemic veins (usually of the abdomen), including the spleen and liver, where most (approximately 70%) of blood is normally found. A compound called a venodilator (e.g., nitroglycerin) dilates the veins of the abdomen (increases capacitance), blood is stolen from the lungs to fill up the abdominal veins, pressure within the lungs falls, and the left ventricular PL—and force of contraction—fall. Of course, another factor important to PL is the blood volume (BV). The greater the BV, the greater the PL, and vice versa. And remember, all else being equal, force of contraction is related to PL. BV is determined by a balance between water intake and urine output. Thus, after a day of vomiting and diarrhea in which a great deal of water and BV has been lost, the force of contraction of the ventricle may become feeble.

How well the ventricle removes blood from the lungs depends on its health (i.e., its contractility), and how much interference is produced by the systemic vasculature. If the ventricle weakens, it pumps less blood into and through the arteries, and the blood it did not pump remains in the lungs. Thus the feeble ventricle ends up being overfilled with blood. On the contrary, a ventricle that vigorously pumps excess blood into and through the arterial circulation, removes extra blood from the lungs, thus decreasing its PL. (The blood the left ventricle pumps out ultimately returns to the lungs after traversing the peripheral capillaries and veins, and being pumped into the lungs by the right ventricle.)

The PL is determined by the difference in pressure between the blood inside the chamber (the EDP) minus the pleural pressure (P_{PL}), and since the P_{PL} is normally subatmospheric, it also helps fill the ventricles. Finally, PL depends on how stiff (i.e., the elasticity modulus) the ventricular wall is. That depends on the histologic structure (is there fibrosis or edema, is the pericardium stiff or is the pericardial sac tight with fluid) as well as the rate with which calcium ions are resequestered by the sarcoplasmic reticulum. This resequestration permits relaxation; it is an energy-consuming process in which energy is derived from hydrolysis of ATP (the ultimate source of energy for both contraction and relaxation).

8. What is contractility and how is it related to the force of ventricular contraction?

The rate of cycling of heavy meromyosin heads, also termed myocardial contractility or the inotropic state, is a prime determinant of force of contraction because it is that cycling which is responsible for generating contraction. Contractility is often denoted by the symbol V_{max}. The rate of energy release through the ATP hydrolysis, which governs the force of contraction if all else (e.g., PL) is constant, governs contractility. Sympathetic stimulation produces the neurotransmitter norepinephrine that, along with other catecholamines and digitalis, is termed **positive inotrope**. Positive inotropes increase the rate of cycling of the heavy meromyosin heads, probably by increasing the rate of ATP hydrolysis and the release of energy.

9. Can contractility be measured in living patients?

The force of contraction can be estimated by (1) how high the peak systolic arterial BP is; (2) how high the cardiac output is; (3) the left ventricular fractional shortening obtained from an echocardiogram; or (4) the ratio of the duration of left ventricular ejection to the time from the onset of contraction until the aortic valve opens, known as LVET/LVPEP (where LVET is left ventricular ejection time and LVPEP is left ventricular pre-ejection period). The best method, however, is by measuring the maximal rate of rise of the intraventricular pressure termed dP/dt_{max}. Since this point always exists just before the ventricle begins to eject, dP/dt_{max} is relatively unaffected by features (e.g., what goes on in the arterial tree) other than the rate of force development.

10. What is afterload and how is it related to the force of contraction and cardiac performance?

No matter how great PL and contractility may be, the ventricle can still generate no force if there is no resistance to ejection of blood. The resistance to ejection of blood "perceived" by the left ventricle is termed the afterload (AL). The AL is actually the peak tension in the wall of the ventricle, and that peak tension almost always occurs the instant before the aortic valve opens. If we consider the ventricle to be approximated as a thick-walled sphere, the peak tension (according to the law of Laplace) is equal to the peak value of pressure (inside) times the radius of the ventricle, all divided by the wall thickness. Since radius is a function of volume, we may substitute PL for radius, and since the instant the aortic valve opens is equal to the arterial diastolic BP, we can estimate the AL (peak tension) as aortic BP times PL, all divided by the wall thickness. (Interestingly, because AL is *peak* tension, even though ventricular pressure continues to elevate after the aortic valve opens, AL decreases because the ventricle gets smaller and the wall gets thicker. It is also interesting—and of great clinical importance—that even though arterial diastolic pressure may *decrease*, AL may *increase* because PL may have increased and the wall may have become thinner.)

11. What factors determine the afterload?

The interference perceived by the left ventricle to the flow of blood into and throughout the systemic arterial tree is termed the afterload; however, it is important to discuss two features that contribute to the AL: impedance and systemic vascular resistance. The left ventricle ejects a stroke volume into the initial portion of the aorta (see figure below), into a region not much greater than from the aortic valve to the initial portion of the descending aorta. Thus, the stiffness of this initial portion of the aorta interferes with ejection. This interference is termed impedance (Z) and it is usually estimated as the ratio of pulse pressure (systolic minus diastolic pressure) to stroke volume (cardiac output divided by HR). The Z value depends on the degree of contraction or relaxation of the smooth muscle comprising the middle layer of the aorta. The greater the degree of smooth muscle contraction, the stiffer the aorta and the greater the Z. The more relaxed the aortic smooth muscle, the less stiff the aorta and the lesser the Z. Normally Z accounts for approximately 5–15% of the work of the ventricle, so it is not crucially important unless the heart is at the threshold of failing, when even 1% added interference may be lethal.

The systemic vascular resistance (SVR) is the interference to flow attributable to the sum total of the apertures of the arterioles. Much of the blood flows through the SVR because of the recoil of the proximal portion of the aorta while the ventricle is relaxed and filling in preparation for the next beat. The SVR, like Z, depends on the degree of contraction or relaxation of the arteriolar smooth muscle. Since both aortic and arteriolar smooth muscle are generally controlled by the same neuroendocrine factors (e.g., sympathetic nervous system, vasopressin, angiotensin II), they usually change in the same direction, although possibly not quantitatively the same. Oftentimes when the left ventricle is sick, you may want to decrease both Z and SVR so that the ventricle will not have to eject into such an interfering system.

The vascular smooth muscle determining both Z and SVR is under neuroendocrine control. A partial list of vasodilators (smooth muscle relaxants) and vasoconstrictors (smooth muscle constrictors) is shown in the table below.

VASOCONSTRICTOR	VASODILATOR	VASODILATOR OR VASOCONSTRICTOR
Norepinephrine	Isoproterenol	Epinephrine (A1, A2, B1, B2)
Endothelin	Nitric oxide	Dopamine/Dobutamine
Angiotensin II	Adenosine	
Thromboxane	Prostacyclin	
Vasopressin/ADH	Bradykinin	
Neuropeptide Y	Acetylcholine	
	O_2 debt	
	EDRF/EDHF	
	Blood flow	
	ANF	
	VIP	
	H^+, CO_2, K^+	

EDRF, endothelium-derived relaxing factor; EDHF, endothelium-derived hyperpolarizing factor; ANF, atrial natriuretic factor; VIP, vasoactive intestinal peptide.

12. The myocardium requires oxygen in order to release energy required for contraction. What factors determine the amount of oxygen presented to the working tissues of the heart?

Because oxygen is essential for the production of ATP, the source of fuel for all biological activity, the amount of oxygen present in the myocardium is an important determinant of cardiac performance. The amount of oxygen consumed by the myocardium in 1 minute (MVO_2) is determined principally by the HR, V_{max}, and AL. Since AL is the product of PL and arterial diastolic pressure divided by wall thickness, these three parameters also determine MVO_2. Thus, any factor (e.g., catecholamines, digitalis) that affects V_{max}, any factor that affects AL (e.g., PL, wall thickness), or any factor that affects HR (e.g., atropine, exercise, excitement) will increase MVO_2.

The heart owes the coronary circulation to its oxygen, since all oxygen is delivered by the hemoglobin on the red cells within the blood. Of course, the lung must function adequately to provide enough oxygen to the hemoglobin, and there must be enough hemoglobin. The coronary blood flow is driven by the pressure gradient between the aorta, from which the coronary arteries arise, and the right atrium, into which the coronary veins drain. Since the left ventricle is responsible for sustaining aortic pressure and the right ventricle for keeping right atrial pressure low, the heart helps its own coronary blood flow by sustaining an aortic–right atrial pressure gradient. The coronary blood flow is impeded by the degree of constriction or relaxation of the coronary arteries, and—of greatest importance—by the heart beating itself. While the heart is contracting, the left ventricular wall becomes very tense, and actually compresses the coronary blood vessels. In fact, left ventricular myocardium receives blood flow only when the heart is in diastole—relaxed. The higher the heart rate, the more time the heart spends contracted, the less time relaxed, and the lower the coronary blood flow. (It is crucial to remember that elevation of heart rate increases myocardial oxygen consumption, but it also decreases the delivery of oxygen by the coronary arteries. Thus, elevation of heart rate may lead to oxygen debt and to inadequate oxidative production of ATP.)

13. How does myocardial stiffness affect cardiac performance?

Myocardial stiffness along with EDP and PPL are important determinants of ventricular filling; therefore, the filling of the ventricle and cardiac performance will be impaired by increased myocardial stiffness. The myocardium may be inappropriately and dangerously stiff if it is fibrotic, or it may by stiff because the myocardial fibrils (the smallest linear units of heart muscle) fail to relax properly. Relaxation is an active process that occurs when energy, derived from the hydrolysis of ATP, drives calcium from the contractile machinery into the sarcoplasmic reticulum (SR), minute sacs within the myocardial cells. Because calcium is concentrated in the SR, the re-sequestration in the SR consumes significant energy. (Thus you can see that lack of oxygen, producing lack of ATP, results in the myocardium becoming both stiff and weak.)

14. What is cardiac output and how does it relate to factors that interfere with blood flow?

The amount of blood pumped by the heart each minute is termed the cardiac output, usually marked by the letter Q. Of course, this parameter of cardiovascular function is the most important one, since oxygen and nutrients, and carbon dioxide and wastes are ferried in the blood between the cells of the body and the ports of contact with the outside environment: lungs, kidneys, skin, GI tract, etc. The cardiac output may be approximated simply by using the analogy of the well-known Ohm's law for current (I) driven by a voltage difference (E) through a wire of resistance (R):

$$I = E/R$$

The corresponding equation for cardiac output (Q) is:

$$Q = (Pao – Pra)/SVR$$

where P_{ao} is the aortic pressure, P_{ra} is the right atrial pressure, and SVR is the systemic vascular resistance offered by the degree of constriction of the arterioles produced by contraction of smooth muscle in the media of systemic artcrioles, as well as resistance attributable to the viscosity (i.e., thickness) of blood imposed by the packed cell volume. P_{ao} is determined by the ejection of blood from the left ventricle into and through the systemic arterial tree, while P_{ra} is determined by the right ventricle removing blood from the systemic venous tree and pumping it into and through the pulmonary vascular tree. The entire equation for calculating cardiac output includes the length of the blood vessels (l) and the radius (r) of the arterioles and is given in the Poiseuille equation:

$$Q = (P_{ao} - P_{ra})\pi r^4/8 \, ul$$

where r is the sum total of the radii of all the arterioles, u is the viscosity of blood, and l is the length of the tubes through which the blood must flow. If we assume that the l and u are fairly constant, the equation can be further simplified to:

$$Q = (P_{ao} - P_{ra})r^4$$

This is an obvious re-expression of Ohm's law in which, because resistance is inversely proportional to radius, radius is found in the numerator. The differences in pressure between the aorta and right atrium need no discussion; however, the factors that determine the radii of the systemic arterioles and the relative stiffness of the aorta are highly variable and may be affected by disease or drugs. They are important in the pathogenesis of heart failure and must be adjusted as an important aspect of the treatment of heart failure.

BIBLIOGRAPHY

1. Berne R, Levy M: Cardiovascular Physiology, 7th ed. St. Louis, Mosby, 1997.
2. Braunwald E, Ross J, Sonenblick E: Mechanisms of Contraction of the Normal and Failing Heart. Boston, Little, Brown, 1976.
3. Katz A: Physiology of the Heart. New York, Raven Press, 1992.
4. Opie L: The Heart: Physiology from Cell to Circulation. Philadelphia, Lippincott-Raven, 1998.
5. Shepherd J, Vanhoutte P: The Human Cardiovascular System. New York, Raven Press, 1979.

2. PATHOPHYSIOLOGY OF HEART FAILURE

David H. Knight, D.V.M., M.Med.Sc., and Margaret M. Sleeper, V.M.D.

1. Why should I struggle through the scientific details discussed in this chapter and not proceed directly to the chapter on heart failure therapy, which covers what I really need to know to treat heart disease?

Facts in the abstract are difficult to retain and in themselves are not necessarily enlightening. Accordingly, functional knowledge is not derived simply from compiling facts but from an appreciation of concepts, which once grasped become the framework for reconstructing, integrating and prioritizing information in a manner that enables us to advance our understanding. Good clinicians assess the circumstances of each patient and are able to operate beyond the algorithms that may suffice for the mythical textbook case but shroud critical analysis in a cloak of generalization. We get better at what we do by engaging in thought-provoking challenges. Technicians can perform complicated procedures when the task is clearly defined and repetitious. As clinicians, we must be problem solvers capable of making order out of situations we never may have encountered before in quite the same way. Entire books are devoted to heart failure. The scope of this brief discussion is a synopsis of information and explanations the authors find useful in the conduct of their clinical practice and student mentoring.

2. Define heart failure from a pathophysiologic perspective.

The heart's primary function is to collect the venous drainage returning from capillary beds and pump it back out into the arterial circulation. When for any reason the cardiac output, generally equated with output from the left heart, is unable to match the body's circulatory demands over an extended period, heart failure exists. This is the classic paradigm of heart failure which focuses on the peripheral circulatory complications rather than the heart. However, at the root of these hemodynamic alterations are abnormalities in cardiac mechanics and energetics. Thus a second paradigm refocuses attention from organ physiology to cell biochemistry by emphasizing reduced contractility and/or impaired relaxation of the ventricular myocardium, the two principal functional abnormalities causing the heart to fail. The contemporary view of heart failure now includes a third, more elementary, paradigm of gene expression at the molecular level that addresses the inexorable deterioration of myocardial cells, which accounts for the dismal prognosis of patients suffering from chronic overload of the heart.

Correspondence between cardiac output and heart rate in response to metabolic demand. An inverse relationship prevails between heart rate and stroke volume. The effectiveness of increasing cardiac output is a function of the ability of stroke volume to compensate for fewer cardiac cycles at very slow heart rates, and the adequacy of ventricular filling at high heart rates. At each extreme, the product of heart rate and stroke volume may not match demand for cardiac output.

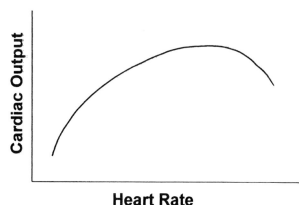

3. What are the primary determinants of the cardiac and stroke outputs?

Cardiac output (total volume ejected/minute) is the product of stroke output (stroke volume) of the left ventricle and heart rate. Although generally a direct relationship exists between the heart rate and cardiac output, an inverse relationship exists between heart rate and stroke volume. Therefore, when all other variables remain unchanged, cardiac output is eventually compromised as heart rate accelerates, if the decline in stroke volume is not compensated by the increase in heart rate (see figure above).

The other variables affecting stroke volume are ventricular loading conditions and myocardial contractility. The relationships of these variables to ventricular stroke volume are expressed in the following proportionality:

$$\text{Stroke Volume} \approx (\text{Preload} \times \text{Contractility}) \div \text{Afterload}$$

The interplay of these variables is illustrated throughout this chapter with ventricular pressure/volume loop diagrams (see figure below), rather than with pressure pulse curves.

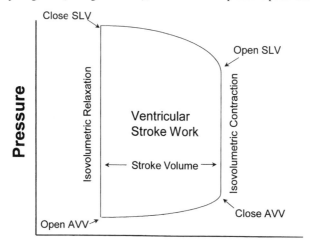

Phases of the cardiac cycle schematically depicted by a generic ventricular pressure–volume loop diagram. The actual magnitude of the pressure changes depends on which ventricle is illustrated, and the sequence of events follows a counterclockwise progression. Ventricular filling begins when the atrioventricular valve (AVV) is pushed open as ventricular pressure drops below atrial pressure. The slope of the pressure–volume relationship during diastole depends on the distensibility (lusitropic) properties of the ventricle and reflects the state of diastolic function. Normally, filling pressure rises only a few mm Hg at end-diastole and exerts a low preload on the relaxed ventricle. As soon as systole begins, the pressure gradient across the AVV reverses, closing the valve. A brief period of isovolumetric contraction follows until the rising ventricular pressure pushes open the semilunar valve (SLV) and ejection begins. Ventricular pressure continues to rise while chamber volume is reduced toward the end-systolic pressure–volume point, which represents the peak elastance (stiffness) attainable at the existing state of contractility (inotropy) and myocardial fiber (sarcomere) length. The abrupt cessation of contraction (ejection) and pressure reversal in the aortic root close the SLV. Isometric relaxation ensues until the ventricular pressure once again falls below atrial pressure and another cycle begins. Stroke volume is represented by the width of the loop, bounded by the end-diastolic and end-systolic volumes. The useful stroke work performed by the ventricle is approximated by the integral of the pressure and volume changes (∫ PdV) represented by the area within the loop.

Preload. Work performed on the ventricles during diastole and which restores the end-diastolic volume is referred to as the preload. In clinical terms, it is equated to ventricular filling pressure. Therefore, the length to which the sarcomere functional subunits of the myocytes are stretched as the ventricles fill in preparation for the next contraction is produced by the preload, and the amount of force that can be generated during systole is directly proportional to sarcomere length. Consequently, preload has a positive effect on stroke volume. This length–active tension relationship is a fundamental property of cardiac muscle, and is referred to as Starling's law of the heart. The primary significance of this relationship is that it provides a mechanism for the two ventricles to independently adapt to phasic disparities in venous return and thereby balance the outputs of each over the course of several beats. The pressure–volume relationship during filling defines the lusitropic (distensibility) properties of the ventricles. Filling at lower pressures indicates improved ventricular diastolic function (lusitropy) (see figure below).

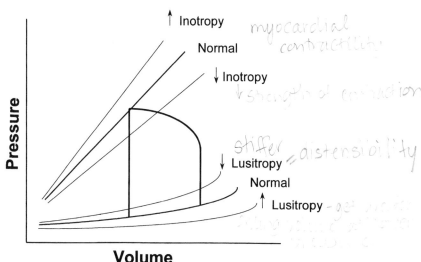

A pressure–volume loop for a normal ventricle is bounded by its end-diastolic and end-systolic pressure–volume relationships (dark lines). The systolic and diastolic properties are represented by families of curves. A positive lusitropic effect shifts the end-diastolic pressure–volume relationship down and to the right, indicating a more compliant ventricle (↑ΔV/↓ΔP), capable of greater filling at lower pressure. A shift of this relationship up and to the left reflects a stiffer ventricle requiring higher filling pressure. The end-systolic pressure–volume relationship is a function of the contractile state of the myocardium and represents the peak force that can be generated at that volume (fiber length). A negative inotropic effect shifts the end-systolic pressure–volume relationship down and to the right, causing end-systolic volume to increase, and a positive inotropic effect shifts it up and to the left, reducing end-systolic volume.

Contractility. In the broadest sense of the term, contractility is the ability of muscle to perform work. For the myocardium, the Frank-Starling length–active tension relationship defines the inotropic state (contractility) encompassed by all of the factors affecting the interaction of the contractile proteins. Although a precise definition of myocardial contractility is thwarted by the complexity of contributing variables, what constitutes a change in contractility is specifically defined by a shift in the amount of work performed from the same end-diastolic chamber volume (sarcomere length). When more pressure or volume work is performed starting from the same sarcomere length, a positive inotropic response has occurred. The slope of the myocardial length–active tension relationship becomes steeper and is shifted to the left as contractility improves, but is flattened and shifted to the right when contractility is depressed. The positive relationship between contractility and stroke volume makes it possible for the ventricles to empty more completely during systole. By decreasing end-systolic volume, the same stroke volume can be delivered from a lower end-diastolic volume, which facilitates venous return at a lower preload (see figure at top of next page).

Afterload. The myocardium is not exposed to the wall tension opposing myocyte shortening until contraction begins, hence the origin of the term afterload. This variable occurs in the denominator of the stroke volume equation because of its negative (inverse) effect. The analogs of afterload are arterial blood pressure and vascular impedance, to which ventricular chamber radius may become a significant contributing factor in dilated ventricles, consistent with the Laplace relationship for thick-walled chambers:

Wall Tension = (Internal Pressure × Chamber Radius) ÷ Wall Thickness

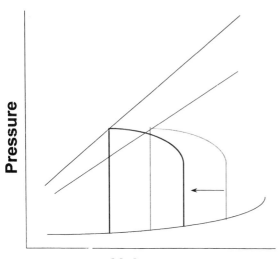

Effect of a positive inotropic intervention (dark loop) during which afterload and venous return are held constant. Since the ventricle is now able to empty more completely, the same stroke volume can be ejected from a lower end-diastolic volume and filling pressure, thereby reducing preload. In reality, by operating at this smaller end-diastolic volume on the lower portion of the ventricular diastolic function curve, an increase in venous return could be achieved. Only a slightly greater filling pressure would be needed to further increase stroke volume, without substantially raising filling pressure and causing congestion.

The ventricular end-systolic pressure/volume relationship or point of peak elastance (stiffness) represents the maximum afterload that can be borne at the corresponding chamber volume (sarcomere length) and contractility. This is a measure of ventricular systolic function that reflects the match between contractility and afterload (see figure below). In heart failure, a mismatch exists due to disproportionately high afterload relative to ventricular contractility, and reduces stroke output.

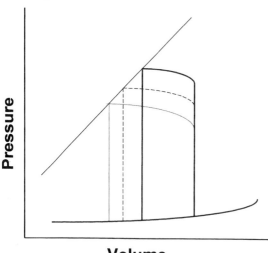

Effect of increasing afterload without altering contractility or preload. As afterload is progressively increased, the peak end-systolic pressure– volume relationship at which active tension at the existing myocardial fiber length is maximum (peak elastance) is shifted upward and to the right, enlarging the end-systolic volume. Since in this example, preload and end-diastolic volume are fixed, stroke volume is reduced. Conversely, afterload reduction augments stroke volume.

4. What hemodynamic abnormalities are the signature features in the pathogenesis of all causes of heart failure?

For the heart to perform its indispensable function of pumping nutrients to the entire body, it is essential that the effective arterial blood volume and perfusion pressure be maintained. This is achieved by balancing cardiac output and systemic vascular resistance. When mechanoreceptors located in the left ventricle, the carotid sinuses, aortic arch and afferent renal arterioles detect so-called "underfilling" of the arterial vascular compartment, they are partially deactivated and trigger positive feedback loop servo-responses. These regulatory responses are designed to maintain homeostasis by increasing central nervous system sympathetic activity, activating the renin-angiotensin-aldosterone system, initiating nonosmotic retention of solute-free water and increasing water consumption by stimulating thirst. The consequence of these adjustments is expansion of total vascular fluid volume in an effort to at least temporarily restore effective arterial blood volume. The obligatory volume expansion of the venous vascular component also leads to an increase in ventricular filling pressure. Therefore, the core features of heart failure are: (1) decreased effective arterial blood volume; (2) increased total body fluid volume; and (3) increased ventricular filling pressure.

↓ arterial blood volume → fluid retention/thirst → Avent. fill P.

5. What does the cardiovascular system most closely conserve, cardiac output or systemic arterial blood pressure?

The hydraulic force required to circulate blood is provided by the perfusion pressure (arterial–venous pressure gradient). The adequacy of the perfusion pressure equates to the effective arterial blood volume. Increases in arterial pressure and/or decreases in vascular impedance (resistance) facilitate flow by increasing perfusion pressure. The perfusion pressure must exceed hydrostatic pressure equivalent to a column of blood corresponding to the height a peripheral vascular bed rises above heart level, for antegrade blood flow to continue. Therefore, postural (orthostatic) relationships have a critical effect on peripheral perfusion. The brain, which ordinarily is above the level of the heart, is particularly vulnerable to reductions in perfusion pressure. The function of systemic arterioles is to preserve perfusion pressure by controlling peripheral vascular impedance. In this way, a declining cardiac output can be conserved through preferential redistribution to organs with the highest metabolic requirements, by individually controlled vasomotor responses in regional vascular beds. Consequently, flow to some organs (kidney, skin, nonexercising skeletal muscle for example) may be redistributed where it is needed most (brain, heart, exercising skeletal muscle). Therefore, in attempting to maintain circulatory homeostasis, conservation of systemic arterial blood pressure is prioritized, even if as a consequence, there is a further decline in cardiac output (see SV equation in question 3), and as will be discussed later in greater detail (see question 17), deleterious side effects result.

6. How does the cardiovascular system adjust to declining cardiac function?

Neural responses. The immediate compensatory responses to acute heart failure and acute hemorrhage are similar. Adrenergic stimulation of the heart and peripheral vessels produces tachycardia and peripheral arterial and venous constriction (see figure below), the primary benefit of which is maintenance of systemic blood pressure and ventricular preload. Arteriolar constriction, particularly of vascular beds with less critical need for blood flow, improves the effective arterial blood volume and preserves flow to vital organs such as the brain and heart. Venoconstriction facilitates venous return by maintaining or even increasing ventricular filling pressure (preload), which is critical to supporting total contractile force via the length–active tension (Frank-Starling) relationship. These reflexes are well adapted for making short-term adjustments, but like all compensatory mechanisms, lead to deleterious side effects if homeostasis is not restored. In the face of declining cardiac function, increased peripheral vascular resistance (impedance) creates an afterload mismatch for the failing heart. Therefore, increased pressure work and an initial sympathetically mediated positive inotropic response raise the energy expenditure by the failing heart, as estimated by the blood pressure–heart rate index (see question 14). As the double product index increases, cardiac efficiency declines (see question 13).

Hormonal responses. If circulatory homeostasis is not promptly restored by the acute neural reflexes, slower developing, more persistent hormonal responses are evoked. Stretch receptors in the afferent arterioles of the renal glomeruli initiate a cascade of enzyme-induced peptide conversions beginning with the release of renin and ending with production of angiotensin II, a potent vasoconstrictor. Angiotensin II further increases sympathetically mediated arteriovenous

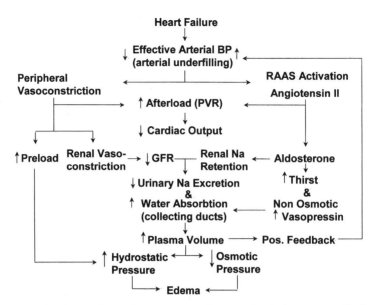

Flow chart integrating the neurohumoral compensatory adjustments invoked to preserve effective systemic arterial blood pressure in the presence of heart failure. The net effect of the compensatory responses is expansion of plasma volume, which is beneficial in preserving perfusion pressure to the brain, heart and other organs with high metabolic requirements, but also promotes edema formation.

constriction and stimulates the release of the adrenocortical sodium conserving hormone, aldosterone (see figure above). As sodium is being reabsorbed from the distal renal tubules, aldosterone also stimulates the release of antidiuretic hormone from the pituitary gland. This causes reabsorption of water from the renal collecting ducts and maintains plasma osmolality. Angiotensin II also triggers increased thirst to ensure that water intake keeps pace with reabsorption. The net effect is expansion of plasma volume to ensure adequate ventricular filling and arterial perfusion pressure. If a new hemodynamic balance is not achieved, the feedback loops of the servo mechanisms controlling salt and water retention do not close and volume expansion will continue (see figure above). This process is limitless so long as nominal organ function is preserved, and accounts for the huge volume of extravascular edema that can collect in some heart failure patients.

Structural adaptations. Myocardial hypertrophy is a second chronic adaptive mechanism. Up to a point, hypertrophy is effective in lowering fiber (myocyte) tension during systole by creating additional functional subunits called sarcomeres. This process is particularly apparent for concentric ventricular hypertrophy, which increases wall thickness relative to chamber size. Since the tension borne by each myofibril is reduced, less energy is utilized during systole and contraction becomes more efficient. However, as myocardial cells hypertrophy, the distance nutrients must diffuse into the cells increases. Since there is not a compensatory increase in capillary density, myocardial ischemia and fibrosis may develop in the overloaded, hypertrophied myocardium and contribute to a reduction in ventricular compliance ($\downarrow\Delta V/\uparrow\Delta P$), i.e., worsening ventricular diastolic function. The relationship between energy consumption and work performed is also affected by a preferential synthesis of the myosin heavy chain isoform, which slows the rate of contraction but improves energy efficiency. Thus the vigor of contraction in pathologically hypertrophied myocardium is reduced, even though total force development may increase temporarily.

7. Are there counter-regulatory mechanisms modulating these homeostatic responses?
In the normal ebb and flow of homeostatic adjustments, the flux of triggering events stimulates reciprocal responses. A stimulus is withdrawn with restoration of balance, and the effector response subsides. This stimulus-response pattern does not pertain when the appropriate adjustment

is inadequate, as is typical of chronic heart failure. Under these circumstances, the response intensifies, eventually reaching a state of diminishing benefit to the point that deleterious side effects predominate (see question 17). Prior to entering this cycle of progressive deterioration, the body makes adjustments designed to counter responses that in the extreme, have the potential to exacerbate adverse clinical signs.

Beta-adrenergic receptor desensitization. A wide array of cardiovascular compensatory responses (heart rate acceleration, increased myocardial contractility, vasomotor contributions to afterload and preload, myocardial hypertrophy, activation of the renin-angiotensin-aldosterone system, nonosmotic vasopressin release and proximal renal tubular retention of sodium and water) are controlled through baroreceptor-mediated sympathetic stimulation. Catecholamines circulate at high levels reflecting the severity of heart failure and this chronic overstimulation has particularly damaging effects on the myocardium. Persistent, intense beta-adrenergic stimulation decreases the number of functional beta-receptors. This desensitization of the beta-receptors for their agonist, referred to as down-regulation, protects the myocardium from Ca^{++} overload and subsequent deterioration. Down-regulation of alpha-receptors found predominantly in vascular smooth muscle also blunts their response to overstimulation and the adverse effects of excessive vasoconstriction.

Atrial natriuretic peptide. Within atrial and to a lesser extent overloaded ventricular myocytes are granules containing a diuretic and vasodilatory polypeptide that is released by triggering mechanoreceptors that respond to stretch (chamber distension). The production, storage and release of this atrial natriuretic peptide (ANP) by the cardiac myocytes makes the heart an autoregulating endocrine organ, as well as a pump. In heart failure, ANP and its analogue, brain natriuretic peptide (BNP) cause vasodilation that also affects afferent renal glomerular arterioles and increases renal glomerular filtration, decreases sodium reabsorption from the collecting ducts, inhibits aldosterone secretion and antagonizes angiotensin II. Despite the increase in levels of plasma ANP as the amount of atrial dilation and heart failure worsen, a relative deficiency of ANP exists since despite attenuating the effects of aldosterone and angiotensin II, it cannot overcome them.

Other intrinsic vasoactive agents. Glomerular afferent arteriolar synthesis of the vasodilatory prostaglandins, prostacyclin and prostaglandin E, is stimulated by norepinephrine, renal nerve stimulation and angiotensin II, and partially neutralizes the vasoconstrictor effects of these neurohumoral mediators. However, a decrease in endothelial synthesis of the potent vasodilator, nitric oxide, may occur in heart failure and potentiate the effect of these endogenous vasoconstrictors. In the late stages of heart failure when homeostasis can no longer be preserved, the potent vasoconstrictor, endothelin, exerts its local effect at end-organ sites. The specific contribution of these agents to the pathogenesis of heart failure is difficult to assess but it is apparent that they participate in the process.

8. Do these mechanisms differ from those evoked to maintain circulatory homeostasis in normal individuals?

The same compensatory mechanisms that are operative in maintaining circulatory homeostasis in normal individuals are recruited to support the circulation in the presence of a failing heart. However, where as normal homeostasis is maintained by making proportional adjustments to transient imbalances in cardiac function, heart failure imposes need for a sustained and usually increasing level of support. This progression passes through a series of stages beginning initially with acute failure triggering adjustments leading to compensatory hyperfunction that is eventually followed by a terminal stage of deterioration (cardiomyopathy of overload), during which the myocardium becomes exhausted as cells die.

9. How do sympathoadrenal stimulation and increased preload differ in the manner they increase myocardial contractile performance?

The endogenous catecholamine, norepinephrine, improves cardiac performance by initiating a positive inotropic response. This is achieved by facilitating the movement of Ca^{++} ions from the sarcoplasmic reticulum to the cytosol of the myocytes. The Ca^{++} cations activate the contractile machinery by reversing the inhibitory effect of the regulatory proteins tropomyosin and troponin, allowing interaction of the contractile proteins actin and myosin, thereby completing the final step in the excitation-contraction process. In the short term, an increase in contractility improves cardiac performance by decreasing ventricular end-systolic volume, thereby facilitating stroke output. Although ventricular relaxation (diastolic function) also is improved by increasing contractility of normal myocardium, in failing hearts, cytosolic Ca^{++} overload occurs and produces the opposite (negative lusitropic) effect, which compromises stroke volume by hindering ventricular filling.

The enhanced performance achieved by increasing preload operates through the length–active tension (Frank-Starling) relationship of cardiac muscle, to increase the force of contraction, without altering the load independent maximum velocity of shortening. Since contractility (force development independent of changes in sarcomere length) is unchanged (see question 2), any improvement in stroke volume is achieved by increasing end-diastolic volume, rather than decreasing end-systolic volume (see figure below). The physiologic role of Starling's law of the heart that ensures stroke output matches filling, is to balance the beat to beat variations in stroke output on both sides of the heart that result from phasic imbalances in venous return. Additionally, in the failing heart, preload reserve may augment or help to maintain stroke output.

Since the systolic load (afterload) also affects the extent of muscle shortening, the distinction between the effects of contractility and fiber length dependent determinants of cardiac performance are often unclear. Though it is usually impossible to be certain of the relative influences of preload, afterload and contractility in any particular circumstance, understanding the principles of the interactions between these variables is fundamental to formulating a clinical assessment of cardiac performance.

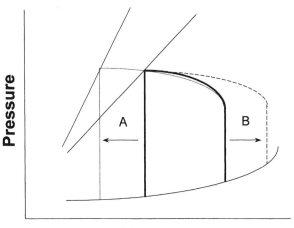

Volume

Ventricular pressure–volume loops illustrating the fundamental difference between increasing cardiac performance by sympathoadrenal stimulation and preload recruitable stroke volume reserve. In this example, afterload is unchanged. Beta-adrenergic stimulation elicits a positive inotropic response that enables the ventricle to reach a smaller end-systolic volume. If preload is maintained, stroke volume will increase by the additional reduction in systolic chamber size (displacement A). In the absence of improved contractility, additional preload will augment effective stroke work by stretching the ventricle to a larger end-diastolic volume. Without changing the original end-systolic volume (contractility unchanged), stroke volume is increased by the additional end-diastolic volume (displacement B). These two mechanisms are complementary and each is counteracted by an increase in afterload.

10. Define the clinical terms used to describe the heart failure syndrome.

A decline in the heart's pumping ability is invariably accompanied by impeded venous return and increased filling pressure of one or both ventricles. Compensatory responses to preserve at least nominal hemodynamic homeostasis have limits and eventually cause deleterious side effects, with clinical manifestations that characterize the syndrome. The clinical signs of heart failure vary in recognized ways depending on the specific nature of the underlying heart disease.

Therefore, since many causes of heart failure exist, no single set of clinical signs describes the syndrome, because despite dependence on the same compensatory mechanisms, the pattern of direct regional vascular involvement differs considerably. The following glossary of terms addresses these clinical differences.

Congestive heart failure. The term congestive relates to the cardinal feature of elevated ventricular (atrial) filling pressure, which is the prerequisite for congestion and edema formation. The terms heart failure and congestive heart failure are generally interchangeable.

Right- and left-sided heart failure. The right/left designation refers to the ventricle or side of the heart into which venous return is impeded, resulting in elevated venous pressure (congestion). Accordingly, right heart failure applies to systemic venous congestion and left heart failure applies to pulmonary venous congestion.

Generalized heart failure. Since the right and left chambers of the heart are arranged in series and share common septa, global failure of the whole heart may exist. Therefore, failure is described as generalized when both systemic and pulmonary circulations are congested, though the clinical manifestations may reflect congestion behind predominantly one side of the heart. Low-output failure states usually are a consequence of generalized heart failure.

Forward (inotropic) and backward (lusitropic) failure. These terms find their origins in the earlier conceptually over simplified view that heart failure is the result of either low cardiac output (inadequate contraction and emptying) or pooling of blood behind one side of the heart or the other (inadequate relaxation and filling). Since blood flows in a circuit, the inflow and outflow of each ventricle must balance within several cardiac cycles. Therefore, forward and backward failure can not exist independently. The terms are seldom used except to emphasize the dominant clinical manifestations of cardiac dysfunction, i.e., poor peripheral perfusion, prerenal azotemia, decreased skeletal muscle mass with forward failure and congestive signs with backward failure.

Acute and chronic heart failure. These terms are frequently combined with the left and right designations. Because of the lower blood volume and tissue pressure in the pulmonary vascular bed, pressure and volume imbalances can lead rapidly to the production of pulmonary edema. Thus the onset of left heart failure and its potentially life threatening consequences may be appropriately termed "acute." If pulmonary edema is tolerable for longer periods of time, it may be classified as chronic. On the other hand, the more insidious accumulation of extravasated fluid from the systemic vascular beds into organs or body cavities is typically a relatively chronic process that can be tolerated for a much longer time.

Compensating heart failure. At this stage, cardiac output still can be maintained in the normal range at rest and during periods of moderate exertion. However, the level of cardiac function is attained at the expense of developing variable degrees of deleterious side effects (see question 17) resulting from over-reliance on physiologic compensatory mechanisms. Use of the term "compensating" in this context ignores whether the short-term clinical trend is toward improvement and reflects only a general functional state in which at least basal cardiac performance can be maintained by support mechanisms, though congestive signs are evident.

Decompensated heart failure. In the decompensated state, cardiac output is inadequate even at rest and can be raised little in response to increased demand, despite the intense application of compensatory mechanisms. This is a terminal condition in which the catabolic state of cardiac cachexia and organ dysfunction compound pre-existing compensatory signs of congestion and edema. As with the preceding definition, this term relates to the existing level of cardiac deterioration, not its progression.

Refractory heart failure. Once clinical signs persist despite aggressive therapy, heart failure has become refractory. Refractory heart failure can be acute or chronic.

11. Is there a meaningful distinction between myocardial failure and heart failure?

The two are not interchangeable since myocardial failure begets heart failure but the converse does not always follow. Myocardial failure explicitly implies loss of contractility and in the case of the dilated cardiomyopathies, may be the sole reason for the heart to fail. However, heart failure is more generic in terms of its pathogenesis and also may develop due to systolic mechanical overloading before contractility is critically reduced, or pure diastolic dysfunction. Eventually, chronic volume or pressure overloading may lead to myocardial failure, which then becomes the pivotal factor determining the heart's ability to respond favorably to therapy, particularly surgical correction of malfunctioning valves or vascular shunts.

12. Categorize the major causes of heart failure.
Cardiovascular diseases that cause heart failure can be categorized in four classes:
I. **Primary contractility deficits.** The inability of the ventricular myocardium to adequately shorten against a load compromises stroke output. Contractility is the primary cause of dysfunction in idiopathic dilated cardiomyopathic hearts and those in which there may have been substantial injury due to ischemia (infarction), toxins, nutritional deficiency (taurine), or persistent tachycardia > 250 bpm. Primary systolic dysfunction frequently develops concurrently with diastolic dysfunction, and mechanical inefficiency due to abnormal valves or vascular shunts, which compound the clinical consequences of depressed contractility.
II. **Chronic systolic mechanical overload.** Two distinct types of systolic mechanical overload are possible, but both contribute in variable degrees to the total ventricular workload:
A. **Pressure overload** exists when ventricular wall tension during systole is excessive due to elevated intraventricular pressure caused by outflow obstruction (pulmonary and aortic stenosis) or high impedance to blood flow through the peripheral vascular bed to which the ventricle is coupled (pulmonary and systemic hypertension). The afterload mismatch under these conditions can be corrected at least partially by a pattern of concentric myocardial hypertrophy. This is accomplished by adding myofibrils in a parallel arrangement, thereby increasing ventricular wall thickness relative to chamber volume and reducing wall tension per cross-sectional area.
B. **Volume overload** occurs when preservation of the effective ventricular stroke output requires maintenance of an abnormally high total stroke output to compensate for the regurgitant fraction of an incompetent atrioventricular or semilunar valve, or the mechanical inefficiency of blood recirculating through a left to right peripheral vascular or intracardiac shunt:

$$\text{Total SV} = \text{Effective SV} + \text{Recirculation Fraction}$$

Volume-overloaded ventricles remodel by adding sarcomeres in series to lengthen myofibrils, and by slippage between myocytes. This eccentric pattern of ventricular hypertrophy increases muscle mass and chamber volume without appreciable thickening of the wall. Ventricles that are dilated purely as a consequence of depressed contractility (dilated cardiomyopathy) but morphologically resemble those of volume overloaded hearts are not actually volume overloaded because the effective and total stroke outputs are essentially equal. Only if a substantial secondary atrioventricular valve regurgitation developed as a consequence of ventricular dilation would such a ventricle become partially volume overloaded.
III. **Diastolic mechanical inhibition.** Ventricular diastolic dysfunction occurs when venous return is impeded due to decreased ventricular wall compliance ($\downarrow\Delta V/\uparrow\Delta P$) and/or rate of active relaxation. Pericardial effusion with tamponade is the classical example of pure diastolic dysfunction causing heart failure. Severe concentric hypertrophy (increased wall thickness relative to chamber volume), particularly if complicated by ischemia and fibrosis also can compromise ventricular filling and lead to compensatory increases in filling pressure. Tachycardia may further complicate diastolic function by decreasing filling time and slowing ventricular relaxation. Diastolic dysfunction is thought to play a pivotal role in the pathogenesis of heart failure due to ventricular pressure overload, and primary hypertrophic and restrictive cardiomyopathies. Since a decline in contractility interferes with relaxation, ventricular diastolic dysfunction is to some extent a contributing factor in all cases in which contractility is reduced.
IV. **Hyperkinetic circulation.** Hyperkinetic circulation is rarely sufficient in the absence of preexisting heart disease to cause heart failure, despite significantly increasing the cardiac workload. In such instances, a reduction in peripheral vascular resistance imposes ventricular volume overloading by forcing a compensatory increase in cardiac output, in order to maintain the perfusion pressure. Conditions that can substantially raise cardiac output are thyrotoxicosis, pregnancy, fever and chronic anemia.

13. Is the heart any better able to cope with the increased workload imposed by pressure or volume overloading?

The volume (flow) and pressure at which blood is ejected are measures of cardiac stroke work. When work is increased by raising pressure, the consumption of energy is greater than when the same amount of work is performed by increasing the volume ejected (stroke volume) (see figure below). Therefore, as a consequence of the reciprocal relationship between afterload and stroke volume, the heart is more efficient pumping larger volumes at lower pressure. Cardiac efficiency improves as the amount of external (useful) work performed increases relative to the amount of internal work, which is liberated purely as heat. During an isovolumetric contraction, no blood is ejected; yet the muscle performs pressure work as it deforms its elastic and viscous elements. In such an instance, only internal work is performed and cardiac efficiency is zero (Efficiency = Useful Work ÷ Total Work). As ejection increases, progressively more external work is performed and efficiency improves, since less energy is wasted as internal work (heat) and more muscle shortening occurs generating flow. The mismatch between afterload and contractility that eventually develops as the myocardium fails results in prolongation of the pre-ejection period, which includes the period of isovolumetric contraction, during which only internal work is performed, and decreases the ejection period, when external work is performed. Therefore, the energetics of pressure overloading are intrinsically more costly as opposed to volume overloading, which can be tolerated longer. Vasoconstriction, which is so vital to preserving perfusion pressure in the short term, is detrimental if sustained at an intense level because the compensatory increase in afterload seriously reduces cardiac efficiency and compromises function.

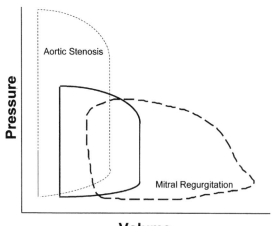

Volume

Ventricular pressure–volume loop diagrams schematically depicting the hemodynamic consequences of aortic stenosis and mitral regurgitation. The heavy loop represents a normal ventricle for comparison. Stroke work for the two pathologic ventricles is approximately equal. The end-systolic pressure–volume point of the pressure overloaded aortic stenosis ventricle is displaced upward and to the left, indicative of a state of hyperfunction. However, in the compensatory stage, during which contractility is essentially normal, systolic wall stress is normalized by concentric hypertrophy, and only later if cardiomyopathy of overload develops, does afterload mismatch occur. Work efficiency is reduced by the proportionately greater amount of pressure work performed during isovolumetric contraction, which is converted into heat rather than ejection of blood. The slope of the diastolic pressure–volume relationship is steeper (decreased lusitropy) due to the loss of wall compliance ($\downarrow\Delta V/\uparrow\Delta P$) resulting from increased ventricular wall thickness and in some cases, myocardial fibrosis secondary to ischemia. In the volume overloaded ventricle with hemodynamically severe mitral regurgitation, there is a conspicuous loss of isovolumetric contraction due to the immediate leakage of blood into the low pressure left atrium. Consequently, this ventricle is afterload reduced and contraction mostly progresses under low wall stress, particularly late in systole when wall thickness has increased and chamber volume is smaller (Laplace relationship). Although mitral regurgitation makes the ventricle mechanically inefficient, the energy cost is not nearly so great as for pressure overloading. Compensatory hypertrophy in volume overloaded ventricles lengthens myofibers by adding sarcomeres serially to accommodate a large stroke volume, rather than develop thicker walls. Diastolic function is well preserved in these ventricles, which allows large end-diastolic volumes to be reached with relatively low preloading, until the late stage of disease.

14. How does heart rate factor into cardiac efficiency?

Minute work (power) incorporates cardiac output (CO = SV × HR) and thereby inserts heart rate into the work calculation:

$$\text{Minute Work} = \text{Ejection Pressure} \times \text{Stroke Volume} \times \text{Heart Rate}$$

The range of effective heart rates is limited by the ability of stroke volume to increase as rate slows, and the adequacy of ventricular filling, as diastole shortens during heart rate acceleration. At each extreme, cardiac output and minute work decline (see question 2). Within the effective range, heart rate acceleration is a partially effective compensatory mechanism in heart failure. However, whatever benefit is derived from tachycardia comes at a substantial incremental cost in energy consumption. A significant portion of this expenditure is wasted doing internal (isovolumetric) work, restoring myocyte plasma membrane ion gradients and pumping Ca^{++} back into the sarcoplasmic reticulum during each cycle. Therefore, cardiac efficiency tends to decline as heart rate increases.

Since pressure work is less efficient than volume work and both are directly influenced by heart rate, the "double product" (pressure × HR) is an effective index for estimating the energy (oxygen) consumed in the production of cardiac work. Since these two variables are easily measured, this index has clinical value.

15. Why do the most dilated hearts usually have the worst cardiac function?

The most extreme cardiac dilation is seen in conjunction with severe primary dilated cardiomyopathies, and chronically heavily volume overloaded hearts. Chamber enlargement is induced by applying a distending force to the wall during filling. This is accomplished through augmenting venous return by venoconstriction and expanding the effective blood volume (see question 6), both of which increase preload. Although this is the mechanism for evoking the Frank-Starling length–active tension relationship and increasing the force of contraction, in the latter stages of heart failure, dilation may impair rather than improve cardiac function. The net effect of dilation on cardiac performance is the relative influence of a physical relationship (Laplace) and a physiological response (Frank-Starling). Wall tension (stress) is directly proportional to the chamber radius (see question 3). Therefore, at the same ejection pressure, a large end-diastolic volume adds to the afterload by necessitating even greater wall tension, thereby partially offsetting the incremental force generated by stretching sarcomeres. If a mismatch exists between afterload and contractility, stroke volume will decline because end-systolic volume rises. Therefore, the ventricle will not experience the same degree of load reduction that would otherwise occur as the chamber becomes smaller during systole.

As contractility declines, the additional force generated through dilation diminishes as the Starling function curve relating cardiac work (output) to end-diastolic chamber volume is shifted to the right and the slope flattens (see figure below). Overfilling of the normal heart is unlikely due to pericardial restraint and viscoelastic forces within the walls, but is more problematic in the failing heart, for which a descending limb on the Starling curve is illustrated classically. At the extreme end-diastolic volumes, the greatly elevated filling pressure impedes venous return just as the inappropriately high afterload reduces stroke output. Once the heart begins to operate this far out on the function curve, the situation becomes very unstable because any further dilation also reduces cardiac output, creating a negative feedback loop and setting in motion the downward spiral of intractable failure.

16. Rank the level of contractile reserve in the late stages of left heart failure due to examples of pure pressure and volume overloading, and primary defects in contractility.

The loading conditions imposed on the heart are the primary determinants of the intrinsic contractile reserve remaining at the end-stage of a chronic cardiac disease. The insidiousness of the process and the extent of ventricular remodeling are moderating factors. A suddenly imposed heavy load can overwhelm even a relatively healthy muscle but given the opportunity to adapt with an appropriate hypertrophic response, compensation may be sustained for a lengthy period.

Subaortic stenosis. In its uncomplicated form, this represents a pure pressure overload that can more than double peak systolic pressure in the left ventricle. The natural history of this anomaly is a progressive narrowing of the left ventricular outflow tract during the first several months of

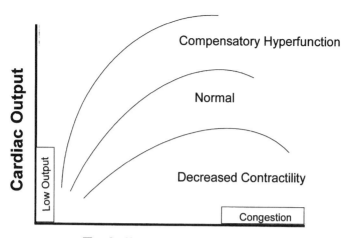

Cardiac function (Starling) curves displaying cardiac output as a function of end-diastolic volume (preload). Each function curve is defined by a particular end-systolic pressure–volume relationship reflecting the state of contractility (inotropy). An entire family of curves representing an array of changes in contractility or loading conditions imposed by therapeutic interventions or natural progression of disease is possible. As contractility declines, the curves are shifted to the right and the slopes flatten, making it progressively more difficult to meet an increased demand for cardiac output, and eventually even to maintain normal output at rest, without necessitating such high filling pressure that congestion and edema develop. The state of compensatory hyperfunction occurs while contractility is still well preserved and ventricular hypertrophy has normalized wall stress (force/cm^2).

life, which allows ample time for compensatory hypertrophy to develop. The pattern of left ventricular hypertrophy is classified as being concentric and is characterized by a thickened wall relative to the volume of the chamber, which may actually be smaller than normal. Consequently, the tremendous systolic wall stress (force/cm^2) that would otherwise be exerted on individual myocardial cells is normalized by distributing the force across the thickened wall. Consistent with the Laplace relationship, the normal to small chamber radius and thickened walls minimize the wall stress required to contain the left ventricular peak systolic pressure. Therefore, contractile dysfunction ordinarily is not a limiting factor, except perhaps at high cardiac output when afterload becomes extreme ($\uparrow$Pressure = $\uparrow$Flow × Fixed Resistance). When "congestive" heart failure is caused by subaortic stenosis, it is diastolic dysfunction due to decreased wall compliance ($\downarrow\Delta V/\uparrow\Delta P$) secondary in large part to myocardial ischemia and fibrosis that is responsible.

Mitral valve regurgitation. Incompetence of the mitral valve produces a pure form of volume overload on the normally pressure adapted left ventricle. In severe cases, the volume of blood regurgitated into the left atrium can more than double the total stroke volume of the left ventricle (Total SV = Effective SV + Regurgitant Fraction). Even when elevated, left atrial pressure is substantially lower than aortic pressure and the regurgitant flow follows the path of least resistance. This effectively reduces afterload on the ventricle. Since regurgitation begins as soon as ventricular pressure exceeds atrial pressure, the ventricle starts unloading early and the energy inefficient period of isovolumetric contraction is eliminated. Although the regurgitant flow reduces cardiac mechanical efficiency, the energy cost is much less than would be the pressure work performed during isovolumetric contraction (see question 13). Furthermore, even though the left ventricular end-diastolic volume eventually becomes very large, the initial reduction in afterload afforded by the low impedance regurgitant flow offsets the increased systolic wall tension that would otherwise be attributable to dilation (Laplace relationship). This allows the left ventricle to achieve a substantial further systolic reduction in volume, though the end-systolic volume still may be larger than normal. Consequently, when mitral regurgitation exists, left ventricular wall tension continues to decrease during systole, as the chamber becomes smaller and the wall thickens.

Ventricular remodeling to accommodate the increased stroke volume imposed by mitral regurgitation is characterized by chamber dilation without appreciable wall thickening (eccentric hypertrophy) since systolic wall stress is minimally increased. Although there is a substantial increase in ventricular mass, wall thickness remains essentially normal and therefore, chamber compliance (diastolic function) is better preserved than in pressure overloaded ventricles. However, left atrial pressure (ventricular preload) can become critically elevated by a large volume of retrograde filling (regurgitant fraction). Since volume overloading entails relatively low energy cost and mitral regurgitation ordinarily progresses gradually, this type of mechanical overload can be sustained for long periods. Eventually, chronic volume overloading severely reduces left ventricular contractility, leaving little contractile reserve by the terminal stage.

Dilated cardiomyopathy. In uncomplicated cases, there is insufficient valvular incompetence to cause significant volume overloading and although peripheral vascular resistance rises, systemic arterial pressure remains in the normal range since cardiac output is relatively low. Therefore, the poor contractile performance secondary to a dilated cardiomyopathy is not initiated by excessive loading but rather it is the inability of a weak myocardium to generate sufficient force to function adequately, even under a normal pressure and reduced volume load (see figure below). A compensatory elevation of ventricular filling pressure increases end-diastolic volume but end-systolic volume also rises because systolic function is progressively declining. Cardiac dilation and eccentric ventricular hypertrophy are hallmarks of this condition and the afterload mismatch is exacerbated by the additional ventricular wall tension that must be generated due to the Laplace relationship. This situation contributes to a vicious cycle of deterioration since a negative feedback loop is established between compensatory ventricular dilation and adequate force generation. As a consequence of the primary deterioration in contractility, the ventricular function curve for a dilated cardiomyopathy is displaced further to the right and the slope is flatter than for either pressure or volume overloading (see figure above). Therefore, at the onset of heart failure the contractile reserve is lowest in dilated cardiomyopathic hearts.

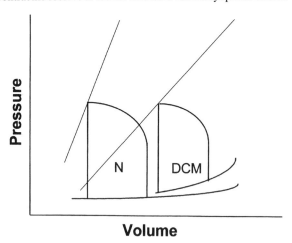

Volume

Ventricular pressure–volume loops for a normal and a dilated cardiomyopathic (DCM) ventricle are displayed schematically for comparison. Although peripheral vascular resistance (actually impedance) eventually becomes very high in the DCM patient, arterial blood pressure remains in the normal range since cardiac output is limited to relatively low levels. For the purpose of this illustration, isovolumetric contraction and relaxation are shown, despite the fact that secondary to extreme ventricular dilation in the later stages, annular dilation results in moderate mitral regurgitation. The depressed slope of the end-systolic pressure volume relationship precludes achieving substantial reduction in end-systolic volume and preload recruitable stroke volume reserve also reaches its limits. Consequently, the ejection fraction (stroke volume as a percent of ventricular end-diastolic volume) is greatly diminished in the terminal stage. As a result of the inability to sustain an adequate compensatory adjustment, ventricular filling pressure becomes progressively higher as the ventricle operates further out on its diastolic function curve (end-diastolic pressure–volume relationship).

17. What clinical signs are commonly associated with heart failure and what is the relationship of these signs to the compensatory processes?

The clinical signs of heart failure reflect primarily impedance of venous return (elevated ventricular filling pressure), and particularly in the later stages, a progressive inability to match cardiac output to metabolic demand. Thus in the early compensatory stages, signs of congestion and edema predominate until under perfusion limits exercise capacity, and in advanced heart failure, causes generalized organ dysfunction.

The clinical signs of heart failure are manifestations of deleterious side effects resulting from chronic overutilization of the same compensatory mechanisms that were beneficial in the early stages. These associations can be grouped accordingly:

1. **Sympathetic overdrive:** tachycardia, sometimes accompanied by ventricular ectopy, generalized vasoconstriction causing pale membranes, slow capillary refill and cool peripheral extremities.

2. **Volume overexpansion:** accentuated third heart sound (gallop rhythm) indicative of elevated ventricular filling pressure, generalized venous distension, hepatomegaly, pleural effusion, ascites and occasionally pitting subcutaneous edema in dependent areas of the body, pulmonary edema and associated signs of respiratory distress (tachypnea, hyperpnea, pulmonary rales, frothy pink tinged sputum, cough).

3. **Excessive myocardial hypertrophy** (eventually contributing to cardiomyopathy of overload): decreased ejection phase indices of myocardial function, ventricular arrhythmia, skeletal muscle weakness, generalized muscle atrophy (cardiac cachexia), and renal insufficiency.

18. Can these clinical signs be relied upon to identify the heart failure syndrome?

With the exception of generalized venous engorgement, none of these signs is specific for heart failure. Therefore, before any can be attributed to heart failure, definite signs of heart disease must be identified, and the functional significance and severity of the underlying heart disease must be consistent with these clinical signs. For example, pulmonic stenosis could be the etiologic explanation for signs resembling right-sided heart failure (ascites, pleural effusion) but is an improbable explanation for pulmonary alveolar disease resembling pulmonary edema.

Signs considered reliable evidence of heart disease in small domestic animals include:
• Grade III/V or greater systolic murmur in the absence of anemia (hemoglobin < 6 gm/ml)
• Gallop rhythm (transient diastolic extra sound) due to accentuated third heart sound
• Echocardiographic evidence of structural disease and cardiac dysfunction
• Radiographic evidence of cardiomegaly
• Certain dysrhythmias, such as atrial fibrillation, complete heart block, and high-grade ventricular ectopy in the absence of a noncardiac cause

19. How is the severity of heart failure staged?

As heart failure progresses, therapy must become more aggressive and the prognosis for continued survival worsens. Therefore, classifying the stage of heart failure can be useful as a means of tracking the natural history of a patient's condition and for making clinical comparisons, particularly when evaluating therapeutic protocols.

The level of exertion that can be achieved before congestive signs become incapacitating is the basis of the functional method of assessing heart failure severity, patterned on the classical New York Heart Association classification.
• Class I: Capable of strenuous exercise short of high level athletic performance
• Class II: Moderate levels of exertion tolerated
• Class III: Comfortable at rest but even mild exertion cannot be sustained
• Class IV: Clinically compromised even at rest

Since the level of exertion considered representative of normal capacity is highly individualized, and assessment is subjective, this classification provides only an approximation of heart failure severity. Nonetheless, since it is based on functional status, it has utility.

BIBLIOGRAPHY

1. Katz AM: Physiology of the Heart, 2nd ed. New York, Raven Press, 1992.
2. Knight DH: Pathophysiology of heart failure and clinical evaluation of heart failure. In Ettinger SJ, Feldman EC (eds): Textbook of Veterinary Internal Medicine: Diseases of the Dog and Cat, 4th ed. Philadelphia, W.B. Saunders, 1995, pp 844–867.
3. Little WC, Braunwald E: Pathophysiology of heart failure. In Braunwald E (ed): Heart Disease: A Textbook of Cardiovascular Medicine, 5th ed. Philadelphia, W.B. Saunders, 1997.
4. Opie LH: The Heart, Physiology and Metabolism, 2nd ed. New York, Raven Press, 1991.
5. Schrier RW, Abraham, WT: Mechanisms of disease: Hormones and hemodynamics in heart failure. N Engl J Med 341:577–585, 1999.
6. Stephenson RB: Cardiovascular physiology. In Cunningham JG (ed): Textbook of Veterinary Physiology, 2nd ed. Philadelphia, W.B. Saunders, 1997, pp 127–260.
7. Swenson MJ, Reece WO (eds): Dukes' Physiology of Domestic Animals. 11th ed. Part I: Blood, circulation and the cardiovascular system (multiple authors). Ithaca, NY, Cornell University Press, 1993, pp 1–162.

3. SYNCOPE AND SUDDEN CARDIAC DEATH

Jonathan A. Abbott, D.V.M.

1. What is syncope?

The terms syncope and fainting are synonymous. Syncope is a transient loss of consciousness and it is the transient nature of syncope that distinguishes it from stupor, coma, and other more protracted changes in mentation.

2. What are the basic pathophysiologic mechanisms that lead to syncope?

In general, syncope results when the parts of the brain that maintain arousal are starved of the metabolic substrates required for oxidative metabolism. Usually, syncope is due to a precipitous but transient decline in cerebral perfusion. Hypoglycemia can lead to syncope but it more commonly results in seizure activity. Hypoxia resulting from respiratory tract disease can also be responsible for syncope.

The cardiovascular causes of syncope generally fall into one of three basic categories: (1) reflex-mediated vasomotor instability; (2) orthostatic or postural hypotension (most commonly resulting from hypovolemia or vasodilating drugs); and (3) cardiac disorders, including arrhythmias and structural heart diseases that result in abrupt decline in cardiac performance.

Vasomotor instability refers to situations in which the body is unable to maintain normal systemic vascular resistance. Recall that blood pressure is related to both cardiac output (flow) and vascular resistance. If vascular resistance falls due to excessive and widespread vasodilation, perfusion pressure decreases even if cardiac output is maintained. If the brain's reticulated activating system is deprived of adequate blood supply, loss of consciousness can result.

3. What kind of cardiovascular disorders can result in syncope?

Arrhythmias are commonly associated with syncope. Bradyarrhythmias, specifically high-grade second-degree AV block or third-degree AV block and sinus node dysfunction (sick sinus syndrome), are perhaps the rhythm disturbances most likely to cause fainting. However, tachyarrhythmias including rapid supraventricular tachycardia and ventricular tachycardia can also be responsible for episodes of weakness and fainting.

Structural cardiac diseases of virtually any type can also explain syncope. It is important to recognize that cardiac disease must cause an abrupt and usually dramatic decrease in cardiac output or perfusion pressure in order to result in syncope. Therefore, when cardiovascular syncope occurs in the absence of pathologic arrhythmia, it is often associated with exercise. When cardiac disease is present, cardiac output may be adequate at rest but cannot increase to meet the demands of exercise. Patients with pulmonary hypertension due, for example, to heartworm disease fairly commonly faint during exercise. Similarly, congenital cardiac malformations such as aortic stenosis and pulmonic stenosis can be responsible for syncope.

In aortic stenosis and probably other cardiac diseases, a form of vasomotor instability known as neurocardiogenic syncope can also contribute to the pathogenesis of syncope.

4. What is neurocardiogenic syncope?

Neurocardiogenic syncope is a form of acute autonomic dysfunction that can result in reflex-mediated bradycardia and/or hypotension. Neurocardiogenic syncope is a newer term that refers to the common faint that is observed in people: the vasovagal event. The pathogenesis of some fainting episodes in animals is likely similar.

5. What is the pathogenesis of neurocardiogenic syncope?

The pathogenesis of neurocardiogenic syncope is imperfectly understood. However, in some susceptible individuals, vigorous ventricular contractions associated with increases in adrenergic tone stimulate mechanoreceptors within the ventricles. Stimulation of these receptors is more likely to occur when venous return is decreased. Afferent impulses from the mechanoreceptors are conveyed via unmyelinated C fibers to the brain, which triggers vagally mediated bradycardia and/or hypotension. This phenomenon is analogous to the Bezold-Jarisch reflex that is described in physiologic models.

This form of syncope is one explanation for fainting in the setting of aortic stenosis. High pressures generated within the left ventricle during exercise result in stimulation of mechanoreceptors and reflex bradycardia/hypotension. Bradycardia in the absence of sinus node disease has been documented as a cause of syncope in Doberman pinschers with dilated cardiomyopathy and the pathogenesis in this syndrome may relate to stimulation of ventricular mechanoreceptors.

6. How is the patient history used to differentiate syncope from seizures?

Typically, syncope is brief and results in unconsciousness and flaccid paralysis. In contrast, seizures, at least in the most common form, result in tonic or clonic contractions of the skeletal muscles. However, overlap is definitely observed and some syncopal patients will demonstrate muscular activity or even void. The patient's activity following the event is helpful in making the distinction between syncope and seizures. Usually, the recovery following a syncopal episode is rapid. In contrast, patients that have experienced a seizure are often confused and may be ataxic, blind, or have other residual neurologic deficits.

7. Is the patient signalment helpful in the diagnosis of syncope?

Breed predispositions for disorders that result in syncope are recognized and the patient signalment is occasionally helpful in the diagnosis of syncope. Sinus node dysfunction (sick sinus syndrome) is commonly observed in the miniature schnauzer, cocker spaniel, and terriers. Large-breed dogs, including the boxer dog and Doberman pinscher, are predisposed to the development of myocardial disease. Syncope associated with ventricular tachyarrhythmia is observed in both boxer dogs and Doberman pinschers and can occur in the absence of radiographically obvious cardiac disease. Bradycardia that has a pathogenesis that is likely similar to neurocardiogenic syncope has been documented in Doberman pinschers.

8. What is situational syncope?

Syncope that is consistently associated with specific circumstances is referred to as situational syncope. Examples include micturition syncope, defecation syncope and deglutition syncope. Some susceptible animals faint following a vigorous bout of coughing; this is referred to as tussive syncope or, sometimes, the "cough-drop syndrome." Tussive syncope is observed fairly commonly in dogs that cough as a consequence of mitral valve endocardiosis. The pathogenesis of tussive syncope is not known with certainty, although elevations in intrathoracic pressures related to coughing may precipitate a reflex-mediated bradycardia that is similar to neurocardiogenic syncope.

9. What diagnostic evaluation is appropriate for patients that have had episodes of weakness or syncope?

The diagnosis of syncope poses a considerable challenge. The appropriate diagnostic plan depends very much on the patient history and the results of physical examination. Conscientious neglect is likely a safe and suitable approach when a single fainting episode is observed in an apparently healthy patient in which a careful physical examination, resting electrocardiogram, thoracic radiographs, and blood glucose fail to reveal abnormalities. When syncopal episodes are recurrent or abnormalities are detected on physical examination, further diagnostic evaluation is indicated. A resting electrocardiogram, thoracic radiographs, complete laboratory data, and an echocardiographic examination would represent a suitable initial diagnostic approach to the patient with syncope.

The presence or absence of structural heart disease is a clinically useful way of categorizing potential causes of syncope. This basic determination provides diagnostic direction and sometimes

BIBLIOGRAPHY

1. Calvert CA, Meurs KM: CVT update: Doberman pinscher occult cardiomyopathy. In Bonagura JD (ed): Kirk's Current Veterinary Therapy XIII: Small Animal Practice. Philadelphia, W.B. Saunders, 2000, pp 756–760.
2. Calvert CA, Jacobs GJ, Pickus-CW: Bradycardia-associated episodic weakness, syncope, and aborted sudden death in cardiomyopathic Doberman pinschers. J Vet Intern Med 10: 88–93, 1996.
3. Calvert CA, Hall G, Jacobs G, et al: Clinical and pathologic findings in Doberman pinschers with occult cardiomyopthy that died suddenly or developed congestive heart failure: 54 cases (1984–1991). J Am Vet Med Assoc 210:505–511, 1997.
4. Kapoor WN: Syncope and hypotension. In Braunwald E (ed): Heart Disease: A Textbook of Cardiovascular Medicine, 4th ed. Philadelphia, W.B. Saunders, 1997, pp 840–863.
5. Kittleson MD: Syncope. In Kittleson MD, Kienle RD (eds): Small Animal Cardiovascular Medicine. St. Louis, Mosby, 1998, pp 495–501.
6. Moisie NS, et al: Inherited ventricular arrhythmias and sudden death in German shepherd dogs. J Am Coll Cardiol 24:233–243, 1994.
7. Myerburg RJ, Castellanos A: Cardiac arrest and sudden death. In Braunwald E (ed): Heart Disease: A Textbook of Cardiovascular Medicine, 4th ed. Philadelphia, W.B. Saunders, 1997, pp 742–779.
8. Rush JE: Syncope and episodic weakness: Myocardial diseases of dogs. In Fox PR, Sisson D, Moise NS (eds): Textbook of Canine and Feline Cardiology: Principles and Clinical Practice. Philadelphia, W.B. Saunders, 1999, pp 446–454.

4. SHOCK

Paolo Porzio, D.V.M., M.Vet.Sci.

1. What is shock?

Shock is the acute failure of the cardiovascular system to provide adequate tissue oxygenation. The fundamental abnormality of this diverse clinical syndrome is impaired perfusion of the body tissues. Shock is a final common pathway for pathophysiologic events that are common to many disorders. It is important to recognize that shock is a syndrome. The clinical picture reflects the sum of the effects of each disorder on each system and the clinical presentation varies. However, regardless of the nature of the underlying disease, shock is characterized by an acute generalized disturbance in the normal circulatory pattern, resulting in hypoperfusion and dysfunction of critical organs.

2. How is shock classified?

Various schemes for the classification of shock have been proposed and each has its limitations. The following classification has a pathophysiologic basis and is therefore clinically useful:

Hypovolemic shock. Hypovolemic shock can result from hemorrhagic and nonhemorrhagic causes. Hemorrhagic etiologies include trauma, ruptured malignancies (hemangiosarcoma), and coagulopathies, while nonhemorrhagic causes lead to extracellular fluid volume contraction and hypovolemia. The latter include gastrointestinal losses (vomiting and diarrhea), renal losses (diuretics, diabetes insipidus), and burns.

Distributive shock. Distributive shock usually involves a combination of mechanisms leading to an abnormal distribution of the extracellular fluid; most commonly, an inappropriate decrease in vascular resistance results from generalized vasodilation. Initially, cardiac output may be preserved or even enhanced—as in the hyperdynamic phase of septic shock—however, loss of fluid from the intravascular space and myocardial depression ultimately decrease cardiac performance. Types of distributive shock include septic, anaphylactic, toxic and neurogenic shock.

Cardiogenic shock. Shock that results primarily from cardiac dysfunction is known as cardiogenic shock. Cardiogenic shock can result from myocardial dysfunction, valvular dysfunction, and arrhythmias.

Obstructive shock. This term refers to causes of shock that include cardiac tamponade, massive pulmonary embolism, and other disorders that cause obstruction to the flow of blood.

3. What are the important pathophysiologic mechanisms in shock?

The vital organs most commonly affected by shock are the brain, heart, and kidneys. Brain hypoperfusion can be responsible for mental status changes including stupor or even coma. The effect of shock on the cardiovascular system is particularly important because cardiac dysfunction resulting from myocardial ischemia can perpetuate shock. Clinically, the most obvious manifestation of cardiovascular dysfunction is tachycardia. This is primarily due to a reflex sympathoadrenal response to impaired cardiac performance.

As the body attempts to improve perfusion to the vital organs, arteriolar vasoconstriction in the skin, muscle, kidney, spleen, and gastrointestinal tract allows blood to be shunted centrally to the brain and heart. In shock, however, this compensatory response may be inadequate. The functions of the kidney are critically dependent on perfusion and oliguria is a common manifestation of shock. Activation of the coagulation cascade is common, although disseminated intravascular coagulation is not often clinically evident at initial presentation. Two other common systemic manifestations of shock are metabolic acidosis secondary to tissue hypoxia and arterial hypotension.

4. What abnormalities are detected on physical examination?

In hypovolemic, cardiogenic, and advanced distributive shock the patient may have cool extremities, pallor, hypotension, and tachycardia. In the initial phase of distributive shock, patients may have warm extremities, hyperemic mucous membranes, variable systemic blood pressure (hypotension to normotension), and tachycardia. The character of peripheral pulses is an important component of the physical examination of the shock patient. Femoral pulses are usually hypokinetic in most cases of shock but can be hyperkinetic (bounding pulses) in the hyperdynamic phases of septic shock.

5. How is noncardiogenic shock managed?

Strategies to improve perfusion are the cornerstone of shock therapy. Fluids should be administered intravenously. Recommended infusion rates are up to 90 ml/kg/hr in dogs and 45 ml/kg/hr in cats. The most commonly infused fluid types are crystalloids such as 0.9% NaCl, Ringer's lactate, Normosol-R (Baxter, Deerfield, IL), and P148 (Abbott, Abbott Park, IL).

Colloid osmotic pressure is critical in the management of shock. In fact, the maintenance of colloid osmotic pressure via administration of colloids improves perfusion and is indicated in noncardiogenic shock states. Whole blood transfusions may be necessary to manage severe hemorrhagic shock and antibiotics are indicated in septic shock patients.

6. Compare and contrast the use of colloids and crystalloids in the management of shock states.

Sodium is the major component of crystalloid fluids and its distribution determines the distribution of the infused fluids. Sodium is the principal solute of the extracellular space and 80% of this space is extravascular. Therefore, infused sodium will reside primarily outside the vascular compartment. In fact, crystalloid fluids are designed to expand the interstitial space, not the vascular space. Only 20% of infused sodium chloride solutions that are isotonic to the patient will remain in the vascular space.

Colloids have a large molecular weight and do not diffuse readily across capillary walls. Colloids are more effective than crystalloids for increasing vascular volume and most protocols for volume resuscitation combine colloid and crystalloid fluids to expand both vascular and interstitial volume. Among the colloids, plasma is not a very effective plasma expander since its albumin content and infused volume are not sufficient to produce a significant and long-lasting rise in colloid osmotic pressure. Moreover, over 50% of the body albumin resides outside the vascular space. The infused albumin passes into the interstitial space and is either returned to the bloodstream via the lymph or is metabolized for energy. Commonly used colloids include hydroxyethyl starch and dextrans, while 5% and 25% human serum albumin preparations deserve consideration but are not widely available to veterinarians.

7. How is cardiogenic shock managed?

The management of cardiogenic shock is directed towards the improvement of cardiac performance. Specific strategies are dictated by the nature of the causative disease. In general, treatment modalities are directed towards the optimization of systolic and diastolic performance, improvement of oxygen delivery to the myocardium, and the correction of rhythm disturbances when indicated.

8. How are patients with shock monitored?

Noninvasive monitoring of the vital signs, cardiac rhythm, and urinary output is recommended for all patients suffering from shock. In many circumstances, invasive hemodynamic monitoring is appropriate and may include the placement of intraarterial and central venous catheters, or even pulmonary artery floatation catheters.

9. What is central venous pressure?

Central venous pressure (CVP) is the pressure within the lumen of the venae cavae. Its principal determinants are intravascular volume, right heart function, and venous tone. The CVP can be measured in cmH_2O through a simple plastic water column attached to the end of a central venous catheter positioned just cranial to the right atrium. The expected CVP in most dogs and cats is 0–6 cmH_2O. Negative values suggest hypovolemia, while increased values suggest right-sided congestive heart failure, caval obstruction, or iatrogenic volume overload. Interpreting changes in pressure over time rather than interpreting single measurements increases the diagnostic utility of CVP measurement.

BIBLIOGRAPHY

1. Civetta JM, Taylor RW, Kirby RR (eds): Critical Care. Philadelphia, J.B. Lippincott, 1997.
2. Fox PR (ed): Canine and Feline Cardiology. New York, Churchill Livingstone, 1988.
3. Grenvik A, Ayres SM, Holbrook PR, Shoemaker WC (eds): Textbook of Critical Care, 4th ed. Philadelphia, W.B. Saunders, 2000.
4. Marino PL (ed): The ICU Book. Baltimore, Williams & Wilkins, 1998.

5. PULMONARY EDEMA

Marilyn Dunn, D.M.V., M.V.Sc.

1. What is pulmonary edema?

Pulmonary edema is defined as the accumulation of excessive extravascular fluid within the peribronchial, interstitial, or alveolar spaces. Pulmonary edema should be considered a manifestation of disease rather than a disease in itself.

2. How does pulmonary edema develop?

Pulmonary edema develops when the rate of fluid flux across the capillary endothelium exceeds the ability of the lymphatics to drain it. Capillary endothelial cells, located in alveolar septa, have pores allowing fluid to flow passively into the interstitium. This fluid is rapidly absorbed by interstitial lymphatic vessels and then enters the systemic circulation. In the presence of excess fluid, the interstitium protects gas exchange in the alveola by acting as a "sink." The interstitium can hold a large amount of fluid until pressure exceeds 2 mmHg relative to atmospheric pressure. At this point, alveolar epithelial cells break down, allowing fluid to leak into the alveola (see figure below).

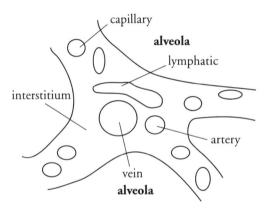

3. Name the four pathophysiologic mechanisms that can lead to the development of pulmonary edema.

1. **Increased pulmonary capillary hydrostatic pressure.** This is the most common cause of pulmonary edema in small animals and usually results from left-sided heart failure.

2. **Increased alveolocapillary membrane permeability.** Various syndromes result in damage to the alveolar capillary membrane and can be referred to as adult respiratory distress syndrome (ARDS).

3. **Decreased colloid oncotic pressure.** Hypoalbuminemia is the most common cause. Decreased oncotic pressure alone rarely causes pulmonary edema; however, it may contribute to edema development in the presence of elevated capillary hydrostatic pressure or altered alveolocapillary permeability.

4. **Pulmonary lymphatic insufficiency.** This is usually the result of neoplasia. It is an uncommon cause of pulmonary edema in small animals.

In clinical practice, pulmonary edema falls into one of two broad categories: (1) cardiogenic or high-pressure edema, and (2) noncardiogenic or permeability edema.

4. What are the four stages in the development of pulmonary edema?
One description of the sequence of lung edema formation follows:
Stage 1: The passage of fluid into the interstitium exceeds the capacity of the pulmonary lymphatic system to absorb it, resulting in fluid accumulation around bronchioles.
Stage 2: Continued fluid accumulation results in alveolar septal swelling.
Stage 3: Beginning of fluid accumulation within the alveola.
Stage 4: Complete alveolar filling occurs.
It should be recognized that small volumes of lung liquid are not necessarily visible radiographically and the correlation between radiographic appearance and the stages of edema formation listed above is imperfect. However, stages 2 and 3 are likely to be manifest radiographically by the presence of interstitial pulmonary opacities. The appearance of air bronchograms, the radiographic hallmark of an alveolar pulmonary pattern, indicates stage 4 of edema formation, the filling of the alveoli.

5. Name two common causes of high-pressure pulmonary edema.
• **Left-sided heart failure.** Left-sided heart failure results in a rise in left atrial pressures, which is reflected upon the pulmonary venous circulation; this, in turn, causes an increase in pulmonary capillary pressures and the development of high-pressure edema. The tendency for the formation of frank edema depends in part upon the speed with which atrial pressure rises. Pulmonary edema develops in normal dogs if left atrial pressures exceed 23 mmHg. In chronic heart disease, however, the rate of pulmonary lymphatic drainage increases and left atrial pressures may exceed this value before edema becomes evident. Thus patients with chronic heart disease and gradually increasing left atrial pressures may tolerate marked elevations in left atrial pressures prior to the development of radiographically visible pulmonary edema.
• **Iatrogenic volume overload due to overly aggressive intravenous fluid therapy.** The infusion of excessive volumes of crystalloids, colloids, or blood products can cause an increase in ventricular filling pressures that results in edema formation. In the case of crystalloid infusion, the development of dilutional hypoalbuminemia probably contributes to edema formation.

6. What is ARDS? Name some conditions commonly associated with ARDS.
ARDS is an acronym that stands for adult (or acute) respiratory distress syndrome. This syndrome is well recognized in critically ill human patients. ARDS refers to a noncardiogenic permeability edema that can complicate the presentation of many pulmonary and extrapulmonary diseases.
Factors predisposing to ARDS can be pulmonary, including
• Bacterial and aspiration pneumonia
• Pulmonary contusions
Nonpulmonary causes include:
• Sepsis
• Shock
• Pancreatitis
• Disseminated intravascular coagulation
• Head trauma, seizures (neurogenic)
• Upper airway obstruction

7. How can so many different diseases result in ARDS?
The response of the lung in ARDS is relatively consistent and is independent of the initiating stimulus. An intense inflammatory response occurs and results in alveolar and capillary endothelial damage, increased vascular permeability, increased lung water and protein, and decreased gas exchange.

8. What clinical signs are found in patients with acute pulmonary edema?
• Dyspnea
• Shallow breathing

- Cough (rarely in cats)
- Open-mouth breathing
- Cyanosis
- Expectoration of foamy, occasionally blood-tinged, fluid

9. What clinical features distinguish cardiogenic edema from noncardiogenic edema?

Historical information and the presence of concurrent disease may aid in their differentiation. The patient should be evaluated for cardiac disease initially (cardiac auscultation, ECG, thoracic radiographs, and/or echocardiography). If clinical evidence of cardiac disease is lacking, the patient should be evaluated for concurrent disease that may have led to noncardiogenic edema (complete blood count, serum biochemistry, urinalysis, abdominal radiography, and ultrasound). If the cause remains elusive, more invasive methods (pulmonary vascular catheterization for measurement of pulmonary artery and wedge pressures) may help in differentiating high pressure from permeability edema.

10. Should drugs be used to minimize anxiety in dyspneic patients?

Morphine, at a dose of 0.05 to 0.1 mg/kg subcutaneously, is the sedative of choice in dogs with moderate to severe dyspnea due to pulmonary edema. Morphine not only relieves anxiety but also causes depression of the respiratory centers and venodilation. Some degree of respiratory depression may be beneficial as it changes the character of the breathing from rapid and shallow to slower deeper breaths. However, morphine can increase intracranial pressure and is not indicated in animals with neurogenic edema. The effects of morphine in the cat are unpredictable and this drug should probably be avoided in this species.

11. How do I treat ARDS?

The goals of therapy are to alleviate hypoxemia, provide cardiovascular support, and treat the underlying condition.

- **Oxygen.** Oxygen should be administered by the least stressful method possible (face mask, nasal oxygen line, oxygen cage). Mechanical ventilation may be required.
- **Maintenance of cardiovascular support.** Cardiac output can be maintained by intravascular volume expansion and the use of inotropes (dobutamine, dopamine). Therapy should be aimed at maintaining pulmonary perfusion but avoiding volume overload, which could worsen the edema.

Identification and treatment of the underlying disorder is the major objective.

12. Should ARDS patients receive diuretics?

The use of diuretics in pulmonary edema is controversial. Diuretics will lower capillary hydrostatic pressure, therefore slowing the transudation of fluid into the pulmonary interstitium. Diuretics should be used cautiously in these patients.

13. Should ARDS patients receive corticosteroids?

Corticosteroids have theoretical benefits (decreasing inflammation and subsequent fibrosis), but their efficacy has not been proven.

14. Are there new therapies currently being investigated in the treatment of ARDS?

Yes, some examples of these are free radical scavengers, cyclooxygenase/lipooxygenase inhibitors, complement inhibitors, nitric oxide, and the administration of exogenous surfactant.

15. How do I decide when my patient needs mechanical ventilation?

Indications for positive pressure ventilation include an arterial oxygen tension of less than 50 mmHg in an animal breathing 100% oxygen or a progressive increase in arterial CO_2 (signalling ventilatory failure). Positive end-expiratory pressure (PEEP) is the most effective way to ventilate an ARDS patient. PEEP improves functional residual capacity, may reverse hypoxemia, and prevents alveolar and small airway collapse between breaths. Hemodynamic monitoring is essential as PEEP can dramatically reduce cardiac output.

16. What is the prognosis for a patient with ARDS?

Prognosis for ARDS is dependent on the underlying disease process. If the disease (e.g., sepsis) can be controlled then the prognosis is improved. Despite advances in therapy in both human and veterinary medicine, ARDS has a high mortality rate (70–100%) and those animals that recover may have persistent pulmonary dysfunction caused by irreversible fibrosis.

BIBLIOGRAPHY

1. Drobatz KJ, Concannon K: Noncardiogenic pulmonary edema. Comp Cont Educ Pract Vet 15:1011–1030, 1994.
2. Fowler AA, Hamman RF, et al: Adult respiratory distress syndrome: Risk with common predispositions. Ann Intern Med 98:593–597, 1983.
3. Harpster N: Pulmonary edema. In Kirk JW, Bonagura JD (eds): Kirk's Current Veterinary Therapy. Philadelphia, W.B. Saunders, 1989, pp 385–392.
4. Hawkins EC: Disease of the lower respiratory tract. In Ettinger SJ, Feldman EC (eds): Textbook of Veterinary Internal Medicine. Philadelphia, W.B. Saunders, 1995, pp 800–803.
5. Kuehn NF, Roudebush P: Pulmonary edema. In Allen DG, Kruth SA, Garvey MS (eds): Small Animal Medicine. Philadelphia, J.B. Lippincott, 1991, pp 433–443.
6. Olivier NB: Pulmonary edema. Vet Clin North Am Small Anim Pract 15:1011–1029, 1992.
7. Parent C, King L et al: Clinical and clinicopathologic findings in dogs with acute respiratory distress syndrome: 19 cases (1985-1993). J Am Vet Med Assoc 208:1419–1428, 1996.
8. Parent C, King L, et al: Respiratory function and treatment in dogs with acute respiratory distress syndrome: 19 cases (1985-1993). J Am Vet Med Assoc 208:1428–1433, 1996.
9. Trottier JT, Taylor RW: Adult respiratory distress syndrome. In Shoemaker WC (ed): Textbook of Critical Care, 3rd ed. Philadelphia, W.B. Saunders, 1995, pp 811–835.

6. ASCITES

Julie Armstrong, D.V.M.

1. What is ascites?

Ascites is the accumulation of free fluid in the peritoneal cavity. The fluid is generally described as a transudate or an exudate but can consist of blood, bile, urine, or chyle. Ascites is a clinical finding and not a disease in itself.

2. How do you tell on physical examination if a distended abdomen is due to ascites?

Ballottement of the abdomen often reveals a fluid wave. With one hand on either side of the abdomen, gently tap the abdominal wall with the fingers on one side. The other hand will feel the fluid wave. If only a small volume of fluid is present, the clinician may get the impression on abdominal palpation that the intestines feel "slippery."

3. What are the differential diagnoses for a distended abdomen in the absence of fluid?

Differential diagnoses include obesity, pregnancy, gastric dilation, obstipation, bladder distention, neoplasia, hyperadrenocorticism, and organomegaly. Organomegaly may involve the spleen, liver, kidney, or a nongravid uterus, i.e., pyometra, mucometra, or neoplasia.

4. What are Starling's forces? How are they important in the formation of ascites?

Starling's forces are the hydrostatic and oncotic forces that determine the direction of fluid movement across the permeable capillary wall. Hydrostatic pressure is the mechanical force exerted by a fluid related to area; in health, intracapillary hydrostatic pressure exceeds interstital hydrostatic pressure and this favors capillary filtration. Colloids, more specifically proteins within the capillary and in the interstitium are responsible for oncotic pressure. In addition to Starling's forces, capillary permeability and lymphatic pressure are two factors that determine whether or not there is net accumulation of interstitial fluid.

If these variables are altered to a degree that compensatory mechanisms (e.g., increased lymphatic flow and collateral vessel development) become overwhelmed, ascites will develop. Increases in intracapillary hydrostatic pressure favor the transudation of fluid and can result in the development of ascites; the causes include right-sided congestive heart failure. Plasma oncotic pressure is a force that retains fluid within the capillary. Reductions in plasma oncotic pressure can therefore lead to the development of ascites. The main determinant of plasma oncotic pressure is albumin. Ascites secondary to hypoalbuminemia is unlikely to occur unless the albumin is less than 15 g/L. Lymphatic obstruction due to trauma, inflammation, or neoplasia will lead to increased pressure and therefore leakage of fluid. Diffuse increases in vessel permeability can also result in interstitial fluid accumulation. The most common cause of increased vessel permeability is inflammation.

5. Which conditions commonly lead to the development of ascites?

Conditions that can lead to ascites include portal hypertension (prehepatic, hepatic and posthepatic), hypoproteinemia, inflammatory peritoneal or visceral disease (abdominal neoplasia or peritonitis), sodium or water retention states, coagulopathies, trauma, and obstructive or traumatic rupture of lymphatics or obstruction to lymphatic (peritoneal or subperitoneal) drainage.

6. How is portal hypertension categorized?

Portal hypertension is a cause of elevated hydrostatic pressure in splanchnic capillaries. It can be categorized as prehepatic (or presinusoidal), hepatic, or posthepatic (or postsinusoidal). Prehepatic portal hypertension results when there is compression or obstruction of portal venous

flow, such as can occur in portal vein stenosis, thrombosis, or intravascular or extravascular obstructive neoplasia. Prehepatic portal hypertension rarely results in ascites because collateral vessels quickly develop between the portal vein and the vena cava. These collateral vessels decrease
hydrostatic pressure, and lymph flow from the intestinal tract is increased in order to compensate
for increased portal venous pressure. Together, these factors limit the development of ascites.

Hepatic portal hypertension most commonly results from fibrosis and scarring of the liver.
Other causes include metastatic neoplasia, intrahepatic vein thrombosis, cholangiohepatitis (cat),
intrahepatic arteriovenous shunting, and hepatic vein atresia.

Posthepatic causes of portal hypertension include right heart failure, pericardial tamponade,
constrictive pericarditis, intracardiac neoplasia, heartworm disease, and compression or obstruction of the caudal vena cava.

7. What are the major systemic effects of ascites?
- Large volumes of fluid can increase intra-abdominal pressure leading to a decrease in
  venous return and therefore decreased cardiac output.
- Increased abdominal pressure also impairs the movement of the diaphragm and can cause
  hypoventilation or panting.
- If the fluid accumulation occurs quickly there will be an inadequate time for plasma
  volume equilibration, and cardiovascular collapse and shock can ensue. Most commonly,
  this is caused by hemorrhage. Severely exudative peritonitis can also cause a large loss of
  fluid and protein leading to circulatory collapse, hypoproteinemia, and edema formation.
- In addition, cytokines, vasoactive amines, or eicosanoids present in the fluid can contribute
  to circulatory collapse. Inflammatory mediators can also activate the coagulation cascade,
  which can lead to coagulopathies or disseminated intravascular coagulation.
- Increases in abdominal pressure cause discomfort and inflammation of the peritoneum can
  exacerbate this pain.

8. Besides history and physical exam, what are additional diagnostic tools that can identify ascites?
- Radiographs can be suggestive of ascites if a moderate to large volume of fluid is present.
  The fluid causes a loss of abdominal detail. If there is a large volume, all detail is lost and
  the entire abdomen will take on a radiographic appearance consistent with soft tissue.
  Radiographs should be taken before abdominal paracentesis to avoid the iatrogenic entry of
  air that can cause a diagnostic dilemma if free air is visible in the peritoneal cavity.
- Ultrasound is more sensitive than radiographs for the detection of abdominal fluid; it can
  detect small volumes of clinically unrecognizable fluid. Ultrasound can also be used to
  guide the selection of the site for abdominal paracentesis.
- Abdominal paracentesis is the third means of diagnosing abdominal fluid.

9. When and why is abdominal paracentesis performed?
Abdominal paracentesis can be both diagnostic and therapeutic. The technique is used to
obtain a sample of fluid when ascites is known to be present, when fluid is suspected (e.g., suspected postoperative dehiscence, suspected hemorrhage in a trauma patient nonresponsive to
shock therapy), or if an animal presents for an "acute" painful abdomen.

In addition, abdominocentesis may be part of the management plan. If the animal is dyspneic
and/or in pain due to excessive abdominal pressure, fluid removal is necessary to allow for comfortable respiration as well as to relieve pain.

Abdominocentesis may also be necessary to allow for organ biopsy, radiographs, or ultrasonography when a large volume of fluid is interfering with these diagnostic tests.

10. Do I need restraint to perform abdominal paracentesis?
In most cases manual restraint is all that is needed. If necessary, local anesthesia (lidocaine),
low-dose oxymorphone and acepromazine (0.1 mg/kg and 0.025–0.05 mg/kg, respectively, IV),

or low-dose oxymorphone and midazolam (0.1 mg/kg and 0.2 mg/kg, respectively, IV; use 0.1 mg/kg midazolam in cats) can be used. If the ascites is due to right-sided heart failure, low-dose opioid and benzodiazepine-derivative drugs are considered to have the least adverse hemodymamic effects of drugs commonly used for sedation.

11. What equipment do I need for abdominal paracentesis?

Paracentesis may be performed using a simple needle, a butterfly catheter, an intravenous catheter, or a peritoneal dialysis catheter. For simple needle paracentesis a one-inch 22-gauge needle or butterfly catheter is used. A 16–18 gauge needle and a stopcock can be used for large-volume drainage. A 60-cc syringe can be directly attached to the butterfly or an extension set can be attached directly to the needle. When using an intravenous catheter, the stylet is removed once the abdomen is punctured. Additional holes can be cut into the catheter to increase the likelihood of aspirating fluid. If a peritoneal dialysis catheter is used, local anesthesia is recommended in advance to facilitate a stab incision through the skin with a number 11 or 15 scalpel blade. Once the skin is incised then the peritoneal catheter is inserted. Once the peritoneal catheter penetrates the abdomen the trocar should be pulled back into the catheter. The entire unit is then advanced a short distance more into the abdomen and the catheter is threaded over the trocar into the abdomen.

12. How should the patient be positioned for abdominal paracentesis?

The patient can be placed in left lateral recumbency to avoid puncture of the spleen or the animal can remain standing. When placing a peritoneal catheter some prefer to place the animal in dorsal recumbency and direct the catheter in a dorsal-caudal direction. Sedation may be required for this position and is recommended if lavage is necessary.

13. Where do I insert the needle for abdominal paracentesis?

Initially a 4 × 4-cm area of the abdomen just caudal to the umbilicus is shaved and aseptically prepared. The needle or catheter is inserted 2–4 cm caudal to the umbilicus on the midline or just laterally. The needle should be inserted to a depth where fluid is first obtained. Scars should be avoided due to the increased chance of associated omental adhesions. A quadrant approach can also be used. Four quadrants can be created by using the linea alba as one line and then bisecting that line by drawing a line through the umbilicus. The needle is inserted into each quadrant, 2–4 cm from each imaginary line, after aseptic preparation. Gentle aspiration is necessary to prevent suction of omentum or fat against the needle.

14. What do I do if I don't aspirate any fluid during abdominal paracentesis?

• Withdraw the needle and repeat the procedure in a different quadrant.
• Use a larger gauge needle or use a large gauge catheter with extra holes.
• If the animal was lying in lateral recumbency, try a standing position. If the patient is cooperative the front legs can be elevated and/or the abdomen can be gently massaged or ballotement performed.
• Ensure that the syringe and aspiration technique is not creating too much suction such that omentum may be blocking the flow of fluid.
• If ultrasound is available, abdominal paracentesis can be guided by ultrasonography.
• If a small volume of fluid is suspected, then a diagnostic peritoneal lavage can be performed to increase the likelihood of obtaining a sample.

15. How is diagnostic peritoneal lavage performed?

A peritoneal catheter or a peritoneal dialysis catheter is inserted into the abdomen as described above. The catheter is attached to an infusion delivery system and 20 ml/kg of warmed lactated Ringer's solution or 0.9% saline is infused into the abdomen. The animal is gently rocked from side to side and the abdomen is gently massaged. Once the volume has been delivered, one can try to collect the fluid by allowing gravity to fill the infusion set or by gentle aspiration with a 6-cc syringe. In general only 30–50% of the fluid will be recovered.

16. What are the contraindications to performing abdominal paracentesis?

Abnormal hemostasis is a relative contraindication. Other concerns would be organomegaly, suspected body wall adhesions, or suspected diaphragmatic hernia.

17. What are some possible complications of abdominal paracentesis?

The main concern with needle paracentesis is laceration of abdominal organs. Catheter paracentesis can cause perforation of the viscera and spread of infection from localized sites of inflammation as well as vessel puncture and iatrogenic hemorrhage. Complications can result in a false-positive tap especially when the spleen, liver, a vessel, the intestines, the bladder, or the gallbladder is punctured iatrogenically. Furthermore, puncture of these sites can lead to iatrogenic infection.

It is not uncommon to have mild leakage of fluid into the subcutaneous site of paracentesis or a small hematoma, but these complications are self-limiting.

18. Does it matter how much fluid is removed?

The risks associated with large-volume rapid drainage are protein depletion and possibly circulatory shock secondary to rapid reaccumulation of fluid and hypovolemia. However, "rapid" removal of fluid does not usually cause immediate changes in blood pressure, heart rate, hematocrit, or electrolytes. There can be rapid reaccumulation within 2–3 days; therefore, ongoing medical therapy should be instituted following abdominocentesis. Electrolytes and protein should be monitored frequently if multiple abdominocentesis procedures have been performed or if diuretics are included in medical therapy.

19. What are the principles behind the management of ascites?

Ascites is not a disease in itself; therefore, management must be directed at the underlying disorder. For example, ascites secondary to a ruptured bladder, a splenic hemangiosarcoma, or a ruptured viscus needs to be handled surgically. Bacterial cultures should be taken and antibiotic therapy implemented when appropriate. Blood transfusions may be lifesaving in addition to exploratory surgery if the effusion is hemorrhagic and is secondary to trauma causing laceration of a major blood vessel. If the effusion is due to hypoalbuminemia, initial supportive care may include plasma transfusion and or colloids for cardiovascular support. Large volumes of plasma are necessary to cause any significant increase in plasma protein and the effects are only temporary, once again emphasizing the need to treat the underlying cause of protein loss. Sodium restriction and specific medical therapy may be of benefit in those diseases such as heart failure and liver disease where there is activation of the renin-angiotensin system.

Management of Ascites

TYPE OF FLUID	ANCILLARY TESTS USEFUL IN SELECTED CASES	COMMON DIFFERENTIAL DIAGNOSES
Transudate (protein < 2.5 g/dl)	CBC, chemistry, urinalysis Urine protein: creatinine ratio Serum B_{12}, folate, and TLI Intestinal biopsy Bile acids, ammonia tolerance Liver biopsy, abdominal radiographs, and ultrasound	Protein-losing enteropathy Protein-losing nephropathy Liver failure Intrahepatic arteriovenous fistula Hepatic and prehepatic portal hypertension Neoplasia (lymphoma) Burns Obstructing lymphatic drainage
Modified transudate (protein > 2.5 g/dl)	Chest radiographs Echocardiography ECG, CVP, heartworm test Angiocardiogram	Right heart failure Vena cava disease Budd-Chiari syndrome Posthepatic and occasionally hepatic or prehepatic portal hypertension Neoplasia (obstructing lymphatics and blood vessels), carcinoma, and sarcoma

Table continued on facing page

Management of Ascites (Continued)

TYPE OF FLUID	ANCILLARY TESTS USEFUL IN SELECTED CASES	COMMON DIFFERENTIAL DIAGNOSES
Exudate (protein > 2.5 g/dl inflammatory)	Ascites albumin:globulin ratio FIP antibody titer CBC, chemistry, U/A Ascites bilirubin test Ascitic creatinine measure Ascitic amylase measure Ascitic fluid culture: bacterial and fungal Abdominal radiographs and ultrasound Contrast cystograms	Feline infectious peritonitis Peritonitis: trauma, spontaneous septic, bile, bowel rupture, pancreatitis, pyometra or prostatic abscess rupture, steatitis, bladder rupture Abdominal neoplasia: carcinoma, lymphosarcoma, or sarcoma Diaphragmatic hernia: serosanguinous exudate
Blood	CBC, platelet count, PT, PTT FDP, antithrombin III Abdominal radiographs and ultrasound Chest radiographs	Coagulopathy Trauma or postsurgical: spleen, liver, or vessel Neoplasia eroding a vessel: pheochromocytoma Ruptured hemangiosarcoma Splenic or gastric torsion
Chyle	CBC, serum chemistry Chest radiographs and echocardiography Abdominal radiographs and ultrasound Lymphangiography	Congenital Heart disease: secondary to cardiomyopathy, pericardial effusion, constrictive pericarditis Thoracic duct disease: spontaneous or traumatic Lymphangiectasia/lymphangitis or defective lymphatic development Neoplasia Pancreatitis Pseudochylus Chronic fluid accumulation Chronic infection

BIBLIOGRAPHY

1. Allen DG: Ascites. In Allen DG, Garvey MS, Kruth SA (eds): Small Animal Medicine. Philadelphia, J.B. Lippincott, 1991, pp 105–114.
2. Ettinger SJ, Barrett KA: Ascites, peritonitis and other causes of abdominal distention. In Ettinger SJ, Feldman EC (eds): Textbook of Veterinary Internal Medicine. Philadelphia,W.B. Saunders, 1995, pp 64–71.
3. King LG, Gelens HCJ: Ascites. The Compendium 14:1063–1075, 1992.
4. Kristal Orna: Abdominal paracentesis. In Wingfield WE (ed): Veterinary Emergency Medicine Secrets. Philadelphia, Hanley & Belfus, 1997, pp 408–413.
5. Paddleford RR, Harvey RC: Critical care surgical techniques. Vet Clin North Am Small Anim Pract 19:1079–1094, 1989.

7. EXTRACARDIAC DISEASE AND THE HEART

Rebecca E. Gompf, D.V.M., M.S.

1. How can systemic diseases affect the heart?

Systemic diseases can directly or indirectly affect the heart. Disease processes that alter electrolytes, acid-base balance, or neurohormonal balance of the body can have a direct effect on the electrical and mechanical functions of the heart. Some diseases directly affect the heart by causing the release of cardiac stimulant or cardiac depressant factors. The heart can also be indirectly affected when disease imposes abnormally great demands on the cardiovascular system, such as can occur in chronic and severe anemia.

2. Which diseases will cause electrolyte imbalances that may affect the heart?

The primary electrolyte changes that affect the heart usually involve hypokalemia, hyperkalemia, hypocalcemia, or hypercalcemia. Hypoadrenocorticism (Addison's disease), primary aldosteronism (Conn's syndrome), diabetes mellitus, gastric dilation and volvulus, septic shock, and renal disease can all influence electrolyte balance in the body. Depending on the severity and the rate at which the electrolyte imbalance develops, the heart may be adversely affected.

Other diseases can result in vomiting and diarrhea, which can affect the electrolyte balance. However, the changes are usually gradual and primary cardiac events are unusual.

3. What is hypoadrenocorticism (Addison's disease) and how does it affect the heart?

Addison's disease is a deficiency of either cortisol or mineralocorticoid secretion from the adrenal gland. Cortisol has many effects that are noncardiac. Its cardiac effects include its effect on systemic vasculature and on calcium.

Cortisol helps to maintain blood pressure by preserving vascular integrity and responsiveness to circulating vasoconstrictors; it therefore contributes to the maintenance of vascular tone. The decrease in vascular tone and intravascular volume associated with the lack of cortisol contributes to the hypotension found in patients with Addison's disease.

Cortisol also helps to maintain the normal calcium levels in the body by affecting the renal excretion of calcium. About one third of dogs with Addison's disease are hypercalcemic. The elevated levels of calcium are mild (12.0–14.9 mg/dl) and are correlated with the severity of their dehydration and potassium elevation. Cardiac problems resulting from the elevated calcium levels have not been reported.

Mineralocorticoids maintain the sodium, potassium, and chloride balances in the body. The primary mineralocorticoid is aldosterone. Aldosterone promotes the renal reabsorption of sodium and chloride in exchange for potassium and hydrogen ions. Water is reabsorbed with the sodium and chloride. A lack of aldosterone results in the loss of sodium, chloride, and water. One result is hypovolemia, which in turn reduces cardiac output and contributes to hypotension. One of the classic findings on thoracic radiographs in a patient with Addison's disease is a small heart.

Sodium is necessary for both excitation and contraction in the heart. The low sodium level associated with Addison's disease does affect the heart's normal functions; however, its cardiac effects are overshadowed by the effects of the hyperkalemia and are not recognized as specific clinical signs associated with the heart.

Hyperkalemia due to Addison's disease is potentially life threatening. Its primary effects are on electrical conduction throughout the myocardium and on the strength of contraction.

The severity of the hyperkalemia can be monitored with an electrocardiogram (ECG). When the serum levels of potassium are mildly elevated (5.5–6.5 mEq/L), the ECG may show bradycardia with tall, peaked T-waves. With moderate hyperkalemia (6.6–8.5 mEq/L), the ECG can show decreased P-wave height, and prolonged QRS-, P-wave, and PR-interval duration. When the potassium levels exceed 8.5 mEq/L, the P waves generally disappear (atrial standstill occurs and the atria are not contracting). When potassium levels exceed 11 mEq/L, death can occur due to ventricular asystole or ventricular fibrillation. In clinical cases, the correlation of serum potassium levels to electrocardiographic appearance is imperfect; however, the ECG is an excellent way to monitor the clinical consequences of moderate and severe hyperkalemia.

The overall cardiac effects of Addison's disease include decreased cardiac wall motion, decreased cardiac output, decreased heart rate, and decreased peak left-ventricular work. Most of these changes are due to hypovolemia and hyperkalemia. Stress can cause cardiac collapse and death but congestive heart failure does not occur.

4. How does hyperadrenocorticism (Cushing's disease) affect the heart?

Cushing's disease in people has caused congestive heart failure secondary to the severe hypertension that it causes. The hypertension results from the retention of sodium and water from activation of the renin-angiotensin system, and from the increased sensitivity to vasopressors, which causes vasoconstriction. Fifty percent of dogs with Cushing's disease are hypertensive, but congestive heart failure caused by the hypertension is rare.

It is likely that the only dogs with Cushing's disease that develop congestive heart failure are those with underlying heart disease. Most of the dogs that develop Cushing's disease are those breeds that are also prone to mitral valve endocardiosis. The increased fluid retention in Cushing's disease could result in problems if the dog has significant preexisting heart disease.

The most common side effect of Cushing's disease that indirectly affects the heart is pulmonary embolism. See Chapter 47 for a discussion of this problem.

5. What is primary aldosteronism (Conn's syndrome) and how does it affect the heart?

Primary aldosteronism is an excessive secretion of aldosterone from the adrenal glands, which results in hypernatremia, hypokalemia, and severe systemic hypertension in man. As a result of the hypertension, the left ventricle will hypertrophy and can eventually fail. Also, arrhythmias can occur.

While cardiovascular abnormalities have been observed in small animals with Conn's syndrome, it should be recognized that this disorder is very uncommon, having been reported in only one dog and two cats.

6. How can diabetes mellitus affect the heart?

In people, diabetes mellitus causes hypertension, arrhythmias, and coronary atherosclerosis. As a result, myocardial infarcts (heart attacks) are common in diabetics and result in high morbidity and mortality. Diabetic cardiomyopathy has also been reported in people and is associated with severe, prolonged coronary microvascular disease caused by the diabetes.

Dogs with diabetes have an increased risk of hypertension. However, dogs and cats rarely develop coronary artery disease. Diabetic dogs may develop mildly impaired systolic myocardial function but congestive heart failure is not a problem in diabetic dogs and cats.

Dogs and cats that are being treated for ketoacidotic diabetes may develop profound hypokalemia. Atrioventricular conduction disturbances have been observed in association with severe hypokalemia. However, and perhaps most importantly, hypokalemia predisposes to the development of ventricular arrhythmias including ventricular premature complexes, ventricular tachycardia, and potentially ventricular fibrillation.

7. How does gastric dilation/volvulus (GDV) affect the heart?

GDV affects the heart in several different ways. In experimental GDV, it was found that GDV reduced cardiac output, contractility, mean arterial pressure, total peripheral resistance, coronary perfusion, and myocardial oxygen consumption. After gastric decompression most of these variables return to normal except that the cardiac output and mean arterial pressure remain low. Myocardial contractility increases due to sympathetic stimulation. However, cardiac output remains low because of arrhythmias, decreased preload, and increased afterload.

Most of the above effects are secondary to the hypovolemia that occurs when the enlarged stomach occludes flow in the hepatic portal vein and posterior vena cava. However, endotoxins from congestion of the abdominal viscera activate many inflammatory mediators such as histamines, prostaglandins, and leukotrienes. Also, there is a release of a vasoactive peptide from the pancreas that decreases myocardial contractility and contributes to decreased cardiac output and myocardial hypoperfusion.

Arrhythmias develop in about 40% of the dogs with GDV. Most of these tend to occur one-half to three days after presentation. Ventricular arrhythmias are the most common. They are primarily due to myocardial hypoxia from the hypovolemia and decreased cardiac output. Reperfusion injury, which is caused by the release of accumulated neutrophils and reactive hydroxyl radicals resulting in superoxide radicals plus hypochlorite ions, may also contribute to the ventricular arrhythmias. The hypokalemia, acidosis, and hypoxia that are also associated with the GDV facilitate the ventricular arrhythmias and make them resistant to antiarrhythmic therapy.

8. How do endotoxins from septic shock affect the heart?

Many different factors, including gastric torsion, can contribute to septic shock in animals. In people with septic shock, tumor necrosis factor and interleukin-1 cause myocardial depression. These inflammatory substances cause myocardial depression by causing nitric oxide synthesis, which in turn forms nitric oxide in the myocardium. This same mechanism of myocardial depression is thought to exist in animals with septic shock. Besides myocardial depression, the toxins may also result in atrial and/or ventricular arrhythmias.

9. Do animals with renal failure have cardiac problems?

Toxins that accumulate due to renal failure may have a direct cardiotoxic effect. In man, an uremic cardiomyopathy has been documented, but it has not been documented in animals.

Most of the cardiac complications of renal disease in humans are the results of coronary atherosclerosis, hypertension, lipid abnormalities, and the complications of chronic hemodialysis. These complications can result in congestive heart failure.

Dogs with protein-losing nephropathies are at risk for pulmonary thromboembolism and systemic hypertension can be associated with canine renal disease. However, congestive heart failure resulting from either of these problems has not been reported in the dog or cat.

People with acute or chronic uremia have been reported to have pericardial inflammation, which is probably secondary to the accumulation of uremic toxins causing a pericardial serositis. Uremic pericarditis usually results in the accumulation of a small amount of hemorrhagic pericardial effusion and a few patients develop cardiac tamponade.

Pericardial effusions do occur in animals with renal disease but the effusions are usually small and cardiac tamponade has not been reported. Those animals with pericardial effusion may have a pericardial friction rub on auscultation and a small amount of effusion may be detected on echocardiogram. Other than these findings, there is no other evidence of cardiac disease in these animals.

Cats with lower urinary obstruction can develop significant hyperkalemia. The obstructed cat's ECG is similar to a dog's with hyperkalemia (see Addison's disease above).

10. Do animals develop hypertension and what effect does it have on the heart?

Systemic hypertension is a sustained elevation in systemic arterial pressure. While animals can develop primary, or essential, hypertension, it is more commonly associated with other disorders such as renal disease, hyperadrenocorticism, hyperthyroidism, and diabetes mellitus.

The clinical signs associated with hypertension are those of the underlying disease process. However, with chronic hypertension, other organs such as the retinas, kidneys, and heart can become damaged.

Hypertension causes a chronic pressure overload of the left heart. As a result, the left heart will hypertrophy, but the hypertrophy is seldom severe and heart failure appears to be uncommon. The increased afterload can increase the severity of mitral regurgitation in patients with preexisting heart disease.

11. What is synchronous diaphragmatic flutter and what causes it?

Synchronous diaphragmatic flutter occurs when the diaphragm contracts with every heart-beat. The animal appears to be shaking or twitching and auscultation confirms that the twitches correspond to the heart rate. Fluoroscopy can provide radiographic confirmation of the diagnosis.

The flutter is believed to be caused by excitation of the pericardial segment of the phrenic nerve by the electrical activity of the heart. This problem occurs most commonly in dogs with persistent vomiting. This problem is felt to be the result of either the alkalosis associated with the persistent vomiting or hypocalcemia resulting in hyperirritability of the phrenic nerve. Once these underlying problems are corrected, the flutter disappears.

12. How does a pheochromocytoma affect the heart?

Most of the cardiac problems associated with a pheochromocytoma, which is a functional tumor of the adrenal medulla, are due to the invasion of the tumor into the caudal vena cava or to the effects of increased levels of catecholamines. Neoplastic invasion of the caudal vena cava can obstruct blood returning to the heart, which can cause ascites.

The increased levels of catecholamines cause sinus tachycardia, which is the most common ECG finding; it is observed in 15–54% of the cases. Catecholamines can also sensitize the heart to arrhythmias such as atrial and ventricular premature beats. Ventricular arrhythmias may cause sudden death. Also, 50% of the dogs whose blood pressure is measured are hypertensive, and left ventricular and left atrial enlargement is common in dogs. In one report, 2 out of 15 dogs showed signs of congestive heart failure.

13. How does hypothyroidism affect the heart?

Thyroid hormones have a direct effect on the heart and will increase contractility, stimulate myocardial hypertrophy, and increase the myocardial sensitivity to adrenergic simulation. When hypothyroidism occurs, the number of beta receptors in the heart decreases, which means that the heart cannot respond well to sympathetic stimulation. This results in a bradycardia and decreased contractility. A decrease in the rate of myocardial relaxation may also be observed.

In people, a myxedematous heart is the result of chronic hypothyroidism. The myxedematous heart has the same appearance as the heart with dilated cardiomyopathy, except that with thyroid supplementation the myxedematous heart returns to normal. In dogs, chronic hypothyroidism has not been shown to cause dilated cardiomyopathy. However, some breeds such as the Doberman pinscher, golden retriever, Irish setter, Great Dane, Old English sheepdog, and cocker spaniel are prone to having both problems. By treating the hypothyroidism in dogs with dilated cardiomyopathy, the dogs feel better and their heart disease may be easier to manage.

The common cardiac signs associated with hypothyroidism are bradycardia, weak cardiac apex beat, and arrhythmias. In humans there is an increased incidence of hypertension. With severe hypothyroidism, the dog's ECG may show sinus bradycardia and low-voltage QRS complexes. In experimental dogs, the PR interval is prolonged, which may indicate a problem in the atrioventricular node secondary to the hypothyroidism. Some hypothyroid dogs have had atrial fibrillation or other arrhythmias.

Echocardiographic changes include thinning of the left ventricular posterior wall, decreased shortening fraction due to decreased left ventricular wall excursion, alterations in the systolic and diastolic time intervals, and mildly increased left ventricular systolic diameter.

The cardiac manifestations of canine hypothyroidism are generally of little clinical consequence and resolve after replacement therapy. There have been anecdotal reports of thyroid supplementation causing dogs with dilated cardiomyopathy and hypothyroidism to go back into congestive heart failure by starting them at their normal level of thyroid replacement. Studies in humans have not found any problems with thyroid supplementation at normal levels in people with dilated cardiomyopathy and hypothyroidism. Until such studies are done in dogs with both diseases, dogs with hypothyroidism and dilated cardiomyopathy should be monitored closely for the first few weeks of thyroid supplementation.

14. Can dogs have heart attacks?

Heart attacks in people are caused by the sudden blockage of blood flow through one or more coronary arteries, resulting in hypoxia and death of the areas of the heart perfused by the blocked vessel(s). The underlying cause of the heart attacks is usually atherosclerosis, which is the accumulation of cholesterol plaques that causes gradual obstruction of the vessel(s).

In dogs, atherosclerosis is uncommon but it can occur secondary to chronic hypothyroidism. A major heart attack can occur but is uncommon. More commonly the dog has arrhythmias and decreased contractility of the area of the wall affected by atherosclerosis.

Since major arteriosclerosis causing a heart attack is rare in the dog, the practitioner should refrain from telling a client that an animal has suffered or died from a "heart attack." When cardiac disease is indeed responsible, it is much more likely that the dog died of heart failure or a sudden arrhythmia.

15. What is an arteriovenous (AV) fistula and how does it affect the heart?

An arteriovenous (AV) fistula is an abnormal connection between an artery and a vein in which the blood does not pass through a capillary bed. These shunts can be congenital or acquired. Acquired AV fistulas are usually the result of trauma or perivascular injection of an irritating substance, or are associated with the presence of a neoplasm. Most AV fistulas involve single vessels but occasionally more than one AV fistula can be present in an area.

An AV fistula can be located anywhere in the body, but it is usually located in an extremity. The AV fistula allows oxygenated blood from an artery to enter the venous system directly. This can cause proliferation of the affected vessels, which can increase the number or size of the AV fistulas. The affected area may also be painful and may become edematous due to the increased blood flow. Occasionally the area can develop necrosis and ulceration and sometimes the area develops abnormal pigmentation.

Depending on the size or number of AV fistulas in an area, a continuous murmur may be auscultated over the area. Also, the murmur sometimes can be felt as a "thrill" over the affected area.

If the AV fistula is large and a significant volume of blood flows from the artery into the vein, it can cause a volume overload of the entire heart. On radiographs there is generalized cardiomegaly. Echocardiography confirms generalized cardiomegaly and may show an increased fractional shortening due to the volume overload. In very large shunts, there is an increase in end-diastolic pressure, which can lead to congestive heart failure.

Diagnosis of AV fistulas can be difficult and may require angiography to outline the AV fistula. Once the AV fistula has been identified, surgery is done to ligate it. Once the AV fistula has been ligated, the circulation in the area will return to normal if all of the fistulas have been located and ligated. The heart will also return to normal size and function.

16. How can anemia affect the heart?

In people, anemia is an important cause of high cardiac-output states. The low oxygen-carrying capacity of the blood stimulates a sequence of reactions that results in increased heart rate, increased volume of blood pumped by the heart, and increased cardiac output. The increased volume of blood pumped by the heart is similar to the volume overload due to leaky heart valves or congenital left-to-right shunts such as a patent ductus arteriosus (PDA). The heart will dilate and hypertrophy. Radiographs of an animal with chronic anemia may show generalized cardiomegaly.

Clinical complications of anemia only occur with chronic, severe anemia (packed cell volume less than 20%). Most animals will have a soft systolic murmur. Occasionally an animal may have a gallop rhythm. Many times the precordial impulse of the heart is stronger than normal.

In people, anemia can cause high-output cardiac failure and signs of congestion. In animals, cardiac failure is rare unless the animal has underlying heart disease that is potentiated by the anemia. The symptoms and treatment of the heart disease will depend on which disease is present in those animals with both heart disease and anemia. Heart disease is not a cause of anemia in animals.

17. What causes polycythemia and how does it affect the heart?

Polycythemia, or erythrocytosis, refers to a pathologic increase in red blood cell mass; it must be distinguished from elevations in packed cell volume (PCV) that result from hemoconcentration. The two major causes of polycythemia in small animals are right-to-left cardiac shunts (such as tetralogy of Fallot) and idiopathic polycythemia vera. Chronic congestive heart failure can lead to increases in red cell mass, but this is typically offset by the increase in intravascular volume that results from salt and water retention; thus, the packed cell volume (PCV) in most patients with chronic heart failure is normal.

Pathologic polycythemia (PCV over 60% in dogs) causes an increase in the amount of oxygen carried by the blood, an increase in blood volume, and potentially an increase in cardiac output despite an increase in ventricular afterload. High-output cardiac failure can occur, but is rare in animals. The animals have brick-red mucous membranes. Their other clinical signs and examination findings depend on the cause of their disease. Some animals will present for seizures due to the slow movement or sludging of blood in the brain.

18. How does pancreatitis affect the heart?

When pancreatitis occurs, a myocardial depressant factor is released that can depress myocardial function. Clinically this rarely is significant in animals.

Pancreatitis has also been associated with ventricular arrhythmias in animals. The cause of ventricular arrhythmias in this syndrome has not been identified, although inflammatory mediators, myocardial depressant factor, electrolyte derangements, and acid-base disturbances could potentially have a role in arrhythmogenesis.

BIBLIOGRAPHY

1. Atkins CE: The role of noncardiac disease in the development and precipitation of heart failure. Vet Clin North Am Small Anim Pract 21:1035, 1991.
2. Atkins CE, Engerman RL, Kern TS: Diabetic cardiomyopathy. Proc Am Coll Vet Int Med 2:9, 1988.
3. Chastain CB, Panciera DL: Hypothyroid diseases. In Ettinger SJ, Feldman EC (ed): Textbook of Veterinary Internal Medicine, Philadelphia, W.B. Saunders, 1995.
4. Fox PR, Nicols CER: Cardiac involvement in systemic disease. In Fox PR (ed): Canine and Feline Cardiology, New York, Churchill-Livingstone, 1988.
5. Kittleson MD, Kienle RD: Myocarditis and the effects of systemic disease on the cardiovascular system. In Small Animal Cardiovascular Medicine, St. Louis, Mosby, 1998.
6. Kobayashi DL, Peterson ME, Graves TK, et al: Hypertension in cats with chronic renal failure or hyperthyroidism. J Vet Intern Med 4:58, 1990.
7. Lesser M, Fox PR, Bond BR: Assessment of hypertension in 40 cats with left ventricular hypertrophy by Doppler-shift sphygmomanometry. J Small Anim Pract 33:55, 1992.
8. Miller CW, Boon JA, Soderberg SA, et al: Echocardiographic assessment of cardiac function in beagles with experimentally produced hypothyroidism. J Ultrasound Med 3(Suppl):157, 1984.
9. Nelson RW: Disorders of the thyroid gland. In Nelson RW, Couto CG (eds): Essentials of Small Animal Internal Medicine. Mosby, St. Louis, 1992.
10. Panciera DL: M-mode echocardiographic and electrocardiographic findings before and after levothyroxine treatment in hypothyroid dogs [abstract]. J Vet Intern Med 7:115, 1993.
11. Suter PF: Peripheral vascular disease. In Ettinger SJ (ed): Veterinary Internal Medicine, 3rd ed. Philadelphia, W.B. Saunders, 1989.
12. Williams GH, Braunwald E: Endocrine and nutritional disorders and heart disease. In Braunwald E (ed): Heart Disease: A Textbook of Cardiovascular Medicine. Philadelphia, W.B. Saunders, 1992.

II. Cardiovascular Pharmacology

8. DIURETICS

Darlene R. Blischok, D.V.M.

1. What is a diuretic?

A diuretic is a drug or agent that increases urine production.

2. When is a diuretic indicated?

In the management of congestive heart failure (CHF), diuretics are used to decrease preload. While ancillary vasodilatory effects are produced by specific agents such as furosemide, these drugs are used primarily to increase urine production. This, in turn, serves to reduce intravascular volume and therefore venous pressures. The development of edema in congestive heart failure results from elevation in venous pressures and the resulting derangement of Starling transmural capillary forces. The administration of a diuretic can reverse this abnormality and allow the lymphatic circulation to reabsorb excessive extravascular fluid. Thus, the use of diuretics is exquisitely suited to the treatment of cardiogenic or "high-pressure" edema. Edema that results from other pathophysiologic mechanisms such as lymphatic obstruction or hypoalbuminemia responds less well to diuretic administration.

3. Name the different types of diuretics, describe how they work, and give examples of each.

The diuretic agents in clinical use cause increased salt and water loss by interfering with ion transport within the nephron. This is accomplished through alterations in intracellular ionic entry or uptake; energy generation used for ion transport; or ion transfer from the cell to the peritubular capillaries outside the cell. Those drugs that alter ion transport can affect the nephron in different areas with differing effects. For example, the loop of Henle is the most sensitive to alterations in ion transport, thus it is this region of the nephron that can cause the most salt and water loss.

Loop diuretics are among the most powerful of the diuretics. These drugs inhibit the sodium-potassium-chloride cotransporter located in the luminal membrane of the thick ascending loop of Henle. This pump has high metabolic activity and is capable of resorbing 25% of the total filtered load of ions such as potassium, sodium, and chloride, as well as large amounts of water. Loop diuretics block this pump and thus inhibit the active reabsorption of sodium, chloride and potassium. These electrolytes are left in the urine and they act as osmotic diuretics, preventing further water absorption. This decrease in absorption of ions also lessens the effect of the countercurrent multiplier mechanism used to concentrate urine. Due to these multiple effects, the diuretic capability of these agents is extremely powerful. *Furosemide* is an example of a loop diuretic.

Thiazides interfere with ion transport across renal tubular epithelium at the distal convoluted tubule primarily by altering membrane permeability of sodium, potassium, and chloride. These agents work best when renal blood flow is normal (possibly explaining why they don't work well in those patients with severe heart failure). Moderate amounts of both sodium and potassium are lost to urine, allowing for modest water excretion. *Hydrochlorothiazide* is a common thiazide.

Aldosterone inhibitors competitively inhibit aldosterone in the distal renal tubules. Aldosterone increases the activity of the sodium-potassium pump within the collecting tubule, collecting duct and distal tubule, causing increased sodium reabsorption and potassium excretion. This increased uptake of sodium in turn leads to water retention. Inhibition of aldosterone consequently will decrease the amount of sodium and thus water that is reabsorbed. Decreased amounts of potassium are excreted and so these drugs are said to be *potassium-sparing*. An example of an aldosterone inhibitor is *spironolactone*.

Sodium channel blockers inhibit sodium exchange within the collecting duct and the cortical collecting tubule. They also indirectly inhibit the secretion of potassium, thus allowing them to be labeled potassium-sparing. The diuretic effects of this class are mild, but can be used in combination with drugs from the other classes to achieve desired diuresis. *Amiloride* is an example of a potassium-sparing sodium channel blocker. Magnesium loss is also spared with this class of diuretics.

4. Which of these diuretics are used most often in the management of CHF?

The drugs we rely on the most in CHF are furosemide, spironolactone, hydrochlorothiazide, and amiloride. Other classes of diuretics, such as the carbonic anhydrase inhibitors and osmotic diuretics, are not used in the treatment of congestive heart failure.

5. Should I use just one diuretic or can I combine them?

Furosemide is the most potent of the diuretics, so it is often used as a first-line drug. However, in the management of chronic and severe congestive heart failure, it is appropriate and occasionally necessary to combine diuretics. Because each diuretic works at a different level to prevent sodium and water resorption, the combined effects may control signs of congestion better than one drug alone. Using combined diuretics in this fashion is called "sequential nephron blockade." The use of diuretics with additive or synergistic effects may permit the use of lower doses of the individual agents, which may reduce the risk of adverse effects. In veterinary medicine, the dose of furosemide is often maximized (due to its potency) prior to adding a second diuretic. Some diuretics work better if combined and are more effective than either drug alone. For example, combining spironolactone and hydrochlorothiazide is more effective than either drug by itself.

6. What is triple diuretic therapy?

Triple diuretic therapy combines three different classes of diuretics to achieve a desired effect. One of the commonly used triple diuretic combinations is furosemide, hydrochlorothiazide, and spironolactone; another is furosemide, hydrochlorothiazide and amiloride. Due to the fact that potassium loss may be substantial with furosemide and hydrochlorothiazide, it is wise to rely on a potassium-sparing diuretic as a third member of the trio of drugs. Careful monitoring of electrolytes, renal function, and clinical parameters (such as attitude and appetite) is recommended when administering combination diuretic therapy.

7. What are the adverse effects of these drugs?

The most common side effects associated with diuretic use are dehydration and/or electrolyte disturbances.

8. Diuretics are used to reduce intravascular volume; why is volume depletion considered an adverse effect?

Although the goal in using diuretics is to decrease preload, excessive preload reduction is to be avoided because of the danger of reducing cardiac output. Stroke volume is related to end-diastolic volume through the Frank-Starling law of the heart. Because patients that have congestive heart failure due to systolic dysfunction have enlarged cardiac chambers and a "flat" Frank-Starling relationship, judicious diuresis decreases ventricular filling pressures but affects cardiac output only minimally. However, excessive diuresis may lead to decreased renal blood flow, causing azotemia. Azotemia can then lead to clinical signs of lethargy, anorexia, and vomiting.

9. Is diuretic use associated with any other adverse effects?

Uncommonly, gastrointestinal disturbances, weakness, restlessness, ototoxicity (seen with high IV doses in cats), or CNS changes may be seen.

10. How often does hypokalemia complicate diuretic use? Is potassium supplementation necessary for animals receiving diuretics?

Hypokalemia is the most common electrolyte abnormality associated with diuretic use. Sodium and chloride levels are less likely to become abnormal, although they certainly can. Maintaining potassium levels is more difficult in those patients that have depressed appetites. This problem results from a combination of diuretic-driven potassium loss and reduced intake. Cats are especially sensitive to this phenomenon and serum electrolytes must be carefully monitored. Dogs that are on furosemide and have good appetites very rarely have a problem with hypokalemia. In general, potassium supplementation is not recommended unless hypokalemia has been documented through the measurement of serum potassium levels.

11. How (and how often) do I monitor patients who are on diuretics?

Serum electrolytes (especially sodium, potassium and chloride), renal function (BUN, and creatinine), and hydration (total solids) should be monitored. These parameters should be documented prior to initiation of treatment. When starting diuretics, these parameters should be rechecked approximately 7 days after initiation of therapy. Once stabilized, monitoring can be done every several months. If azotemia is preexistent and mild congestive failure is seen, low-dose diuretics may be enough to control signs without further offending the kidneys. Uncommonly, preexisting azotemia may resolve with treatment of congestive heart failure if renal blood flow improves. If azotemia develops during diuretic usage, decreasing the dose or switching to a less potent diuretic may be enough to return kidney values to normal and still control signs of congestive failure.

12. Is there a limit to how much diuretic I can use?

In cases of fulminant failure, dogs may tolerate initial doses of 1–6 mg/kg IV. Furosemide's duration of action following intravenous administration is about 2 hours. Clinical signs will then dictate dose and frequency of the medication. Lower doses are generally used in cats.

13. When do you start a second diuretic?

If high doses of furosemide are not enough to control signs of congestive heart failure, multiple diuretic therapy can be considered. When adding differing diuretics together, it is advisable to decrease the dose of the original diuretic initially. For example, if furosemide can no longer be tolerated at 4 mg/kg 3 times/day and congestive heart failure is still present, consider adding a combination diuretic, such as aldactazide (spironolactone and hydrochlorothiazide) or adding both hydrochlorothiazide and amiloride together with furosemide. When using multiple diuretics, decreasing the furosemide to 2 mg/kg 3 times/day may be sufficient. Clinical signs and monitoring the above mentioned parameters will help dictate when to increase or decrease the drugs.

14. What about cats?

Cats are more sensitive to the effects of diuretics, so caution must be used. Starting furosemide at 1 mg/kg IV every 2–4 hours as needed in severe congestive failure is a reasonable starting dose. As breathing becomes less labored and room air is tolerated, the diuretic can be switched to an oral formulation and decreased to a 1, 2, or 3 times/day dosing schedule. In those cats who are mildly tachypneic, one dose of 1mg/kg subcutaneously or intravenously with an oral dose of 1 mg/kg 2 times/day may be enough. Again, dose and frequency will depend on the cat's clinical signs. If high doses are needed to control signs of congestive heart failure, you may need to monitor renal function and electrolytes more closely than would be necesssary for a dog. High doses of diuretics in cats with hypertrophic or restrictive cardiomyopathy may be detrimental due to the fact that excessive reductions in preload may cause left atrial pressures to drop precipitously, further impairing ventricular filling.

15. What do I do if the patient does not tolerate a needed dose of a diuretic to control signs of congestive heart failure?

There are several things we can try to limit the side effects of diuretics. Combining medications will often allow you to use a lower dose of the offending diuretic, possibly avoiding such side effects as hypokalemia or azotemia. Utilizing other cardiac medications to their fullest potential may aid in controlling congestive heart failure (i.e., increasing the dose of an ACE inhibitor or adding digoxin). If all cardiac medications are being used to their potential and the patient does not tolerate doses of diuretics that control life-threatening pulmonary edema, an endpoint may be reached; this is one definition of medically refractory congestive heart failure.

16. Are different diuretics better at controlling different types of fluid formation seen with congestive heart failure?

In a word, no. Diuretics function at the level of the kidney and not within specific body cavities. Diuretics decrease preload by causing salt and water loss from the systemic circulation. Fluid that is formed in body cavities (both ascites and pleural effusion) is already "lost" to systemic circulation, making it difficult to mobilize with diuretics. While diuretics can slow or prevent the accumulation of ascites or pleural effusion, they are seldom able to mobilize large volumes of cavitary effusion. Indeed, centesis is the appropriate therapy when large effusions result in clinical signs; the temptation to treat only with diuretics should be resisted. For example, overly aggressive diuresis in a cat with pleural effusion can result in hypovolemia and reduced cardiac output before there is reduction in the volume pleural fluid. On presentation, the patient may be dyspneic due to pleural effusion; however, after inappropriately brisk diuresis, the patient may be both dyspneic *and* volume depleted.

17. List doses of diuretics.

The following are typical starting doses.

DRUG	DOSE FOR DOGS	DOSE FOR CATS
Aldactazide (combination of spirono- lactone and hydrochlorothiazide)	2 mg/kg 1 or 2 times/day	
Amiloride	1.25 mg/10 kg daily	
Furosemide	1–4 mg/kg 2 or 3 times/day	0.5–1.0 mg/kg 2 times/day
Hydrochlorothiazide	2–4 mg/kg 1 or 2 times/day	
Spironolactone	1–2 mg/kg 2 times/day	2–4 mg/kg/day

Keep in mind that when initially combining diuretics, start with a lower dose and titrate up to effect.

REFERENCES

1. Bonagura JD: Congestive heart failure in the dog and cat: Medical management. Lecture given to Metropolitan New Jersey Veterinary Medical Association, October 1996.
2. Ganong WF: Review of Medical Physiology, 18th ed. Stamford CT, Appleton & Lange, 1997, pp 653–681.
3. Guyton AC, Hall JE: Integration of renal mechanisms for control of blood volume and extracellular fluid volume: Renal regulation of potassium, calcium, phosphate, and magnesium. In Guyton AC, Hall JE (eds): Textbook of Medical Physiology, 9th ed. Philadelphia, W.B. Saunders, 1996, pp 367–383.
4. Guyton AC, Hall JE: Micturition, diuretics, and kidney diseases. In Guyton AC, Hall JE (eds): Textbook of Medical Physiology, 9th ed. Philadelphia, W.B. Saunders, 1996, pp 408–410.
5. Hamlin RL: Evidence for or against clinical efficacy of preload reducers. Vet Clin North Am Small Anim Pract 21:936–944, 1991.
6. Kittleson MD: Pathophysiology and treatment of congestive heart failure. In Miller MS, Tilley LP (eds): Manual of Canine and Feline Cardiology, 2nd ed. Philadelphia, W.B. Saunders, 1995, pp 355–369.
7. Opie LH, Kaplan NM, Poole-Wilson PA: Diuretics. In Opie LH (ed): Drugs for the Heart, 4th ed. Philadelphia, W.B. Saunders, 1997, pp 83–104.
8. Plumb DC: Veterinary Drug Handbook, 3rd ed. Ames, Iowa State University Press, 1999, pp 27–30, 345–348, 380–381, 531–533, 670–672.
9. Rodkey SM, Young JB: The cardiovascular use of diuretics. In Crawford MH (ed): The Cardiology Clinics Annual of Drug Therapy, vol 1. Philadelphia, W.B. Saunders, 1997, pp 63–80.
10. Sisson D, Kittleson MD: Management of heart failure: Principles of treatment, therapeutic strategies, and pharmacology. In Fox PR, Sisson D, Moise NS (eds): Textbook of Canine and Feline Radiology: Principles and Clinical Practices, 2nd ed. Philadelphia, W.B. Saunders, 1999, pp 235–237.

9. INOTROPES

Matthew S. Mellema, D.V.M.

1. Define inotropy.

Inotropy or the inotropic state is difficult to define precisely. Inotropy is used as an alternative term for contractility. Changes in the inotropic state refer to alterations in the velocity of contraction and the development of peak tension independent of variations in heart rate, afterload, or preload. At the level of the sarcomere, an increase in inotropy results from an enhancement of the interaction of calcium with the contractile proteins in a load-independent fashion. Increases in inotropy may result from increased adrenergic stimulation or the administration of digitalis or other inotropic agents. Decreases in the inotropic state may result from intrinsic myocardial dysfunction (e.g., cardiomyopathies), circulating mediators (e.g., cytokines), electrolyte imbalances, or the administration of negative inotropic agents (e.g., calcium channel blockers or beta-adrenergic antagonists).

2. What classes of positive inotropes are available in clinical veterinary practice?

- Glycosides (e.g., digoxin and digitoxin; see Chapter 14)
- Sympathomimetic amines (e.g., dopamine, dobutamine, epinephrine, norepinephrine, and isoproterenol)
- Phosphodiesterase (PDE) inhibitors (e.g., amrinone and milrinone)
- Calcium sensitizers (e.g., pimobendan)

3. Excluding digoxin, do the remaining inotropic agents differ in their final effects at the cellular level?

Yes. The calcium-sensitizing agents act via a novel mechanism. Agents such as pimobendan produce an increase in the inotropic state by increasing the sensitivity of the contractile elements to calcium ions. Some of the calcium-sensitizing agents also possess PDE-inhibiting properties as well. The sympathomimetic amines and PDE inhibitors produce the same end-effect via different mechanisms. The action of these agents on the myocardium results in a rise in intracellular cAMP that, in turn, leads to higher cytosolic calcium ion levels during systole. The rise in cytosolic calcium ion levels during systole leads to greater force generation independent of load.

4. By what mechanism do the sympathomimetic amines produce a rise in cytosolic calcium levels?

Sympathomimetic amines with beta-adrenergic affinity are capable of activating a cascade of second messenger systems that is initiated by the binding of the agent with the beta-adrenergic receptors on the cell surface. Upon binding a ligand, the beta-receptor activates a trimeric complex of G proteins associated with the cytosolic surface of the cell membrane. Once activated, the G proteins subsequently increase the activity of adenylate cyclase, the enzyme that catalyzes the conversion of ATP to cyclic AMP (cAMP). Increased levels of cAMP within the cytosol lead to increased activity of protein kinase A, which, in turn, results in the phosphorylation of cell membrane calcium channels. The phosphorylation of these channels thereby alters them in such a way that upon membrane depolarization the transmembrane flux of calcium is greater. The influx of more calcium from the external environment triggers the release of greater quantities of calcium from the sarcoplasmic reticulum during systole.

5. By what mechanism do the PDE inhibitors produce a rise in cytosolic calcium levels?

PDE inhibitors produce the same end-result as the sympathomimetic amines by blocking the activity of the enzyme responsible for the breakdown of cAMP. This inhibition of PDE activity results in rise in cytosolic cAMP levels and a rise in cytosolic calcium levels via the mechanisms described above. Some of the PDE inhibitors also act to block the action of adenosine on the myocardium. Adenosine inhibits adenylate cyclase activity and blocking this effect would also tend to lead to higher cAMP levels within the cell.

6. Which of the non-glycoside inotropic agents are currently available for use in clinical practice?

Digitalis glycosides are currently the only positive inotropes widely used for long-term oral administration. Milrinone, an orally active PDE inhibitor, was available briefly while undergoing clinical trials but was withdrawn due to intolerable adverse effects in humans. Despite data that suggest that milrinone appears to be a better drug in dogs than in humans, the agent remains unavailable in clinical practice. Amrinone, a similar PDE inhibitor, is still available as an intravenous preparation. The sympathomimetic amines are available for parenteral use but are considered unsuitable for chronic oral therapy in part due to their rapid first-pass metabolism by the liver. Pimobendan, a calcium sensitizer with PDE-inhibiting properties, is unavailable for clinical use in North America but is currently approved for use in Germany.

7. Why are the less expensive PDE inhibitors such as aminophylline and theophylline not used as inotropic agents more frequently?

All PDE inhibitors are not equal. Amrinone and milrinone are more specific for the PDE isoform they inhibit. Amrinone and milrinone specifically inhibit PDE III, the third isoform of PDE and the one that predominates within the myocardium. Agents such as theophylline and aminophylline are nonspecific PDE inhibitors and inhibit all the isoforms. This lack of specificity tends to lead to intolerable side effects when they are used at dosages at which they would become clinically relevant positive inotropes.

8. Why are there so few positive inotropes available for long-term use?

Over the years several new agents have been developed and tested in clinical trials. Many of these agents have been shown to be effective at increasing contractility and reducing the signs of congestive and/or forward heart failure, but an increased risk of sudden death has also typically been identified upon completion of larger clinical trials. One example is the agent vesnarinone, which was found to have a dose-dependent risk of sudden death associated with its administration. Unfortunately, many of these agents might have proven to be more useful in small animals than humans but remain unavailable.

9. What are the indications for the administration of non-glycoside positive inotropes?

Sympathomimetic amines and PDE inhibitors are generally reserved for use in fulminant congestive heart failure. These agents are rarely used in the treatment of chronic heart failure except as short-term support in acute exacerbations while one is awaiting the effect of more long-term support (e.g., digoxin) to become apparent. There is a small body of literature that suggests a short-term (48–72 hours) infusion of dobutamine may have some beneficial effects on myocardial performance that last for up to several weeks, but these findings have not been tested in the veterinary clinical setting.

The rationale for the use of inotropes is either to enhance forward blood flow at lower filling pressures, to support mean arterial blood pressure and coronary blood flow, or both. Non-glycoside inotropes are more often used in the treatment of dilated cardiomyopathy than in primary valvular insufficiency. This is due to the fact that mitral valve insufficiency tends to occur in smaller-breed dogs and in these small breeds systolic function tends to be preserved until quite late in the course of the disease. Inotropes are rarely used in the management of hypertrophic cardiomyopathy as the increase in heart rate and ejection velocity may lead to worsening of diastolic ventricular performance and more severe dynamic outflow obstruction, respectively.

Depression of myocardial function secondary to systemic disease may warrant the use of inotropic agents. The preferred agent will vary with the underlying etiology. In sepsis, a growing body of literature suggests that beta-adrenergic receptor dysfunction may limit the utility of sympathomimetics as inotropes in this setting. The responsiveness of septic patients' hearts to PDE inhibition appears to be preserved and these agents may be the better choice in the septic animal.

Sympathomimetics remain one of the mainstays of drug therapy in cardiopulmonary resuscitation (CPR). The goals of sympathomimetic amine administration in this setting are to increase mean arterial pressure and coronary/cerebral blood flow as well as re-establish a viable cardiac rhythm. Agents with affinity for both alpha- and beta-adrenergic receptors (e.g., epinephrine) are preferred in this setting.

10. What types of adrenergic receptors exist and what is the effect of their activation?

There are five main types of adrenergic receptors that are relevant to veterinary cardiology:

1. Alpha-1 receptors: activation of alpha-1 adrenergic receptors results in arterial vasoconstriction.

2. Alpha-2 receptors: the effect of alpha-2 receptor activation is complex and the physiologic role of these receptors is not well defined; presynaptic receptors inhibit norepinephrine release, while stimulation of postsynaptic receptors results in vasoconstriction.

3. Beta-1 receptors: activation of beta-1 adrenorcceptors results in increases in contractility, increased heart rate, and accelerated AV node conduction.

4. Beta-2 receptors: activation of beta-2 adrenoreceptors results in bronchodilation and arterial vasodilation in systemic musculature.

5. Dopaminergic receptors: activation of dopaminergic receptors results in norepinephrine release from sympathetic nerve fiber endings in the heart as well as vasodilation of coronary, renal, mesenteric, and cerebral arteries.

11. How do the different sympathomimetic amines differ in their selectivity for the various adrenergic receptors?

- Epinephrine: alpha = beta-1 > beta-2, no dopaminergic activity
- Norepinephrine: alpha = beta-1, no beta-2 or dopaminergic activity
- Dobutamine: beta-1 > beta-2 > alpha, no dopaminergic activity
- Dopamine: dopaminergic > beta-1 > beta-2 > alpha
- Isoproterenol: beta-1 > beta-2, no alpha or dopaminergic activity

12. Does dopamine have dose-dependent effects?

Yes. The effects of dopamine vary with dosage due to the different affinities of the adrenergic receptors for this agent. Due to its short half-life, dopamine is typically administered as a constant-rate infusion and the clinical response will vary with the infusion rate as follows:

- 0.5–3.0 µg/kg/min: coronary, splanchnic and renal arteriolar dilation
- 3.0–10.0 µg/kg/min: increased heart rate, stroke volume and cardiac output; little change in systemic vascular resistance
- > 10.0 µg/kg/min: increased arterial blood pressure, reduced blood flow, increased cardiac filling pressures

13. Do cats have renal arteriolar dopamine receptors?

Evidence suggests that cats, unlike dogs, do not express dopaminergic receptors in any significant quantity in their afferent renal arteriolar beds. However, cats may still experience a diuresis following dopamine administration via other mechanisms.

14. Over what time period do sympathomimetic amines maintain their effectiveness as positive inotropes?

With time most patients treated with sympathomimetic amines (that possess beta-adrenergic activity) will demonstrate a diminished inotropic response to these agents. Over the course of 1 or 2 days of sympathomimetic administration, a decreasing responsiveness of the myocardium (to about 50% of baseline response) to these agents is observed. Generally, sympathomimetics are suitable for use over a period of 2–3 days before a period of withdrawal is recommended.

This reduction in efficacy is the result of desensitization of the beta-receptors subsequent to chronic stimulation. This desensitization response may have evolved as a mechanism to combat cytosolic calcium overload.

15. Do PDE inhibitors lose their efficacy over time?

It has been proposed that chronic administration of PDE inhibitors does not result in a progressive loss of efficacy as is seen with the administration of beta-adrenergic agonists. Recent studies, however, suggest that the myocyte may in fact develop a reduced responsiveness to these agents over time.

16. Does the failing myocardium exhibit an altered responsiveness to beta-adrenergic agonists?

The beta-adrenergic/adenylate cyclase system is down-regulated in severe heart failure. Circulating catecholamine levels are elevated in the syndrome of heart failure and with time the myocardium initiates mechanisms to ward against cytosolic calcium overload secondary to chronic adrenergic stimulation. Beta-adrenergic receptor density may be altered and the ratio of beta-1 to beta-2 receptors on the cell surface may change as well. In addition, phosphorylation of the receptors may lead to decreased sensitivity of the beta-adrenergic system to stimulation with exogenous or endogenous catecholamines.

17. What adverse side effect might be noted following the administration of positive inotropes?

If one excludes the calcium-sensitizing agents (e.g., pimobendan), each of the remaining classes of non-glycoside inotropes increases contractility by increasing cytosolic calcium levels. This increase in cytosolic calcium may lead to arrhythmias. An increase in heart rate might be noted in the absence of arrhythmias. This increase in heart rate may lead to both an increase in myocardial oxygen consumption and decreased diastolic filling. The increase in heart rate is generally regarded as an undesirable effect of these agents. In addition, AV node conduction velocity may increase and result in a rise in the ventricular response rate in some forms of atrial tachyarrhythmias (e.g., atrial fibrillation). Again, this increase in ventricular rate is often considered undesirable unless the ventricular rates were judged to be too low prior to administering the agent. Myocardial necrosis may result from prolonged excessive catecholamine administration. The cardiomyopathy associated with pheochromocytomas is thought to be the result of excessive endogenous catecholamine production.

Agents with significant affinity for the alpha-adrenergic receptors may cause a clinically important rise in systemic vascular resistance and a detrimental increase in afterload. Prolonged administration of these agents may cause a reduction in renal blood flow, resulting in fluid overload and electrolyte disorders, which may adversely affect the myocardium and lead to edema formation. Filling pressures may also rise with administration of these agents, exacerbating edema formation.

18. How do the different inotropes compare in regards to their proarrhythmic effects?

Studies in humans and animals have shown that dopamine is more likely to result in sinus tachycardia and ventricular arrhythmias compared to dobutamine or PDE inhibitors when doses are controlled to produce similar rises in cardiac output. Dobutamine, dopamine, and PDE inhibitors appear to be similar in their propensity to cause supraventricular arrhythmias. Each agent is more likely to cause ventricular than supraventricular arrhythmias. The sympathomimetic amines all appear to have similar proarrhythmic effects in the anesthetized animal. None of the agents is thought to cause bradyarrhythmias. In the normal animal excessive hypertension may result in slowing of the heart rate via a baroreceptor reflex. In chronic heart failure, baroreceptor sensitivity may be diminished and this response may be blunted. Dobutamine has been shown to have a dose-dependent effect on heart rate. Dopamine's dose-dependent effects have been described above. Both the PDE inhibitors and calcium-sensitizing agents appear to increase the heart rate. The proarrhythmic effects of the calcium sensitizing agents in dogs and cats have not yet been well documented.

19. How do the different inotropes compare in their ability to raise arterial blood pressure?

Dobutamine typically does not affect mean arterial blood pressure to a large degree. Due to its largely beta-adrenergic–mediated effects, this agent generally increases cardiac output with little change in systemic blood pressure. At high doses dopamine can significantly increase arterial blood pressure and is often used as a first-line pressor agent. Norepinephrine and phenylephrine are both potent alpha-adrenergic agonists and can cause significant elevations in blood pressure, often at the cost of reduced flow. The PDE inhibitors, such as dobutamine, might be termed "inodilators" because they increase contractility while causing arteriolar dilation. Similarly, the calcium-sensitizing agents appear to increase contractility while causing arteriolar and venous dilation.

20. If excessive vasoconstriction is noted with the administration of an inotrope, how might this effect be reduced?

The simultaneous infusion of nitroprusside may help to alleviate excessive vasoconstriction in this setting. Alternatively, administration of a pure arteriolar dilator such as hydralazine could be considered. Close monitoring of arterial blood pressure is advised should these agents be given. Hypotension would warrant discontinuing the vasodilator or reducing the dosage.

BIBLIOGRAPHY

1. Adams HR: New perspectives in cardiopulmonary therapeutics: Receptor-selective adrenergic drugs. J Am Vet Med Assoc 185:966, 1984.
2. Bednarski RM, Muir WW: Catecholamine infusion in vagotomized dogs during thiamylal-halothane and pentobarbital anesthesia. Cornell Vet 75:512, 1985.
3. Hosgood G: Pharmacologic features and physiologic effects of dopamine. J Am Vet Med Assoc 197:1209, 1990.
4. Kittleson MD: The efficacy and safety of milrinone for treating heart failure in dogs. Vet Clin North Am Small Anim Pract 21:905, 1991.
5. Kittleson MD: Dobutamine. J Am Vet Med Assoc 177:642, 1980.
6. Marcus FI: Digitalis and acute inotropes. In Opie LH (ed): Drugs for the Heart, 4th ed. Philadelphia, W.B. Saunders, 1997, pp 145–176.
7. Pagel PS, Hettrick DA, Waltier DC: Comparison of the effects of levosimendan, pimobendan, and milrinone on canine left ventricular-arterial coupling and mechanical efficiency. Basic Res Cardiol 91:4, 1996.
8. Tisdale JE, Patel R, Webb CR, et al: Electrophysiologic and proarrhythmic effects of intravenous inotropic agents. Prog Cardiovasc Dis 38:167, 1995.

10. VASODILATORS

Matthew S. Mellema, D.V.M.

1. What classes of vasodilators are in common use in small animal clinical practice?

CLASS	DRUG
ACE inhibitors	Enalapril
	Lisinopril
	Captopril
	Benazepril
Calcium channel blockers	Nifedipine
	Amlodipine
	Diltiazem
Nitric oxide donors	Nitroprusside
	Nitroglycerin
	Isosorbide
Direct smooth muscle relaxants	Hydralazine
Alpha-adrenergic blockers	Prazosin

The angiotensin-converting enzyme (ACE) inhibitors are discussed separately in this book (see Chapter 11).

2. What is the rationale for the use of vasodilators in the treatment of patients with congestive heart failure secondary to systolic dysfunction?

In patients with heart disease, blood pressure may be maintained in the face of reduced cardiac output via constriction of systemic arterioles. This arteriolar constriction can contribute to increased afterload and further reduce cardiac output. Thus, systemic blood pressure may be preserved at the expense of reduced blood flow. Peripheral systemic venoconstriction may also be present in patients with heart disease. This increase in venous tone acts to shift venous blood volume away from the periphery and toward the central compartment. The increase in central blood volume acts to increase preload, promote volume overload–induced cardiac hypertrophy, and increase stroke volume. As heart disease progresses, these alterations in vasomotor tone may be to the patient's detriment. A point may be reached where reduced blood flow and elevated venous pressures lead to signs of congestive heart failure, forward failure, and increases in myocardial workload. In this setting the rationale for the use of vasodilators is to reduce afterload, promote forward blood flow, reduce venous pressures and edema formation, reduce regurgitant fraction, and reduce flow through shunting lesions.

3. Do vasodilators affect fluid and electrolyte balance?

Yes. If one excludes the ACE inhibitors, it can be said that each of the remaining classes of clinically used vasodilators have the potential to cause activation of the renin-angiotensin-aldosterone system (RAAS). A reduction in blood pressure and renal perfusion can result in increased renin release from the kidneys. Renin initiates a cascade of events leading to increased generation of angiotensin II, a potent vasoconstrictor, and aldosterone, which promotes sodium and water reabsorption. The expansion of the extracellular fluid volume that results can promote further venous hypertension and edema formation. It should be noted that diuretics could lead to a similar activation of the RAAS when used alone or in combination of non-ACE inhibitor vasodilators.

4. Is the activation of the RAAS thought to have clinical significance in the setting of congestive heart failure treatment?

Yes. It has been shown in humans that non-ACE inhibitor vasodilators are less effective at reducing long-term mortality than ACE inhibitors. In dogs, the results of the Long-term Investigation of Veterinary Enalapril (LIVE) study suggest that canine patients may derive similar benefits from ACE inhibitors, but further study appears warranted before definitive conclusions about long-term survival may be reached. In human patients, some vasodilators such as prazosin perform no better than placebo in regards to long-term mortality reduction. The activation of the RAAS may lead to worsened long-term survival via sodium and water retention or perhaps secondary to the influence of angiotensin II on myocardial remodeling and hypertrophy.

5. In what settings are vasodilators typically used in clinical practice?

Vasodilators are often used in the management of patients with fulminant heart failure that are refractory to stabilization with oxygen and diuretics (and perhaps intravenous inotropic agents) alone. Patients with chronic refractory heart failure may derive some benefit from vasodilators when these agents are used in combination with standard therapies for the management of chronic heart failure. Patients with mitral valve insufficiency or aortic insufficiency may benefit from the addition of a vasodilator if a reduction of regurgitant fraction and venous pressures can be obtained. Patients with dilated cardiomyopathy may derive some benefit from afterload reduction and lowered venous pressure. In patients with shunting defects, such as patent ductus arteriosus (PDA) or ventricular septal defects (VSD), a reduction in flow through the shunt may be noted after the addition of a vasodilator. Patients with refractory congestive signs due to diastolic dysfunction (e.g., cats with hypertrophic cardiomyopathy) may benefit from reduction of venous pressures when a venodilator is added to their treatment regimen. Arteriolar or balanced vasodilators can be essential in the management of systemic hypertension when the primary cause is not readily correctable or cannot be identified. Vasodilators may play a role in the management of pulmonary hypertension but the response to the vasodilators currently available in clinical practice is limited or unpredictable at best.

6. In what settings are vasodilators contraindicated?

Vasodilators are generally not recommended in the management of patients with fixed obstructive lesions such as subaortic stenosis. In these patients the stroke volume may be relatively fixed and arteriolar constriction is necessary to maintain adequate blood pressure. Vasodilation in this setting may cause overt hypotension or reduced coronary blood flow. Similar arguments may be made against the use of vasodilators in the management of patients with hypertrophic cardiomyopathy, particularly those with dynamic obstruction of the left ventricular outflow tract. It should be noted that this generalization does not hold true across all classes of vasodilators. Pure venodilators such as low-dose nitroglycerin would not result in arteriolar dilation. In addition, the use of ACE inhibitors that are themselves mild vasodilators is favored by some veterinary cardiologists as part of the management of hypertrophic cardiomyopathy in cats. Lastly, vasodilators are clearly contraindicated in the presence of hypotension.

7. What is the mechanism of action of the nitric oxide donor vasodilators?

Some of the nitric oxide donor vasodilators are organic nitrates, which are esters of nitric oxide. Examples include nitroglycerin and isosorbide dinitrate. The organic nitrates are converted to nitric oxide within vascular smooth muscle cells via a reduction reaction with sulfhydryl groups on cytosolic cysteine. The nitric oxide interacts with cytosolic guanylate cyclase, resulting in increased formation of cyclic GMP within the cell. Increases in cyclic GMP lead to decreased interaction of calcium with contractile proteins via the action of protein kinases and ultimately results in smooth muscle relaxation. Nitroprusside is a nitric oxide donor vasodilator that releases nitric oxide by a nonenzymatic pathway and nitrate tolerance is less likely to develop with this agent.

8. What is nitrate tolerance and how does it develop?

Nitrate tolerance is an observed loss of efficacy noted with the long-term use of nitrates without a nitrate-free interval. The phenomenon was first noted nearly a century ago, when it was observed that munitions workers reported headaches each Monday after having been away from work for a few days. The headaches and fatigue resolved within hours to days after returning to repeated exposure to nitrates. Clinically nitrate tolerance manifests as a need for progressively increasing doses of nitrates to achieve the same therapeutic endpoints when the agents are given continuously. Nitrate tolerance is lost over a period of time when administration is discontinued and the agents can then be readministered at a lower dose. Unfortunately, during this period of drug withdrawal the beneficial effects are also lacking. The exact mechanism of nitrate tolerance development is uncertain, but the depletion of available sulfhydryl groups to act as substrate for the nitric oxide–releasing reduction reaction appears to be of central importance.

9. Why do some nitrates appear to be selective venodilators while others are balanced vasodilators?

At low doses nitrates primarily act as venodilators. When higher serum levels are obtained, a balanced dilation of both veins and arterioles is noted. The venodilation observed with topical nitroglycerine ointment is likely a reflection of the low serum levels achieved with this route of administration. Nitroprusside acts as a balanced vasodilator and is typically administered as a constant-rate intravenous infusion that maintains higher serum levels.

10. What adverse effects may be noted with the administration of nitric oxide donor vasodilators?

Nitrate tolerance as discussed above may develop with time. Hypotension may occur with the administration of any of the clinically available vasodilators and it is recommended that arterial blood pressure be monitored during the initial institution of nitrate therapy. Orthostatic hypotension may be noted as well. In addition, nitroprusside is metabolized to a cyanide-containing compound that may build up with time and result in signs of cyanide toxicity. These signs include venous hyperoxemia (bright red venous blood), lactic acidosis, and dyspnea. Signs of cyanide toxicity are more likely to occur in patients with reduced glomerular filtration rates.

11. What potentially beneficial effects may result from nitrate administration in addition to vasodilation?

Nitric oxide also acts to inhibit platelet function and nitric oxide donor vasodilators may also inhibit thrombogenesis or reduce the rate at which pre-existing thrombi enlarge. This action may be of particular benefit in patients with cardiac disease suffering from thromboembolic complications (e.g., saddle thrombus cats).

12. What is the mechanism of action of hydralazine?

Hydralazine is a direct-acting arteriolar dilator. It has no effect on systemic venous tone. Its exact mechanism of action is unclear, but it is thought to act via the local release of prostacyclin, a vasodilatory product of the arachidonic acid cascade.

13. What is the relative efficacy of the available vasodilators in the treatment of acute heart failure?

Intravenous nitroprusside is very efficacious in the reduction of venous pressures and the promotion of forward blood flow. Its clinical utility is hampered by the need for arterial pressure monitoring and requirement that it be administered as a constant-rate infusion. Hydralazine is very efficacious in the treatment of acute congestive signs resulting from mitral regurgitation, less so for those due to dilated cardiomyopathy. However, this is true for vasodilators in general and is not necessarily specific to hydralazine. Topical nitroglycerin is generally considered less efficient than the other vasodilators due to the low serum levels achieved and minimal to absent clinical response noted.

14. What is the relative efficacy of the available vasodilators in the chronic treatment of congestive heart failure?

The available evidence suggests that ACE inhibitors are superior to the other available classes of vasodilators for the chronic systolic failure. ACE inhibitors are generally the recommended agents for all patients in which they are tolerated. Hydralazine may be comparatively efficient in the management of patients with mitral regurgitation, less so in patients with dilated cardiomyopathy. The relative efficacy of orally administered nitrates in this setting is uncertain at this time. The potential of orally administered nitrates for the management of chronic heart failure in veterinary patients continues to be researched. The development of nitrate tolerance may reduce their relative efficacy; however, in some patients these agents seem to be of great benefit. Alpha-adrenergic antagonist agents such as prazosin have largely been replaced in veterinary cardiology by the other classes of vasodilators. The efficacy of prazosin has been shown to decrease with subsequent doses in humans and experimental animals and this observation has led to a decrease in its use as a therapeutic agent. The calcium channel blockers are of uncertain utility in the management of chronic heart failure in dogs. Many of the newer agents possess balanced vasodilatory properties with minimal direct chronotropic or inotropic effects. Further study is required before the role of these agents will be clear in the management of chronic congestive heart failure in dogs and cats.

15. Which vasodilators are preferred in the management of systemic arterial hypertension in dogs and cats?

Amlodipine, an orally active calcium channel blocker, has been shown to be effective in reducing arterial blood pressure in cats with renal disease. It is currently one of the most popular agents for the treatment of hypertension in this setting. An oral dose of 0.625–1.25 mg q24h has been shown to result in an average reduction in systolic blood pressure of about 40 mmHg. The efficacy of this agent in the treatment of systemic hypertension in dogs remains to be established. In hypertensive patients with significant urinary protein losses, ACE inhibitors may act to reduce blood pressure as well as reduce the magnitude of proteinuria. Increased filtration of plasma proteins has been implicated in the mechanism underlying progression of renal disease. The reduction of urinary protein loss may be of considerable benefit to patients experiencing hypertension secondary to renal dysfunction. However, in most patients ACE inhibitors afford only a modest reduction (~ 10 mmHg) in arterial blood pressure and often need to be combined with other agents to achieve the desired result. Prazosin and hydralazine also may be effective in controlling arterial hypertension in dogs and cats. Concurrent administration of beta-adrenergic blockers may improve blood pressure control in patients exhibiting a significant increase in heart rate following institution of vasodilator therapy.

BIBLIOGRAPHY

1. Anderson TJ, Meredith IT, Ganz P, et al: Nitric oxide and nitrovasodilators: Similarities, differences, and potential interactions. J Am Coll Cardiol 24:555, 1994.
2. Brown SA, Walton CL, Crawford P, et al: Long-term effects of antihypertensive regimens on renal hemodynamics and proteinuria. Kidney Int 43:1210, 1993.
3. Cohn JN, Archibald DG, Ziesche S, et al: Effect of vasodilator therapy on mortality in chronic congestive heart failure: Results of a Veterans Administration cooperative study. N Engl J Med 314:1547, 1986.
4. Elkayam U, Mehra A, Avraham S, Osprzega E: Possible mechanisms of nitrate tolerance. Am J Cardiol 70:496, 1992.
5. Ettinger SJ, Benitz AM, Ericsson GF: Relationships of enalapril with other congestive heart failure treatment modalities. Proc Ann Vet Med Forum, p 251, 1994.
6. Kittleson MD, Eyster GE, Olivier NB, et al: Oral hydralazine therapy for chronic mitral regurgitation in the dog. J Am Vet Med Assoc 182:1205, 1983.
7. Snyder PS: Blinded clinical trial of amlodipine in cats with hypertension (abstract). J Vet Intern Med 11:139, 1997.

11. ACE INHIBITORS

Jonathan A. Abbott, D.V.M.

1. What is an ACE inhibitor? Provide examples of drugs in this class.

Angiotensin-converting enzyme (ACE) inhibitors are vasodilators that have important neurohumoral effects in the setting of congestive heart failure. All drugs in this class bind to and inactivate the angiotensin-converting enzyme. The generic names of ACE inhibitors end with the suffix *-pril*. Enalapril, benazepril, and captopril are used fairly commonly in small animal medicine; lisinopril, quinapril, ramipril, and fosinopril are also ACE inhibitors.

2. What are the main components of the renin-angiotensin system? What is the mechanism of the vasodilatory effect of ACE inhibitors?

Circulating renin released from the renal juxtaglomerular apparatus (JGA) acts on the prohormone angiotensinogen, which results in the release of angiotensin I. ACE is a kininase that catalyzes the conversion of angiotensin I to the active octapeptide hormone angiotensin II. Angiotensin II has numerous effects; importantly, it is a potent vasoconstrictor. Pharmacologic inhibition of ACE reduces angiotensin II levels and results in vasodilation.

The magnitude of the vasodilatory effect is partly related to renin levels at the time that the drug is administered. In pathologic states in which renin levels are high, as is the case in congestive heart failure (CHF) and some forms of systemic hypertension, the vasodilatory effect is relatively prominent. In contrast, when renin levels are low, there is little effect on vascular resistance; in fact, ACE inhibitors have little effect on blood pressure in normal, sodium-replete people or animals.

3. What stimuli result in renin release?

Renin is a protease enzyme that is released from the renal JGA in response to diminished renal blood flow or renal hypotension. Specifically, the following stimuli result in the release of renin:

• Decreased sodium chloride reabsorption by the macula densa of the renal JGA
• Adrenergic activity resulting in stimulation of beta receptors within the kidney
• Low intrarenal renal blood pressure sensed by baroreceptors located within the kidney

4. Angiotensin II is a potent vasoconstrictor; what are the other effects of this hormone?

While angiotensin II is indeed a vasoconstrictor, it has numerous other effects and many of these are likely to be of importance in the pathophysiology of congestive heart failure. Angiotensin II has a neuromodulating effect; it augments the release of norepinephrine from adrenergic nerve endings, which tends to further increase vascular resistance. Angiotensin II also induces the release of aldosterone from the adrenal cortex, which in turn contributes to the retention of salt and water in low cardiac output states. In addition, angiotensin II is a dypsogen and it augments the release of antidiuretic hormone (ADH), both of which contribute to the expansion of the intravascular volume. In experimental preparations, angiotensin II has a trophic effect on myocardium and has weak inotropic properties.

5. Why is the renin-angiotensin-aldosterone system (RAAS) important in cardiovascular disease?

When cardiac performance declines due to heart disease, activation of the RAAS is a compensatory mechanism that, at least temporarily, serves to preserve blood pressure through an increase in vascular resistance. The effect of angiotensin II on the adrenergic nervous system contributes further to vasoconstriction. Additionally, the angiotensin II–mediated release of aldosterone results in the renal retention of salt and water; this serves to increase intravascular volume and supports cardiac output through the mechanism of the Frank-Starling law of the heart.

6. Why do vasodilators have a favorable effect in disorders such as dilated cardiomyopathy and mitral valve regurgitation?

Vascular resistance is the hydraulic force that must be overcome in order to maintain flow across a vascular bed. In an approximate fashion, resistance is related to cardiac output and blood pressure through Ohm's law:

$$BP = Q \times SVR$$

where BP is blood pressure, Q is cardiac output, and SVR is systemic vascular resistance. When cardiac disease impairs cardiac performance, reflex mechanisms increase peripheral vascular resistance in order to maintain systemic blood pressure. This increase in vascular resistance allows normal blood pressure to be maintained when cardiac output is low.

Afterload is the sum of forces that oppose myocardial shortening; it is directly related to blood pressure and ventricular radius but inversely related to ventricular wall thickness. A dilated, thin-walled ventricle is therefore subject to increased afterload even when blood pressure is normal; the result is a mismatch between afterload and contractility. Because of this mismatch, a judicious decrease in vascular resistance allows an increase in myocardial shortening and a consequent increase in stroke volume. Ventricular radius is then lower at normal or decreased blood pressure, which lessens afterload and reduces myocardial oxygen demand. When substantial mitral valve regurgitation is present, there is an analogous mismatch between vascular resistance and the resistance imposed by the regurgitant orifice, because stroke volume is limited by abnormally high systemic vascular resistance. In systolic failure, vasodilation reduces vascular resistance and increases cardiac output; because of the relationship described by Ohm's law, blood pressure need not change.

The notion that elevated vascular resistance limits stroke volume in the setting of systolic failure is crucial to an understanding of the effect of vasodilators on cardiac performance. While the favorable effects of ACE inhibition are not related solely to vasodilation, ACE inhibitors are not necessarily effective in all heart diseases. In fact, the efficacy of ACE inhibitors in small animal cardiology is proven only for the approved indications of heart failure due to dilated cardiomyopathy and acquired valvular disease. Vasodilators do not generally cause a large or sustained increase in cardiac output when systolic cardiac performance is normal, because there is little advantage in more exuberant myocardial shortening when end-systolic volume is normal.

7. What is the evidence that ACE inhibitors are effective in the therapy of heart disease in small animals?

In a double-blind placebo controlled trial, enalapril was compared to placebo in a population of dogs that suffered from heart failure due to acquired valvular disease and dilated cardiomyopathy; the subjects enrolled in the study also received furosemide with or without digoxin. The drug was well tolerated and seemed to improve quality of life. The time until death (or euthanasia) was longer in the group that received enalapril, which suggests that mortality is reduced as it is in people with heart failure.

There is experimental evidence and clinical evidence from studies of people with heart disease that suggest that dogs with subclinical heart disease might benefit from ACE inhibition. Proof of this assertion is currently lacking. The efficacy of ACE inhibitors in canine diseases other than dilated cardiomyopathy and acquired valvular disease is unknown.

8. If the RAAS is a compensatory response that maintains blood pressure and cardiac output, why is inhibition of this system used therapeutically ?

Inhibition of the RAAS is important therapeutically because many of the compensatory mechanisms important in heart failure are ultimately maladaptive. Short-term activation of systems that increase vascular resistance and intravascular volume are beneficial; however, chronic elevations in adrenergic tone and angiotensin II levels appear to contribute to the inexorable decline in cardiac function that is a feature of CHF. In people, markers of RAAS and adrenergic nervous system activation are associated with a poor prognosis, but therapies such as ACE inhibitors and beta-adrenergic antagonists that antagonize these effects improve prognosis. The neurohumoral activation that is a feature of heart failure is similar to the body's response to hemorrhage, and it is likely that this is the evolutionary basis for this seemingly maladaptive response. Those that survive injuries long enough to restore circulatory volume can normalize cardiac performance and the compensatory mechanisms are again restrained.

9. What are the indications for ACE inhibitors?
The ACE inhibitors are indicated for the therapy of congestive heart failure resulting from acquired valvular disease or dilated cardiomyopathy in dogs. A double-blind placebo controlled trial demonstrated the efficacy of the ACE inhibitor enalapril in this scenario. Other indications for ACE inhibitors in small animals are less certain. The ACE inhibitors are widely used in people for the management of systemic hypertension and these drugs are occasionally used as antihypertensive agents in both dogs and cats. It is likely that the efficacy of these drugs for this purpose depends on the pathogenesis of the hypertensive state. Patients with "high-renin" hypertension that might complicate renal disease may well respond to ACE inhibitors.

The ACE inhibitors may also have a role in the management of feline myocardial disease, although it is important to recognize that ACE inhibitors are not necessarily beneficial or effective in all heart diseases. While it appears that ACE inhibitors can be safely used in cats with hypertrophic cardiomyopathy, the most common feline myocardial disease, any clinical benefit is likely related to reductions in aldosterone levels or perhaps effects on the local cardiac renin-angiotensin system. Patients with hypertrophic cardiomyopathy generally have normal or even hyperdynamic systolic performance. As discussed earlier, there is no great mechanical advantage to vasodilation when systolic performance is normal.

10. Are the ACE inhibitors potent vasodilators? How does the hemodynamic effect of these drugs compare to other vasodilators such as hydralazine?
The vasodilatory effect of ACE inhibition is relatively modest. Direct-acting vasodilators such as hydralazine and nitroprusside have a more potent effect on vascular resistance. The ACE inhibitors have largely superseded vasodilators such as hydralazine because current clinical evidence favors the view that hemodynamic effects are less important than controlling the body's maladaptive responses. In fact, a large clinical trial conducted in people suffering from heart failure demonstrated reduced mortality in the population receiving enalapril when compared to the group that received a hydralazine-nitrate combination.

11. What adverse effects can result from the administration of ACE inhibitors?
Hypotension and the development of azotemia are potential adverse effects of ACE inhibition. These effects are relatively uncommon; in the veterinary enalapril trial, the incidence of azotemia or hypotension was not significantly higher in the treatment group than it was in the group that received a placebo. Both hypotension and the development of azotemia are adverse effects that are readily explained by the functional properties of the ACE inhibitors. Other adverse effects that are observed on occasion are nonspecific and include vomiting and anorexia.

12. What are the "local" or "tissue-specific" renin-angiotensin systems?
The component hormones of the renin-angiotensin system are found in many organs including the heart, the vasculature, and the brain. The effect on tissue-specific ACE is thought to explain some of the beneficial effects of ACE inhibitors.

13. Are ACE inhibitors nephrotoxic?
ACE inhibitors are not generally thought to have a direct nephrotoxic effect; rather, they alter intrarenal hemodynamics in such a way that some susceptible individuals develop prerenal azotemia. Angiotensin II has a relatively selective effect on the efferent arteriole of the nephron. The reduction in angiotensin II levels that accompanies ACE inhibition causes a decrease in the

pressure gradient across the glomerulus and as a result decreases the glomerular filtration fraction. Glomerular filtration rate (GFR) decreases as a consequence and azotemia can result. Patients with preexisting renal disease, those that are volume depleted due to overly aggressive diuretic therapy, and those with cardiac dysfunction so severe that they are critically dependent on angiotensin II to maintain GFR are at greatest risk for the development of azotemia.

14. How is azotemia addressed when it is observed in patients receiving a diuretic and ACE inhibitors?

The management of this complication is based upon the understanding that vasodilators can increase stroke volume in the setting of systolic failure; diuretics, despite other favorable clinical effects, tend to limit stroke volume. Initially, when faced with this complication, a reduction in the diuretic dose by 50% is appropriate provided the patient does not have overt signs of congestion. If this doesn't result in reduction of the serum creatinine level, the diuretic is discontinued. If azotemia persists, cautious fluid administration with careful observation of respiratory rate and character is initiated. It must be recognized that diuretics are the most effective agents for the removal of cardiogenic edema. Reducing diuretic doses is not advised for patients that have overt congestive heart failure. The development of severe prerenal azotemia in the face of congestion is one definition of medically refractory heart failure.

15. Can ACE inhibitors cause cough?

Cough is an important and use-limiting adverse effect that is observed in people that are receiving ACE inhibitors. The activity of the ACE inhibitor is not specific; the enzyme also accelerates the breakdown of endogenous bradykinin. Bradykinin is a vasodilator and also an inflammatory mediator. Increased bradykinin levels associated with ACE inhibition have been incriminated as a cause of cough, which develops in as many as 15% of people receiving ACE inhibitors. Cough is a common clinical sign in dogs with heart disease and heart failure. For this reason, it is difficult to determine whether or not cough in dogs receiving ACE inhibitors is drug related or simply reflects the disease for which the drug was prescribed. However, informed clients occasionally inquire about this adverse effect and the practitioner should be familiar with the phenomenon of cough associated with the use of ACE inhibitors.

16. What are the contraindications for the use of ACE inhibitors?

Hypersensitivity to ACE inhibitors has not been documented in animals; consequently, contraindications to ACE inhibition in small animals are relative ones. ACE inhibitors are probably best avoided in patients in which cardiac output is limited due to fixed obstructions to blood flow. In the setting of aortic stenosis, for example, cardiac output is limited by the resistance to ventricular ejection that results from the narrowed aortic orifice. In a sense, stroke volume is limited and fixed by the high-resistance aortic orifice; cardiac output can only increase through elevations in heart rate or further increases in ventricular pressure, both of which potentially increase myocardial oxygen demand. In aortic stenosis, therefore, vasodilation will result in either systemic hypotension or a detrimental increase in ventricular pressure or heart rate. Analogous arguments apply when fixed obstruction is present elsewhere in the cardiovascular system.

Therefore, ACE inhibitors should be used with caution, if at all, in heart failure due to aortic stenosis, pulmonic stenosis, mitral stenosis, tricuspid valve stenosis, and possibly heartworm disease. The latter is grouped with anatomical obstructions because the pulmonary vessels in patients with severe pulmonary hypertension due to heartworm disease may have fixed pulmonary vascular resistance and the effect of ACE inhibitors on the systemic vasculature could potentially lead to hypotension and azotemia. These contraindications are, of course, relative ones. Vasodilation is but one effect of ACE inhibition and, in selected cases, the diverse neurohumoral effects of these drugs might shift the risk/benefit in way that favors their use.

17. Is there a "best" ACE inhibitor?

The ACE inhibitors differ primarily in terms of pharmacokinetics. Most, with the exception of captopril and lisinopril, are administered as pro-drugs that must be metabolized to an active form. Captopril was the prototype ACE inhibitor. This drug is distinguished from other ACE inhibitors by the presence of a sulfhydryl group, and by the fact that it is active in its original form but is converted to metabolites that also have ACE-inhibiting properties. The elimination half-life is relatively short in dogs, which necessitates dosing three times per day. The class II ACE inhibitors include enalapril and benazepril. Both of these agents must be metabolized in order to become active. Lisinopril, in class III, is unique among the ACE inhibitors because it does not have to be metabolized to an active form; it is excreted unchanged in the urine.

18. Which ACE inhibitor is preferred when there is preexisting renal dysfunction?
   All ACE inhibitors have an effect on renal hemodynamics such that they can precipitate the development of azotemia in susceptible individuals. Unlike the active metabolites of enalapril, benazepril is excreted by both renal and hepatic routes. It is not necessary to adjust doses if one elects to administer benazepril to a patient with preexisting renal disease. That is not to say that benazepril has a lesser effect on renal function than enalapril, only that enalapril doses should be adjusted in azotemic patients and this is not necessary for benazepril.

BIBLIOGRAPHY

1. The COVE Study Group: Controlled clinical evaluation of enalapril in dogs with heart failure: Results of the Cooperative Veterinary Enalapril Study Group. J Vet Intern Med 9:243–252, 1995.
2. Ettinger SJ, Benitz AM, Ericsson GE, et al: Effects of enalapril maleate on survival times of dogs with naturally acquired heart failure. J Am Vet Med Assoc 213:1573–1577, 1998.
3. Hamlin RL: Pathophysiology of the failing heart. In Fox PR, Sisson D, Moise NS (eds): Textbook of Canine and Feline Cardiology: Principles and Clinical Practice, 2nd ed. Philadelphia, W.B. Saunders, 1999, pp 205–215.
4. Hamlin RL, Nakayama T: Comparison of some pharmacokinetic parameters of 5 angiotensin-converting enzyme inhibitors in normal beagles. J Vet Intern Med 12:93–95, 1998.
5. Lefebvre HP, Laroute V, Concordet D, Toutain P-L: Effects of renal impairment on the disposition of orally administered enalapril, benazepril and their active metabolites. J Vet Intern Med 13:21–27, 1999.
6. Opie LH, Poole-Wilson PA, Sonnenblick EH, Chatterjee K: Angiotensin-converting enzyme inhibitors and conventional vasodilators. In Opie LH (ed): Drugs for the Heart, 4th ed. Philadelphia, W.B. Saunders, 1997, pp 105–144.
7. Packer M, Cohn JN (eds): Consensus recommendations for the management of chronic heart failure. Am J Cardiol 83:1A–38A, 1999.
8. Sabbah HN, Shimoyama H, Kono T, et al: Effects of long-term monotherapy with enalapril, metoprolol, and digoxin on the progression of left ventricular dysfunction and dilation in dogs with reduced ejection fraction. Circulation 89:2852–2859, 1994.
9. Sisson D, Kittleson MD: Management of heart failure: Principles of treatment, therapeutic strategies and pharmacology. In Fox PR, Sisson D, Moise NS (eds): Textbook of Canine and Feline Cardiology: Principles and Clinical Practice, 2nd ed. Philadelphia, W.B. Saunders, 1999, pp 216–250.
10. Ware WA, Keene BW: Outpatient management of chronic heart failure. In Bonagura JD (ed): Kirk's Current Veterinary Therapy XIII: Small Animal Practice. Philadelphia, W.B Saunders, 2000, pp 748–752.

12. CALCIUM CHANNEL ANTAGONISTS

Francis W. K. Smith, Jr., D.V.M.

1. What are the two major classes of calcium channel antagonists and examples of drugs within these classes?

1. **Dihydropyridine calcium channel antagonists.** The prototype dihydropyridine is nifedipine. Newer, longer-acting agents include amlodipine and felodipine. Amlodipine is the only dihydropyridine calcium channel antagonist commonly used in small animal practice.

2. **Non-dihydropyridine calcium channel antagonists.** Verapamil and diltiazem are the classic non-dihydropyridine calcium channel antagonists. Although these two drugs are structurally different and bind to different portions of the calcium channel, they are often classified together because of their similar cardiovascular effects. Diltiazem is the most commonly prescribed non-dihydropyridine calcium antagonists used in small animal practice.

2. Describe the effects of the different classes of calcium antagonists on myocardial contractility.

Verapamil and diltiazem are negative inotropic drugs, so they depress cardiac contractility. The dihydropyridines (e.g., amlodipine) are minimally cardiodepressing, having much greater vascular selectivity than either verapamil or diltiazem. In general, the vasodilating effects of diltiazem offset the effects of this drug on cardiac contractility, such that cardiac output is not adversely affected. Verapamil is a more potent negative inotrope than diltiazem. All calcium channel antagonists must be used with caution in patients with myocardial failure.

3. Describe the effects of the different classes of calcium antagonists on cardiac conduction.

Verapamil and diltiazem lower automaticity in the sinus node and slow conduction through the AV node. With both drugs the effect on the AV node is more potent than the effect on sinus node. They are often prescribed for the management of supraventricular arrhythmias (e.g., atrial tachycardia, atrial fibrillation) because of their effect on the AV node. Dihydropyridines do not affect cardiac conduction and, as a result of vasodilation, may actually increase the heart rate. Tachycardia is more commonly associated with the use of nifedipine, which has a rapid onset and short duration of action, than with felodipine or amlodipine.

4. Describe the effects of the different classes of calcium antagonists on vascular smooth muscle.

All classes of calcium channel antagonists cause smooth muscle relaxation, resulting in vasodilation. However, the dihydropyridines have much greater vascular selectivity than diltiazem or verapamil. Vascular selectivity and a lesser degree of myocardial depression tend to preserve cardiac output.

5. How do the calcium channel antagonists exert their effects on cardiac and vascular smooth muscle?

Calcium is essential for excitation-contraction coupling in muscle cells. In myocytes, calcium entry into the cell results in release of calcium by the sarcoplasmic reticulum, leading to higher cytosolic calcium levels. Calcium then binds to troponin, exposing binding site on the actin molecule. Actin then binds to myosin, leading to cardiac contraction. In vascular smooth muscle, calcium enters the cytosol, binds to calmodulin and this complex then activates myosin light chain kinase, resulting in smooth muscle contraction. By blocking the influx of calcium into vascular and cardiac muscle, calcium channel antagonists lower intracellular calcium levels and depress contractility.

6. What are the clinical indications for calcium channel antagonists in the management of cardiovascular disease in dogs and cats?
- Control or termination of supraventricular tachycardia and atrial fibrillation
- Treatment of hypertrophic cardiomyopathy
- Treatment of systemic hypertension

7. What is the role of calcium antagonists in the management of arrhythmias?

Verapamil and diltiazem lower automaticity in the sinus node and slow conduction through the AV node. Therefore, they are frequently prescribed for the management of supraventricular arrhythmias. In veterinary cardiology, diltiazem is more commonly prescribed than verapamil. In the setting of supraventricular tachycardia (e.g., atrial or junctional tachycardia) either drug can be administered as a slow IV bolus for rapid termination of the arrhythmia. Verapamil is administered to dogs at a dose of 0.05 mg/kg IV q 10–30 minutes (maximum cumulative dose is 0.15 mg/kg). Diltiazem is administered to dogs at a dose of 0.25 mg/kg IV. For long-term control of a supraventricular tachycardia, diltiazem is more frequently used than verapamil and is administered orally. Dihydropyridines do not affect cardiac conduction and are of no value in arrhythmia control.

Verapamil and diltiazem can also be used for heart rate control in atrial fibrillation. As most patients with atrial fibrillation have advanced heart disease and often myocardial failure, these drugs must be used cautiously. While verapamil is more effective at slowing the heart rate, it is also more potent at depressing contractility. Therefore, diltiazem is the preferred calcium antagonist in this setting. Although diltiazem can be used alone to slow atrial fibrillation, it is generally used in conjunction with digoxin. The author generally prescribes digoxin for initial rate control and inotropic support. If the heart rate is not adequately slowed by digoxin, diltiazem is added.

8. What is the role of calcium channel antagonists in the management of cardiomyopathy?

Verapamil and diltiazem may be beneficial in some patients with hypertrophic cardiomyopathy. Diltiazem appears better tolerated in cats, making it the calcium channel antagonist of choice. The therapeutic effects of diltiazem may be due to improved myocardial relaxation, control of tachycardia, coronary vasodilation, peripheral vasodilation, or antithrombotic effects. There is some evidence to suggest that calcium channel antagonists may act as modulators of myocardial hypertrophy. Other than the control of supraventricular arrhythmias, there is little evidence that calcium channel antagonists are beneficial in the treatment of dilated cardiomyopathy.

9. What is the role of calcium channel antagonists in the management of systemic hypertension?

Blood pressure is equal to the product of cardiac output and peripheral vascular resistance. Calcium channel antagonists cause vascular smooth muscle relaxation, lowering systemic vascular resistance and blood pressure. Verapamil and diltiazem also slow the heart rate, which lowers cardiac output and blood pressure.

In veterinary practice, amlodipine is the most commonly prescribed calcium channel antagonist for control of systemic hypertension in cats. It is neutral in its effect on heart rate, but is a potent vasodilator. The drug is very well tolerated in cats and has a very favorable pharmacokinetic profile, requiring only one daily dosing. The recommended dose in cats is 0.18 mg/kg orally q24h. For cats under 5 kg the dose is ¼ of a 2.5-mg tablet daily. For cats over 2.5 kg, the dose is ½ of a 2.5-mg tablet daily. Amlodipine can be used in dogs, but the pharmacokinetics and pharmacodynamics are not as well established in dogs. The empirical dose in dogs is 0.15–0.25 mg/kg orally q24h.

10. What are the contraindications to the clinical use of calcium channel antagonists?

Verapamil and diltiazem depress sinus node automaticity and AV node conduction, and should be used with caution in animals with sinus node or AV node disease (e.g., sick sinus syndrome, AV block, digoxin toxicity). Verapamil and diltiazem depress cardiac contractility. As a potent negative inotrope, verapamil should not be used in animals with myocardial failure. Diltiazem causes mild myocardial depression and also must be used with caution in animals with myocardial failure. In most animals with myocardial failure and supraventricular arrhythmias, diltiazem is well tolerated. The negative inotropic effects of the drug are offset by the vasodilating effects and the improved cardiac output that results from controlling the excessively rapid heart rate. Because all classes of calcium antagonists relax vascular smooth muscle, they are contraindicated in the setting of systemic hypotension.

11. What are potential side effects of calcium channel antagonists?

Verapamil and diltiazem depress myocardial contractility and consequently can lower cardiac output. In animals with myocardial failure, this effect of calcium antagonists can precipitate heart failure. Signs of heart failure include coughing, dyspnea, ascites, lethargy, exercise intolerance, and syncope.

Gastrointestinal disturbances, predominantly anorexia and vomiting, have been reported with the use of calcium channel antagonists. Fortunately, when prescribed for appropriate indications, these drugs are generally well tolerated by most dogs and cats.

Because all calcium channel antagonists relax vascular smooth muscle, caution should be exercised when using them in conjunction with other drugs that lower blood pressure (e.g., beta-adrenergic blockers, angiotensin-converting enzyme inhibitors, hydralazine, prazosin, and acepromazine). In cases of refractory systemic hypertension, these drugs can be used effectively in combination, with close monitoring of blood pressure.

12. What is the treatment for calcium antagonist overdose?

Overdose of verapamil or diltiazem can be treated with calcium gluconate or calcium chloride to help manage hypotension or heart failure. Vasoconstricting or positive inotropic catecholamines (e.g., dopamine or dobutamine) may be required if there is an inadequate response to intravenous calcium. Glucagon has also been shown to be useful in the management of calcium antagonist overdose. Administration of calcium, however, does little to improve cardiac conduction. Atropine or isoproterenol may be helpful to shorten AV node conduction time.

13. How do the effects of calcium channel antagonists compare to those of beta-adrenergic blockers?

1. **Heart rate:** Beta-adrenergic blockers depress sinus node automaticity and AV node conduction. The calcium channel antagonists verapamil and diltiazem also depress sinus node automaticity and AV node conduction. Amlodipine has no effect on heart rate.

2. **Contractility:** Beta-adrenergic blockers depress myocardial contractility as do verapamil and diltiazem. Diltiazem depresses contractility less than beta-blockers. Amlodipine has high vascular selectivity and negligible effects on cardiac contractility at therapeutic doses.

3. **Vasculature:** Nonselective beta-blockers such as propranolol prevent adrenergically mediated vasodilation that can, in some circumstances, increase systemic vascular resistance; calcium antagonists of all classes cause vasodilation.

4. **Myocardial relaxation:** Calcium channel antagonists have a lusitropic effect, resulting in improved myocardial relaxation. Beta-adrenergic blockers do not improve myocardial relaxation.

BIBLIOGRAPHY

1. Doyon S, Roberts JR: The use of glucagon in a case of calcium channel blocker overdose. Ann Emerg Med 22:1229–1223, 1993.
2. Fox PR: Feline cardiomyopathies. In Fox PR, Sisson D, Moise NS (eds): Textbook of Canine and Feline Cardiology, 2nd ed. Philadelphia, W.B. Saunders, 1999, pp 471–535.
3. Kittleson MD: Electrocardiography. Kittleson MD, Kienle RD (eds): Small Animal Cardiovascular Medicine. St Louis, Mosby, 1998, pp 72–94.
4. Moise NS: Diagnosis and management of canine arrhythmias. In Fox PR, Sisson D, Moise NS (eds): Textbook of Canine and Feline Cardiology, 2nd ed. Philadelphia, W.B. Saunders, 1999, pp 471–535.
5. Opie LH, Frishman WH, Thadani U: Calcium channel antagonists (calcium entry blockers). In Opie LH (ed): Drugs for the Heart, 4th ed. Philadelphia, W.B. Saunders, 1995, pp 50–82.
6. Snyder PS: Amlodipine: A randomized, blinded clinical trial in 9 cats with systemic hypertension. J Vet Intern Med 12:157–162, 1998.
7. Snyder PS: Canine hypertensive disease. Compend Cont Ed Pract Vet 13:1785–1793, 1991.

13. BETA-ADRENERGIC ANTAGONISTS

Jonathan A. Abbott, D.V.M.

1. What are beta-adrenergic antagonists (beta blockers)?

Beta-adrenergic antagonists are drugs that affect the adrenergic arm of the autonomic nervous system. Also known as beta blockers, the beta-adrenergic antagonists bind to the beta receptors of the adrenergic nervous system. The names of beta blockers end with the suffix *-olol*. Propranolol is the prototype beta blocker; atenolol, carvedilol, timolol, esmolol, and many others are also in this class.

2. What are the main divisions of the autonomic nervous system? What are their functions?

The autonomic system is the functional division of the nervous system that regulates involuntary processes. The parasympathetic arm of the autonomic nervous system is primarily responsible for the regulation of vegetative functions. With respect to the cardiovascular system, parasympathetic (vagal) stimulation results primarily in slowing of the heart and a negative inotropic effect. The receptors on the effector organs are stimulated by acetylcholine, and the activity of the parasympathetic nervous system is blocked by drugs such as atropine and glycopryolate.

Anatomically, the *adrenergic* (sympathetic) nervous system is comprised of the thoracolumbar outflow, which gives rise to the sympathetic trunk. In general, the adrenergic nervous system is responsible for the "fight or flight" response. The adrenergic receptors are located presynaptically and on effector organs and bind to the catecholamines (epinephrine and norepinephrine). Based upon structural and functional differences, adrenergic receptors are classified as alpha or beta receptors. Stimulation of the alpha-1 receptors results in vasoconstriction of the systemic arterioles. The functional role of the alpha-2 receptors is less well defined; stimulation of presynaptic receptors inhibits norepinephrine release, while stimulation of postsynaptic receptors results in vasoconstriction.

The beta-adrenergic receptors are located throughout the vascular system, the heart, and the bronchioles. Stimulation of beta-1 receptors within the myocardium and specialized conduction system of the heart results in increases in heart rate, AV nodal conduction velocity, and the strength of myocardial contraction. Beta-2 agonism results in vasodilation in skeletal muscles; this effect is most important during exertion and is partly responsible for the fall in systemic vascular resistance that accompanies exercise. Importantly, beta-2 receptors are also found throughout the airways; stimulation of the pulmonary beta-2 receptors results in bronchodilation.

3. What are the main cardiovascular effects of beta-blocking drugs?

Blockade of the beta receptors neutralizes the effects of adrenergic stimulation. Underlying parasympathetic activity is unmasked and in general beta-blockade results in the following effects:

- Slowing of the heart rate—a negatively chronotropic effect
- A reduction in myocardial contractility—a negatively inotropic effect
- Slowing of conduction velocity through the specialized conduction system of the heart—a negatively dromotropic effect

At any instant, the effect of the autonomic nervous system on the heart and blood vessels represents the sum of opposing parasympathetic and sympathetic influences. Thus the clinical importance of the drug effects listed above depends partly on the relationship between sympathetic and parasympathetic tone at the time beta blockade is initiated. For example, some patients with dilated cardiomyopathy are critically dependent upon elevations in adrenergic tone in order to maintain cardiac output and perfusion pressure. In this setting, the negatively inotropic effect of beta blockers can be profound, and as a result the injudicious use of beta blockers may have dire clinical consequences. In contrast, the effects of beta blockade are likely to be less noticeable in a resting athlete.

4. What are the main uses of beta blockers in small animal cardiovascular medicine?
The beta blockers are used most often in the treatment of pathologic tachyarrhythmia and in the management of feline hypertrophic cardiomyopathy.

Antiarrhythmic effects. BAA have a profound effect on conduction velocities within the AV node and this can be of benefit in the setting of supraventricular tachyarrhythmia. Specifically, these agents can be used to slow the ventricular response rate in atrial fibrillation and can slow heart rate in rapid atrial tachycardias by causing AV block. When supraventricular tachycardias are maintained by reentry loops in which the AV node or bundle is a crucial anatomic component, beta blockade can restore normal sinus rhythm (see Chapter 30).

Beta blockers do not directly affect the action potential of cardiomyocytes as do the antiarrhythmic agents that block specific ion channels; however, the electrophysiologic properties of cardiac muscle cells are profoundly affected by changes in autonomic tone. Specifically, high adrenergic tone shortens action potential duration and refractory periods, which may predispose to ventricular arrhythmias such as premature ventricular complexes and ventricular tachycardia. In addition, high adrenergic tone decreases the fibrillation threshold. Because of this, beta blockade can lessen the chances of a patient developing the lethal arrhythmia of ventricular fibrillation. Therefore the beta blockers can control adrenergically mediated ventricular arrhythmias and might have a role in the prevention of sudden cardiac death.

Some caution is warranted, however; not all ventricular tachycardias are adrenergically mediated. If a beta blocker is administered to a patient suffering from a rapid ventricular tachycardia and it fails to effect conversion to sinus rhythm, the negatively inotropic effect of the drug can be problematic. Prior to drug administration the patient has an abnormal and rapid rhythm originating from the ventricles; afterward, the patient must contend with a rapid rate and iatrogenic myocardial dysfunction.

Hypertrophic cardiomyopathy. Hypertrophic cardiomyopathy (HCM) is an idiopathic myocardial disease that is characterized primarily by diastolic dysfunction. The beta blockers may benefit patients with HCM through a number of mechanisms. Beta blockers have a favorable effect on diastolic performance through their effect on heart rate. Slowing of the heart rate increases diastolic filling time and may therefore improve ventricular filling. In some patients, HCM is complicated by dynamic ventricular outflow tract obstruction resulting from systolic anterior motion (SAM) of the mitral valve. The anterior movement of the mitral leaflets obstructs left ventricular outflow and results in mitral valve regurgitation. This phenomenon is dynamic and is accentuated by interventions that increase the inotropic state, decrease systemic vascular resistance, or reduce preload. The beta blockers are negatively inotropic and have little effect on resting systemic vascular resistance. These drugs may therefore diminish or even abolish systolic anterior motion in patients with HCM.

5. Are there other uses for beta-adrenergic antagonists?
The beta-adrenergic antagonists have a role in the management of feline hyperthyroidism. Patients with hyperthyroidism have a hyperdynamic circulation that results from thyroid hormone excess. Heart rates in affected cats are often high and some suffer from hyperthyroid cardiomyopathy. An abnormally great sensitivity to catecholamines is believed to play an important role in the pathogenesis of this disorder and beta-adrenergic antagonists are potentially useful. The administration of beta blockers effectively slows heart rate and can be used to control pathologic tachyarrhythmia that can complicate the hyperthyroid state. In hyperthyroid people, beta blockers help to control the anxiety that can be associated with thyrotoxicosis; many hyperthyroid cats are visibly anxious and it is possible that they also benefit from the effects of beta blockade on the central nervous system.

Beta-adrenergic antagonists also have a role in the management of some congenital heart diseases. Beta-adrenergic antagonists are sometimes administered to dogs with subaortic stenosis.

These drugs slow the heart rate and decrease inotropic state, therefore reducing myocardial oxygen demand. Additionally, the antiarrhythmic effect of these drugs may be helpful. However, it should be recognized that patients with aortic stenosis develop abnormally high pressures within the left ventricle because they must do so in order to overcome the resistance created by the narrowed aortic orifice. In cases of severe aortic stenosis, aggressive beta blockade can potentially result in systemic hypotension and possibly worsen myocardial ischemia.

Beta-adrenergic antagonists may have a palliative role in right-to-left shunting defects such as tetralogy of Fallot. Affected patients may develop episodic weakness that results from the accentuation of right-to-left shunting that occurs on exercise. Nonselective beta blockers such as propranolol prevent the drop in vascular resistance that is an expected consequence of exercise. This effect, together with a negatively inotropic effect that limits dynamic, exercise-related worsening of the pulmonic stenosis component of the tetralogy, may benefit patients with this congenital malformation.

Although newer agents such as the calcium channel antagonist amlodipine and drugs in the angiotensin-converting enzyme (ACE) inhibitor class are now used more commonly, beta blockers are also used in the management of systemic hypertension.

6. How do beta-adrenergic antagonists decrease abnormally high blood pressure?
The mechanism of blood pressure reduction due to beta blockade is poorly understood. It may result from the combined effects of reduced cardiac output and an inhibition of renin release that results from beta-adrenergic antagonism.

7. Do beta blockers have a role in the management of dilated cardiomyopathy?
The beta blockers are negative inotropes and their use in patients with systolic dysfuntion seems counterintuitive. However, recent clinical studies demonstrate that chronic beta blockade decreases mortality and morbidity in people with CHF due to systolic myocardial dysfunction. The role of beta blockers in the management of canine dilated cardiomyopathy is yet to be determined.

8. How do the available beta blockers differ?
The beta blockers differ primarily in terms of beta-receptor selectivity and pharmacokinetics. The first-generation agents include propranolol, the prototype beta-adrenergic antagonist. Propranolol is a nonselective agent; that is, both beta-1 receptors and beta-2 receptors are blocked by this drug. Blockade of the beta-2 receptors can result in bronchoconstriction or at least it prevents adrenergically mediated bronchodilation in patients that have bronchoconstrictive diseases such as asthma. Antagonism of beta-2 receptors located in skeletal muscle prevents exercise-induced vasodilation and therefore prevents the drop in systemic vascular resistance that usually accompanies exercise.

Atenolol and other second generation beta blockers have relative selectivity for beta-1 receptors. The beta-1 selective agents have advantages when beta blockade is indicated in patients that have concurrent bronchoconstrictive diseases such as asthma. It should be recognized that receptor selectivity is a relative and dose-dependent property. Some stimulation of beta-2 receptors is possible and this becomes more important when higher doses are administered. Metoprolol and esmolol are other examples of beta-1 or cardioselective beta blockers.

The third generation beta-adrenergic antagonists are beta-blockers that have vasodilatory effects. Vasodilation results from either beta-2 agonism, which is known as intrinsic sympathomimetic activity, or results from alpha-adrenergic blockade. These agents are not commonly used in veterinary medicine. However, carvedilol, a combined beta and alpha-1 blocker, has recently been shown to benefit human patients with dilated cardiomyopathy. It is possible that there is a role for this drug in some dogs with this heart disease.

9. Is there a single beta-adrenergic antagonist that is superior to others?
There is no single beta-adrenergic antagonist that is superior to others, and the choice of drug is dictated by clinical circumstances. For example, in the palliation of patients with cyanotic

congenital heart disease, a nonselective agent such as propranolol is likely superior to the more cardioselective beta blockers. In other situations, pharmacokinetics might be the variable that determines drug choice. Atenolol, for example, is a cardioselective agent that is generally given once or twice daily. In contrast, esmolol is an "ultrashort" acting beta-adrenergic antagonist that can be given as a test bolus followed by a constant-rate infusion.

10. Which beta blockers are used most commonly in veterinary medicine?

Propranolol is the prototype beta blocker and it continues to be used widely. It is a nonselective agent and has a relatively short elimination half-life, which necessitates an 8- to 12-hour dosing interval. This drug should probably not be used in patients with confirmed or suspected reactive airway diseases such as asthma.

In many situations, atenolol has some advantages over propranolol. It is a cardioselective beta-adrenergic antagonist and can be given twice daily. Esmolol is an ultrashort acting beta blocker that is used primarily in the critical care setting. It has an elimination half-life that is measured in minutes. It is available only in an injectable formulation. For the most part, it is used as an antiarrhythmic agent. It has the advantage that adverse effects, if observed, are relatively short-lived because the effect of the drug is so brief.

11. What are the potential adverse effects of beta blockade? How is a beta-blocker overdose treated?

Adverse effects of beta blockade are observed when the magnitude of the therapeutic effects is undesirable. The adverse effects of beta-adrenergic antagonists are primarily bradycardia and hypotension. Mood alterations are observed in people that receive beta-adrenergic antagonists and this results from effects on the central nervous system.

Beta-blocker overdose poses a therapeutic challenge. Drugs such as atropine can be administered in hopes of increasing the heart rate. However, this is unlikely to have much effect as these drugs have a permissive rather than a direct effect on heart rate—they increase heart rate to a degree that depends on prevailing adrenergic tone and may have little effect in the face of beta-blocker overdose. Temporary transvenous pacing may be required for patients with profound bradycardia. Dobutamine or even epinephrine can be administered; at high doses these catecholamines will compete with the beta blocker for receptor binding. Inotropic support in the form of glucagon administration is recommended as a treatment for beta-blocker overdose in people. Glucagon has a direct inotropic effect that is independent of beta-adrenergic receptors.

12. What drug interactions are important when beta-adrenergic antagonists are administered?

Other drugs that slow the heart or are negatively inotropic should be used together with beta-adrenergic antagonists only with caution. For example, the calcium channel antagonists share many effects with the beta-adrenergic antagonists. While the digitalis glycosides have a positively inotropic effect, they also slow the heart rate through effects on the cardiac conduction system. That is not to say that these drugs cannot be used together. In fact, the combination of digoxin and a beta blocker or calcium channel antagonist is sometimes required to appropriately slow the ventricular rate in atrial fibrillation associated with dilated cardiomyopathy. It is important that the practitioner be cognizant of drugs that can potentiate the effects of the beta blockers.

13. What are beta-3 receptors? What function do they fulfill?

It has long been known that beta-3 adrenergic receptors play a role in fat metabolism. Recently however, beta-3 receptors were isolated from failing human ventricles. These receptors mediate a negatively inotropic effect. It has been postulated that these receptors might be involved in the pathogenesis of progressive myocardial dysfunction in patients with heart failure.

14. What are the contraindications to the use of beta blockers?

Severe conduction system disease such as complete heart block in the absence of a functioning pacemaker is a contraindication to beta blockade. Other contraindications are relative; beta blockers should only be administered with caution to patients with myocardial dysfunction. As stated previously, nonselective beta blockers such as propranolol should be avoided in patients that have reactive airway diseases, such as asthma.

BIBLIOGRAPHY

1. Adams HR: Adrenergic agonists and antagonists. In Adams HR (ed): Veterinary Pharmacology and Therapeutics, 7th ed. Ames, Iowa State University Press, 1995, pp 87–113.
2. Lefkowitz RJ, Hoffman BB: Catechlamines, sympathomimetic drugs and adrenergic receptor antagonists. In Hardman JG, Limbird LE (eds): Goodman & Gilman's The Pharmacological Basis of Therapeutics, 9th ed. New York, McGraw-Hill, 1996, pp 199–248.
3. Opie LH, Sonnenblick EH, Frishman WH, Thadani U: Beta-blocking agents. In Opie LH (ed): Drugs for the Heart, 4th ed. Philadelphia, W.B. Saunders, 1997, pp 1–30.
4. Packer M, Bristow MR, Cohn JN, et al: The effect of carvedilol on morbidity and mortality in patients with chronic heart failure. N Engl J Med 334:1349–1355, 1996.
5. Quinones M, Dyer DC, Ware WA, Mehvar R: Pharmacokinetics of atenolol in clinically normal cats. Am J Vet Res 57:1050–1053, 1996.

14. DIGITALIS

Clarke E. Atkins, D.V.M.

1. What are the meanings of terms digitalis, digoxin, digitoxin, and cardiac glycosides?

The terminology related to digitalis is somewhat confusing. "Digitalis" and "cardiac glycosides" are general terms for the group of drugs derived from the plant *Digitalis purpurea* (foxglove, digitoxin, gitalin, or digitalis leaf) and the leaf of *Digitalis lanata* (digoxin, lanatoside C, and deslanoside). More specifically, the term "cardiac glycoside" indicates the steroid-lactoneglycoside chemical structure of these drugs. "Digitoxin" and "digoxin" are specific drugs derived from *D. purpurea* and *D. lanata*, respectively; they differ little in structure but possess distinct pharmacologic properties. Oubain, an infrequently used intravenous glycoside, is derived from the seeds of the plant *Strophanthus gratus*.

2. What are the differences between digoxin and digitoxin?

Digoxin is by far the most commonly used cardiac glycoside in veterinary medicine. It is the only form of digitalis used in cats because of the long half-life of digitoxin (100 hours) in this species. Digitoxin does have some utility in dogs, however, particularly when renal dysfunction is present. The characteristics of these drugs as they relate to use in dogs are compared in the table below.

CHARACTERISTIC	DIGOXIN	DIGITOXIN
Bioavailability	~ 75% (elixir) ~ 60% (tablets)	~ 100%
Protein-bound	20%	90%
Dosing frequency	BID	TID
Lipid solubility	No (dose on lean BW)	Yes (dose on total BW)
Metabolism	Hepatic	Hepatic
Excretion	Renal	Hepatic
Half-life	Varies, ~ 24 hours	Varies, ~ 8 hours
Time to steady state (~ 98%)	5 days	2 days
Specific use/problems	Toxicity in renal failure Must dose on lean BW Convenient formulation Useful in cats	Used in renal insufficiency Obesity does not alter dosage Difficult to use in large dogs Not used in cats

BW, body weight.

3. Aren't these drugs old-fashioned and relatively useless today?

Indeed, these drugs have been in use in the management of heart failure for over 200 years (Withering, 1785) and likely had use in ancient Egypt and Rome. Since their most recent introduction in 1785, controversy has surrounded the use of these drugs in regards to efficacy and whether there was an adequate benefit vs. risk profile. Recently, however, large clinical studies in human medicine have shown digoxin to improve quality of life and exercise tolerance, while reducing hospital visits due to heart failure. Importantly, the effect on mortality was neutral. Nevertheless, cardiac glycosides remain the only oral positive inotropes that improve heart rate, exercise capacity, and quality of life without increasing mortality.

4. Are there studies of digitalis efficacy in veterinary medicine?

Unfortunately, controlled studies of efficacy and survival of any drugs in veterinary medi-cine are few. Hamlin et al. demonstrated improved right ventricular contractility based on the measurement of an invasive index of systolic myocardial function (dP/dT) in dogs with heart fail-ure due to heartworm disease. Kittleson et al. showed improved echocardiographic and clinico-pathologic measures of cardiac performance in 4 of 10 dogs with dilated cardiomyopathy. In this study, dogs that responded to digoxin survived longer than those that did not. All dogs, most of which were in atrial fibrillation, responded with a fall in heart rate. Atkins et al. demonstrated a positive inotropic benefit in 4 of 6 cats with dilated cardiomyopathy receiving digoxin, based on echocardiographic parameters of myocardial function. Heart rate did not fall significantly, but PR interval lengthened. None of these studies were placebo-controlled or blinded.

5. Are there any risks associated with use of these drugs?

There is some risk in using digitalis therapy as the toxic and therapeutic blood concentra-tions are not markedly different. The side effects are varied and include gastrointestinal signs (vomiting, diarrhea, anorexia), the development of arrhythmias, and central nervous system (CNS) signs. CNS symptoms may not be recognized in animals but include delirium, fatigue, confusion, dizziness, and visual impairment in humans. Digitalis intoxication is known to pro-duce virtually any arrhythmia, but the most common are junctional and ventricular (often in a bigeminal pattern) premature beats, ventricular tachycardia, sinus bradycardia, and AV nodal conduction disturbances (first- and second-degree AV block). Myocyte damage and both systolic and diastolic dysfunction have also been recognized in digitalis intoxication. The latter findings may have to do with calcium overloading of mitochondria.

6. How do cardiac glycosides produce a beneficial effect?

Primarily, these drugs functions as: (1) **positive inotropes**—as they increase myocardial contractility, and (2) **modulators of the autonomic nervous system**—they increase parasympa-thetic tone while reducing sympathetic tone. Positive inotropy is mediated through poisoning of the Na^+/K^+-ATPase pumps on myocardial cell membranes, reducing the cell's ability to extrude sodium, thereby increasing intracellular sodium concentration. This allows greater exchange of in-tracellular sodium for extracellular calcium through the sodium-calcium exchanger on the cell membrane. Increased intracellular calcium concentration produces the positive inotropic effect. A weak diuresis occurs indirectly through improvement in cardiac output and thus renal perfusion, by reducing release of aldosterone and ADH (which promote sodium and fluid retention), and directly by the effect of digitalis on the renal tubular Na^+/K^+-ATPase pumps that promote sodium retention.

In heart failure, baroreflexes (mediated by baroreceptors in aorta and carotid bodies) become dysfunctional, inappropriately signaling to the CNS that blood pressure is low. This results in in-appropriate sympathetic nervous system discharge with elevated norepinephrine concentrations (arrhythmogenic, vasoconstrictive, and positive chronotropic effects), activation of the renin-angiotensin-aldosterone system, and release of vasopressin, all of which have detrimental effects in heart failure. Digitalis appears to normalize baroreceptor function, probably by its effect on baroreceptor cell membrane Na^+/K^+-ATPase pumps. Overall, the benefits of digitalis therapy in heart failure include improved cardiac performance, normalization of neurohumoral aberration, reduced fluid retention, and lowered heart rate.

7. Describe antiarrhythmic properties of digitalis.

The electrophysiologic effects of digitalis are clinically important, generally slowing heart rate and slowing or abolishing supraventricular tachyarrhythmias. The effects vary with the serum concentration but involve both direct and vagally mediated effects, which are most noticeable on the SA and AV nodes. At clinically appropriate serum digoxin concentrations, normalization of autonomic influence on the heart (reducing sympathetic and enhancing parasympathetic input) reduces automaticity and conduction velocity while increasing resting membrane potential and refractory periods of the SA and AV nodes. This slows the sinus rate and reduces the ventricular response in atrial fibrillation by slowing conduction through the AV node. Other supraventricular tachycardias using a reentrant mechanism may be terminated as the digitalis effect on the AV node breaks the reentrant circuit. Digitalis also has a direct effect on the AV node which enhances its negative dromotropic (conductive) effect.

8. How can the toxic side effects of digitalis therapy be avoided?

Digitalis intoxication can be avoided by starting with the low dosage and titrating it upward to the therapeutic level by monitoring serum digoxin levels (in blood taken at steady state [after about 5 days of treatment in dogs and 2 weeks of treatment in cats] and 8–10 hours post-pill) and adjusting the dosage accordingly. Frequent monitoring of body weight with necessary adjustments in dosage is advisable and may reduce the risk of digitalis intoxication. In addition, the digoxin (but not digitoxin) dosage should be reduced (or the dosing interval increased) in the face of renal insufficiency. A commonly applied rule of thumb is to reduce the dose by 50% for every increase in BUN of 50 mg/dl. Some cardiologists prefer to use digitoxin in this situation.

In cases of congestive heart failure, hypokalemia may develop as a result of overly aggressive diuretic administration and/or anorexia. It is complicated by hypomagnesemia, which may result from similar processes. Hypokalemia sensitizes the heart to digitalis intoxication, increasing the frequency of arrhythmias and making them less amenable to antiarrhythmic therapy. In addition, extreme hypokalemia may reduce renal tubular function, compromising digoxin excretion. Monitoring (and, when necessary, supplementation) of serum potassium (and magnesium) concentrations may be useful, particularly in animals requiring aggressive therapy. Likewise, overexuberant use of diuretics and/or angiotensin-converting enzyme inhibitors may produce dehydration and hypotension, leading to reduced renal function with azotemia, electrolyte disturbances, and increased serum digoxin concentrations with resultant toxicity.

Since digoxin is partially metabolized in the liver (15%), it should be used cautiously in the face of liver disease; digitoxin should be avoided in dogs with significant liver dysfunction. The digoxin dosage is decreased in the very old and cachectic animals (reduced muscle mass and, hence, volume of distribution, so serum concentrations are higher), in the face of ascites (10% for mild, 20% for moderate, and 30% for severe), and when concurrent therapy includes drugs that might increase digoxin serum concentration (quinidine, amiodarone, diltiazem, captopril, aminoglycoside antibiotics, tetracycline, acyclosporine, and NSAIDs).

It is important to educate owners about the signs of intoxication and to alert them to stop treatment if signs are noted. In digitalized patients, arrhythmias or gastrointestinal signs should be considered to be digitalis-related until proven otherwise.

9. What is the desired serum concentration for cardiac glycosides in dogs and cats, when should it be measured, and is it important?

It is very important to monitor serum digoxin and digitoxin concentrations because this allows early detection of toxicity or underdosing, thereby making the achievement of a desirable clinical effect without untoward events more likely. Published therapeutic serum digoxin concentrations are 0.8–2.4 ng/ml. This author prefers to use a range of 1–2 ng/ml with the ideal dosage from 1–1.4 ng/ml. This is based on the belief that the neurohumoral effects of digoxin are of greater clinical importance than the inotropic effect; recent human studies have shown that the neurohumoral benefits can be demonstrated at lower serum concentrations while inotropic benefits are realized at higher serum concentrations (≥ 1.4 ng/ml). Desirable serum digoxin concentrations (measured at steady state [at least 5 days after initiation of therapy in dogs and 10–14 days in cats] 8–10 hours post-pill) in dogs and cats are similar. Serum concentrations may, of course, be evaluated at any time point if intoxication is suspected. The desired serum digitoxin concentration in dogs is 15–35 ng/ml, measured 3–8 hours post-pill, 2 days after initiation of therapy.

10. If signs of toxicity develop, how should they be dealt with?

Prevention of toxicity, as described above, is paramount. Nevertheless, digitalis intoxication does develop and is treated primarily by discontinuing therapy for 48 hours (or until signs and/or serum concentrations normalize) and reinstituting at a lower dosage (based on serum digoxin concentration or by 25–50% when serum concentrations are unknown). Supportive care for gastrointestinal disturbances may be useful and might include cautious repletion of fluids. Arrhythmias need not be treated unless severe. If severe ventricular arrhythmias are recognized, lidocaine, procainamide or possibly diphenylhydantoin can be administered. AV nodal conduction disturbances rarely require specific therapy, though atropine (0.02–0.04 mg/kg SC, IM, IV) can be administered to treat bradyarrhythmias. In extreme circumstances, temporary pacemaker implantation might be necessary.

For severe overdoses, recognized early, oral charcoal may be administered to bind digitalis and delay absorption. More often, time has elapsed and signs are present, requiring more extreme measures. Though quite expensive, intravenous glycoside-specific antibodies (Digibind, Glaxo-Wellcome) may be employed to bind serum digoxin. Reduction in free digoxin concentration in serum allows dissociation of tissue-bound digoxin and rapid reduction in signs of intoxication.

The role of potassium metabolism in the pathogenesis of digitalis toxicosis presents a paradox that complicates its management. Hypokalemia and hypomagnesemia increase the chances of digitalis-induced arrhythmias and lessen the odds of pharmacologic control of these arrhythmias. However, very high serum digoxin levels can displace potassium from the Na^+/K^+ pump and lead to hyperkalemia. Hence, supplementation of potassium and/or magnesium may be indicated, but potassium is used only after ruling out hyperkalemia and only in the absence of severe AV block, which is worsened by excessive potassium supplementation.

11. What are the indications for digitalization in dogs and cats?

Dog. There are at least potential benefits to digitalization in all cases of heart failure due to systolic dysfunction. This includes heart failure due to mitral valve regurgitation and dilated cardiomyopathy as well as other disorders that result in heart failure (e.g., valvular endocarditis). Indications are most obvious when myocardial failure is present, particularly when complicated by supraventricular tachycardia (e.g., dilated cardiomyopathy with atrial fibrillation), and digitalization is least indicated when myocardial function is preserved and the rate and rhythm are normal (e.g., early heart failure due to mitral regurgitation with normal sinus rhythm). Digitalis has potential indication in supraventricular arrhythmias, in the absence of heart failure, but safer drugs (calcium channel blockers and beta blockers) are now available to treat such arrhythmias, thereby rendering digitalis somewhat obsolete in this setting.

Cat. The same logic can be employed in cats. Feline heart diseases that might warrant digitalization include heart failure due to dilated cardiomyopathy (even if taurine-responsive), restrictive cardiomyopathy with echocardiographically documented systolic dysfunction, and end-stage thyrotoxic or hypertensive heart disease.

12. What are the contraindications for digitalization in dogs and cats?

Digitalis is contraindicated in cases of digitalis intoxication (or even elevated serum concentrations without signs), significant intraventricular conduction disturbances (advanced second degree and complete AV block), and heart failure primarily due to diastolic dysfunction (e.g., hypertrophic cardiomyopathy, restrictive pericarditis, and pericardial effusion with tamponade). Significant ventricular arrhythmias are a relative contraindication to digitalization but the decision not to employ cardiac glycoside therapy must be weighed against potential benefits of such therapy. It is generally accepted that ventricular arrhythmias will worsen, remain unchanged, or improve with approximately equal frequency with digitalization. This said, cardiac glycosides should be used very cautiously, and with frequent monitoring, in patients with ventricular arrhythmias.

The use of digitalis in right heart failure due to heartworm disease (and all heart failure due to cor pulmonale) is controversial. Both digoxin and digitoxin have been shown to exert a positive inotropic effect on the right ventricle of dogs with heartworm disease. Nevertheless, this author considers heartworm disease to be a relative contraindication and avoids digoxin in this setting because of the recognized lack of efficacy and proarrhythmic effect in heart failure due to pulmonary hypertension in man, previous reports of excessive adverse effects to digitalization in heartworm disease, and the fact that high doses or parenteral digoxin actually cause pulmonary vasoconstriction in dogs, an effect which would worsen signs of heart failure. I do use digoxin in heartworm disease if heart failure is refractory to treatment or if atrial fibrillation complicates the picture.

13. Are there clinically significant differences in the pharmacokinetic properties of digoxin in dogs and cats?

In both dogs and cats there is marked individual variation, making monitoring of digoxin serum levels mandatory. Elimination of digoxin is much slower in cats (half-life of ~ 40 hours) than in dogs (half-life of ~ 24 hours), which necessitates twice-daily dosing in dogs and only q48hr dosing in cats. Steady state is reached after approximately 5 half-lives. It is at this time that routine digoxin monitoring should be performed (~ 5 days after beginning therapy in dogs and 10–14 days after beginning therapy in cats). In cats, when serum digoxin concentration is measured 8 hours post-pill, the value obtained approximates the average blood concentration for the 48 hours between dosing. It has been shown that the concomitant use of sodium restriction and furosemide in cats markedly increases the half-life (~ 80 hours), but the presence of compensated heart failure does not alter the pharmacokinetic properties in cats. The dosage provided in the table below takes this concomitant therapy into consideration.

14. What are the formulations and starting dosages for digitalis in dogs and cats?

DRUG	FORMULATION	DOSAGE (DOGS)	DOSAGE (CATS)
Digoxin	Tablet 0.125 mg 0.250 mg	0.006–0.008 mg/kg bid* or 0.22 mg/m^2 bid* Rapid oral: calculate above dosage, double first dose, then calculated dose bid thereafter	0.007 mg/kg q48h Rapid oral: n/a
Digoxin	Elixir 0.05 mg/ml 0.15 mg/ml	0.005–0.007 mg/kg bid or 0.18 mg/m^2 bid	0.006 mg/kg q48h**
Digoxin	Injectable 0.1 mg/ml 0.25 mg/ml	0.01–0.02 mg/kg Give ½ slowly IV, repeat with ¼ at 1-hour intervals until desired effect or total dose administered	0.005 mg/kg as for dog
Digitoxin	Tablet 0.05 mg 0.1 mg 0.15 mg 0.2 mg	0.01–0.03 mg/kg tid	n/a
Digitoxin	Injectable	0.01–0.03 mg/kg Give ½ slowly IV, repeat with ¼ at 1-hour intervals until desired effect or total dose administered	n/a

* Dosage for large dogs is less (on per kg basis) than for small dogs. Some use a dose of 0.22 mg/m^2 bid to alleviate this concern. The dosage should generally be rounded off to the lower value and serum digoxin concentrations evaluated once steady state has been reached. The dosage is adjusted based on serum concentration (usually upward). It is generally stated that the total daily dosage should not exceed 0.5 mg; this can be exceeded, if based on serum concentrations, in giant-breed dogs.
** Although many cats will not tolerate the elixir, it can be more accurately dosed in cats that will accept it.

15. At what phase of heart disease should digitalis therapy be instituted?

Recent studies in man indicate greatest benefit of digitalis in more severely affected animals. In the absence of supraventricular arrhythmias, digoxin probably provides little, if any, benefit prior to the onset of heart failure. Because of the inherent risks of digitalization, this author uses cardiac glycosides only after the onset of congestive heart failure in both dogs and cats.

16. Is there a need for intravenous or oral loading digitalization?
With the advent of a larger armamentarium of cardiac therapeutic agents, loading doses of digitalis are infrequently employed. While digoxin is positively inotropic, this effect is relatively weak and other, more potent agents, such as dobutamine, are generally preferred when urgent inotropic support is required. Similarly, newer antiarrhythmic agents, such as injectable diltiazem, have a generally more favorable pharmacologic profile for the rapid control of severe supraventricular tachycarrhythmia. Intravenous loading is indicated when one is contemplating the use of dobutamine, in a patient with heart failure complicated by atrial fibrillation. The reason for this is to blunt the positive dromotropic effect of dobutamine which may enhance AV nodal conduction to a rate that might result in ventricular fibrillation.

Since intravenous loading has been associated with peripheral vasoconstriction (due to effects on vascular smooth muscle), digitalis preparations should be administered slowly (≥ 5 minutes) to patients that might be adversely effected by increased afterload. A less aggressive approach, or one used when intravenous glycosides are unavailable, is a rapid oral loading method described below.

BIBLIOGRAPHY

1. Atkins CE, Snyder PS, Keene BW: Effect of aspirin, furosemide, and low-salt diet on digoxin pharmacokinetic properties in clinically normal cats. J Am Vet Med Assoc 193:1264–1268, 1988.
2. Atkins CE, Snyder PS, Keene BW, et al: Effects of compensated heart failure on digoxin pharmacokinetics in cats. J Am Vet Med Assoc 195:945–950, 1989.
3. Atkins CE, Snyder PS, Keene BW, et al: Effecacy of digoxin for treatment of cats with dilated cardiomyopathy. J Am Vet Med Assoc 196:1463–1469, 1990.
4. Spratt KA, Doherty JE: Principles and practice of digitalis. In Messerli FH (ed): Cardiovascular Drug Therapy, 2nd ed. Philadelphia, W.B. Saunders, 1996, pp 1136–1146.
5. Digitalis Investigation Group: The effect of digoxin on mortality and morbidity in patients with heart failure. N Engl J Med 336:525–533, 1997.
6. Hamlin RH, Saradindu D, Smith CR: Effects of digoxin and digitoxin on ventricular function in normal dogs and dogs with heart failure. J Am Vet Med Assoc 32:1391–1391, 1971.
7. Kelly RA, Smith TW: Pharmacological treatment of heart failure. In Hardman JG, Limbird LE (eds): Goodman & Gillman's The Pharmacological Basis of Therapeutics, 9th ed. New York, McGraw-Hill, 1996, pp 809–838.
8. Keene BW, Rush JE: Therapy of heart failure. In Ettinger SJ, Feldman EC (eds): Textbook of Veterinary Internal Medicine, 4th ed. Philadelphia, W.B. Saunders, 1995, pp 867–892.
9. Kittleson MD, Eyster GE, Knowlen GG: Efficacy of digoxin administration in dogs with idiopathic dilated cardiomyopathy. J Am Vet Med Assoc 186:162–165, 1985.
10. Kittleson MD, Kienle RD: Management of heart failure. In Kittleson MD, Kienle RD: Small Animal Cardiovascular Medicine. St. Louis, Mosby, 1998, pp 149–194.
11. Marcus FI, Opie LH, Sonnenblick EH, et al: Digitalis and acute inotropes. In Opie LH (ed): Drugs for the Heart. Philadelphia, W.B. Saunders, 1995, pp 145–172.
12. Packer M, Gheorghiade M, Young JB, et al: Withdrawal of digoxin from patients with chronic heart failure treated with angiotensin-converting enzyme inhibitors: RADIANCE study. N Engl J Med 329:1–7, 1993.
13. Smith TW, Braunwald E, Kelly RA: The management of heart failure. In Braunwald E (ed): Heart Disease: A Textbook of Cardiovascular Medicine. Philadelphia, W.B. Saunders, 1992, pp 464–519.
14. Snyder PS, Atkins CE: Current uses and hazards of the cardiac glycosides. In Kirk RW, Bonagura JD (eds): Current Veterinary Therapy XI. Philadelphia, W.B. Saunders, 1992, pp 689–693.
15. Uretski BF, Young JB, Shahidi FE, et al: Randomized study assessing the effect of digoxin withdrawl in patients with mild to moderate chronic congestive heart failure: Results of the PROVED trial. J Am Coll Cardiol 22:955–962, 1993.

15. ANTIARRHYTHMIC AGENTS

Andrew W. Beardow, B.V.M.&S., MRCVS

1. What are the fundamental mechanisms of arrhythmogenesis?
Three mechanisms are commonly described in the induction of arrhythmias: (1) reentry, (2) enhanced automaticity, and (3) triggered activity.

Reentry. Loops of cells or tissues with differing conduction properties are established, and disparities of conduction within the loop allow perpetuation of an impulse that otherwise would be extinguished. If the timing is right, such impulses trigger ectopic depolarizations in nonrefractory tissue. The loops may occur at the microscopic, cellular level or the macroscopic level. The microscopic loop consists of Purkinje cells and myocytes and a region of diseased tissue that acts as a unidirectional block in one limb of the loop. As an impulse passes down the conduction pathway, it is blocked from antegrade conduction through the diseased pathway. The impulse continues past this region in other portions of the loop and is then conducted in a retrograde direction in the diseased portion because this limb of the loop was not depolarized and therefore is not refractory. If the timing is correct, the tissue beyond the block is ready to conduct another impulse, setting up a reentry loop.

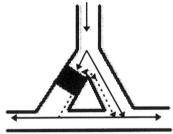

Area of unidirectional block.

Macroreentry loops use larger circuits composed of existing conduction pathways, i.e., reentry loops within the the atrioventricular (AV) node or by an accessory pathway, as in Wolff-Parkinson-White (WPW) syndrome. In humans up to 85% of supraventricular tachyarrhythmias (SVTs) may be due to macroreentry loops utilizing disparity of conduction velocities in the fast and slow pathways through the AV node. These pathways also exist in the canine AV node, but it is unclear how many SVTs in dogs are generated through this mechanism.

Enhanced automaticity. In this mechanism of arrhythmogenesis, either normal pacemaker tissues show abnormal activity or cells that are not usually automatic become so. Automaticity is a property of phase 4 of the action potential. In automatic cells a leakage of ions allows the resting membrane potential to change, moving it toward threshold. When the threshold is reached, depolarization is triggered. The rate of change of this potential determines the rate at which it reaches threshold and hence how frequently the pacemaker will fire. Changes in the membrane or the prevailing autonomic tone may affect this mechanism and hence enhance automaticity. Diseased cells that normally do not show automaticity may start to do so. For example, the membranes of diseased myocardial cells may develop an abnormal permeability to calcium ions. This leak allows the membrane to depolarize spontaneously, reach threshold, and trigger a premature beat.

Triggered activity. As the name indicates, triggered activity does not occur spontaneously but requires one wave of depolarization to trigger another. It is believed that oscillations in the membrane potential following an action potential are responsible for this activity. Disease states or, in some cases, drugs render the membrane unstable and likely to allow such oscillations.

Described as afterdepolarization, these oscillations are further classified, depending on their relationship to the action potential, as either early or late. Late afterdepolarizations are typically cited as causing the arrhythmias induced by digoxin intoxication.

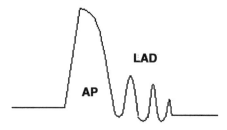

Triggered activity. AP = action potential; LAD = late afterdepolarization.

2. Which steps should be taken to determine the focus of an arrhythmia?

1. Try to identify a normal PQRST, i.e., a complex that originated from the sinoatrial (SA) node, was conducted through the AV node, and depolarized the ventricle with a normal timing and conduction pattern. A normal PQRST may show some abnormalities because of underlying disease, such as abnormal AV nodal conduction, aberrant ventricular conduction, or an abnormally shaped P-wave due to atrial changes. If in doubt, try to identify several complexes that look the same; all of them may have the same abnormality, but in each a P-wave is followed after an appropriate interval by a QRS complex and a T-wave.

2. Compare the normal complex with others on the strip. If the abnormal complexes have only a QRS complex and a T-wave, do they look like the normal QRS-T complex? If so, the arrhythmia most likely arises at or above the AV node and is thus supraventricular in origin. If not, the arrhythmia is probably ventricular in origin.

3. Try to identify any P-waves on the strip. Do they have a temporal relationship to the abnormal QRS complexes? The answer may help to determine whether the source of a supraventricular arrhythmia is atrial or junctional.

3. What is the most important first step in examining the EKG of a patient with tachyarrhythmia?

Try to establish whether the arrhythmia is supraventricular or ventricular in origin. Generally speaking, this distinction is the most useful first step in choosing the most appropriate therapy. Even if you cannot definitively categorize the arrhythmia, first-line therapy has a better chance of success if it is based on your best guess. It is not unusual to have to reassess the diagnosis frequently throughout the management of tachyarrhythmia because of the inappropriate therapeutic response or a change in the underlying arrhythmia.

4. Describe the Vaughan-Williams classification system for antiarrhythmic drugs. Which class(es) do lidocaine, procainamide, diltiazem, and propranolol belong to?

The Vaughan-Williams classification of antiarrhythmic drugs is based on their effect on the action potential of the cardiac myocyte:

Class I drugs, frequently described as membrane stabilizers, block the fast sodium channel. They are subdivided according to their effect on the action potential in terms of automaticity, conductivity, contractility, AV conduction, and fibrillation threshold:

Class IA	Decreased automaticity	Procainamide	SVT
	Decreased conductivity	Quinidine	VT
	Decreased contractility		WPW
Class IB	Decreased automaticity	Lidocaine	VT
	Decreased contractility	Tocainide	
	Increased AV conduction	Mexiletine	
	Increased fibrillation threshold		

Class IC	Decreased automaticity	Flecainide	VT
	Decreased conductivity	Encainide	WPW
	Decreased contractility		
	Decreased AV conduction		

Class II drugs are the beta-blockers, which decrease automaticity and conductivity. They cause variable degrees of depression of both contractility and AV node conduction, depending on the drug in question. Beta-blockers are used to manage supraventricular tachycardia (SVT), ventricular tachycardia (VT), and Wolff-Parkinson-White syndrome (WPW).

Class III drugs block the outward potassium current that is important in repolarization, and in doing so, they prolong repolarization and increase refractory periods. Recently they have received a great deal of attention in the management of arrhythmias refractory to class I drugs. Many have significant side effects that must be taken into consideration. The most commonly used class III drugs are bretylium, amiodarone, and sotalol.

Class IV drugs, which block the slow calcium channel, have the most profound effects on AV node conduction. They also decrease automaticity, conductivity, and contractility, although the magnitude of these effects varies widely across the group. The most commonly used class IV drugs are verapamil and diltiazem.

5. How is the Vaughan-Williams classification used to determine the choice of antiarrhythmic drug?

The ion that carries the action potential differs according to the location of the myocyte. For example, the action potential in the pacemaker cells of the SA and AV nodes is carried principally by the calcium ion. To treat arrhythmias that arise from these tissues or require the AV node for maintenance of the tachycardia (SVTs), a class IV drug (calcium channel blocker) such as diltiazem is appropriate. Class I drugs act principally on the sodium channel and are useful in the management of ventricular tachycardias because the sodium channel carries the depolarization phase of the action potential in working myocytes.

6. What is proarrhythmia?

Proarrhythmia represents a change in or development of arrhythmias during treatment with antiarrhythmic drugs. The clinical importance of this phenomenon first became apparent when a clinical trial demonstrated that class IC antiarrhythmic agents increase mortality relative to placebo in asymptomatic people with ventricular premature complexes. Proarrhythmia must be considered whenever antiarrhythmic drugs are used. All antiarrhythmic drugs affect the myocardial action potential. Although this effect is often beneficial, it may be unpredictable, especially in diseased tissue. Hence drugs that suppress conduction velocity may affect the timing of conduction through reentrant loops in such a way as to "fine-tune" the loop and exacerbate the arrhythmia. Clinicians must consider the risk vs. benefit ratio of such drugs before they are used. Asymptomatic patients with premature ventricular contractions (PVCs) do not invariably need antiarrhythmic therapy.

7. Which medications are often selected for management of acute SVTs in dogs?

The short-acting beta-blocker esmolol, the unclassified agent adenosine, intravenous calcium channel blockers (diltiazem and verapamil), or intravenous digoxin is often selected. Intravenous digoxin is the most difficult to manage and tends to be used less frequently. An exception is the patient with an SVT and suspected dilated cardiomyopathy (DCM); beta-blockers and calcium channel blockers are negative inotropes and should be used with extreme caution in such patients. Digoxin is also appropriate when dobutamine is indicated for the acute management of DCM in patients suspected of atrial fibrillation. Dobutamine increases the rate of conduction through the AV node and the ventricular response rate, thereby exacerbating tachycardia.

Of the calcium channel blockers, diltiazem may cause less myocardial depression than verapamil and may be the better choice. Adenosine is a purine nucleotide found in every cell in the body. When exogenous adenosine is administered, it is presumed to bind to an extracellular purine receptor. It then decreases intracellular levels of the universal second messenger, cyclic adenosine monophosphate (cAMP), by blocking adenylate cyclase. Adenosine has profound inhibitory effects on AV node conduction and depresses SA node and ventricular automaticity.

8. Which characteristics of an arrhythmia are most important in selecting the appropriate antiarrhythmic drug?

Characterizing an arrhythmia is critical if the appropriate antiarrhythmic drug is to be selected. Two important distinctions are whether the arrhythmia is a bradyarrhythmia or a tachyarrhythmia, and whether the arrhythmia arises from the AV node or above (supraventricular) or from the ventricles themselves (ventricular). If an arrhythmia is classified in this way, drug selection can be made as described below:

ARRHYTHMIA CLASSIFICATION	ARRHYTHMIA CHARACTERISTICS	APPROPRIATE MANAGEMENT
Supraventricular tachycardia	Rate > 200 bpm; "normal" QRS; breaks with vagal maneuver	Digoxin; calcium channel blockers; beta-blockers; procainamide for WPW
Supraventricular bradycardia	Rate < 50 bpm; "normal" QRS	Atropine (oral propantheline bromide); nonspecific stimulants of HR (aminophylline, theophylline); pacemaker implantation.
Ventricular bradycardia	Rate < 50 bpm; abnormal QRS	Atropine to stimulate SA node; nonspecific stimulants of HR; pacemaker implantation
Ventricular tachycardia	Rate > 180 bpm; abnormal QRS, hemodynamically unstable; breed predisposition to fatal ventricular arrhythmias (boxers)	Identify and correct underlying cause; acute use parenteral class I drugs (lidocaine); chronic use class I, II, or III

9. If a single antiarrhythmic drug fails to control an arrhythmia, what alternative approaches can be considered?

Combination therapy can be tried but only after the synergistic therapeutic effects and side effects have been considered. For example, a combination of a calcium channel blocker (class IV drug) and a beta-blocker (class II drug) may be necessary to manage a supraventricular tachycardia. While the different mechanisms of action may produce therapeutic synergy, they may also lead to compounding side effects, in this case a negative inotropic effect. Exacerbation of systolic dysfunction may therefore be the net effect of this combination of drugs. It is not uncommon for combinations of antiarrhythmic drugs to be used to control ventricular arrhythmias that are either causing clinical signs in a patient or when the arrhythmia is deemed to be life-threatening. Guidelines for the selection of drugs that can be combined include selecting drugs from different classes. For instance, class IA drugs may be combined with class IB drugs. If a patient with a life-threatening ventricular tachycardia does not respond to parenteral lidocaine, the addition of procainamide (class IA) into the protocol may be beneficial. Class I drugs (lidocaine, procainamide, mexiletine) are frequently combined with class II drugs (beta-blockers) to control the clinical signs associated with a ventricular arrhythmia. This combination may improve not only quality, but also quantity of life due to the beneficial effects of the beta-blocker. This is as yet unproven in veterinary patients, but suggested in humans. Class III drugs should be combined with extreme caution. Many of these drugs already combine the effects of several classes, and the results combining them with other drugs can thus prove unpredictable.

10. How is the efficacy of antiarrhythmic agents determined?

Efficacy can be estimated in a number of ways:

1. Diminution or elimination of clinical signs that have been associated with the arrhythmia. One solid indication for the use of antiarrhythmic drugs is to control clinical signs that are

recognized by the owner or clinician and associated with the arrhythmia. This association can be made by careful clinical observation or recording the arrhythmia while clinical signs are present. This can be challenging, but is facilitated by the use of patient/client-activated or arrhythmia-activated "event recorders." These devices are worn by the patient and constantly record the ECG. The ECG is not "memorized," however, until this unit is activated. Those most commonly used by veterinarians are activated by the client when the clinical sign is seen, but more sophisticated devices can be programmed to become activated when an arrhythmia is detected. The use of owner-activated devices makes sense when trying to correlate "events" that cause the owner concern with the concurrent ECG changes. Having correlated an arrhythmia to clinical signs allows us to use control of those signs as an indication of control of the arrhythmia and hence to judge the efficacy of our therapeutic protocol.

2. A decrease in the frequency of the arrhythmia. Ideally, this method should be used when no or limited clinical signs are seen, but when the clinician is concerned that the arrhythmia is likely to progress and become life-threatening. When no clinical signs are seen, one of the best ways to judge efficacy is an 85% decrease in the frequency of the arrhythmia when quantified by sequential 24-hour Holter monitoring. This is the standard used to judge the efficacy of arrhythmia management in human medicine.

3. A decrease in the frequency of the arrhythmia on a standard 1, 6 or 10 lead ECG. This is the method most frequently used because of its simplicity. While conclusions can be drawn, one should bear in mind the limitations of this method. The likelihood of drawing inaccurate conclusions about the frequency of an arrhythmia increases as the length of the recording of the ECG decreases. Hence quantification of the arrhythmia is limited when only a 1- or 2-minute time frame is reviewed. Increasing the length of recording will help in assessing efficacy, but will never approach the accuracy of 24-hour Holter recordings. This should be borne in mind when making judgements in the asymptomatic patient, because support for your conclusions does not come from resolution of clinical signs.

4. An improvement in clinical signs when the arrhythmia is judged severe enough to have caused those signs but where direct correlation is not possible. Again, this is a technique frequently used in veterinary medicine when the clinician may be limited by the resources of the pet owner, or accessibility to more sophisticated testing. It is reasonable to suppose that if a patient has an arrhythmia deemed severe enough to cause clinical signs and is showing those signs, that resolution of those signs suggests efficacy of the drug. The limitations of this technique are, obviously, that arrhythmias will respond spontaneously, as will clinical signs. Therefore, the danger of this technique is that an animal will be kept on expensive and potentially dangerous drugs that are not contributing to control of clinical signs either because the arrhythmia has resolved spontaneously or because it was not causing these signs in the first place.

11. Lidocaine has a very short half-life when administered intravenously. What is the reason for this and how should I set up a lidocaine infusion?

Lidocaine is often the antiarrhythmic drug of choice for controlling rapid ventricular tachycardias. It has to be administered parenterally because it undergoes extensive first-pass metabolism when administered orally. A single intravenous bolus has a half-life of 10–20 minutes and therefore its effects will not be sustained. In order to sustain therapeutic blood levels, it is necessary to administer lidocaine as a constant-rate infusion (CRI). However, it takes hours for a CRI alone to raise blood levels to therapeutic levels; therefore, a bolus/infusion combination is required. There should be minimal delay between the bolus and the initiation of the CRI. Starting the CRI before giving the bolus prevents inadequate blood levels leading to decreased efficacy. We typically use a dose of 50 μg/kg/min. The table on the next page provides a reference to assist in setting up these infusions. A formula for calculating the amount of a drug to be added to a bag of fluids for CRIs follows:

Body weight (kg) × required dose (μg/kg/min) = amount of drug (mg) to be added to a 250-ml bag of fluids when the fluid/drug mix is administered at 15 ml/hr

For example, for a 20-kg dog that requires 50 µg/kg/min of a drug, the calculation is:

$$20 \times 50 = 1000 \text{ mg of drug that should be added to a 250-ml bag}$$
and administered at 15 ml/hr

If you wish to administer the fluid more rapidly, simply divide the amount of drug by the ratio of the new infusion rate to the old infusion rate. For example, to administer the fluid at 30 ml/hr instead of 15 ml/hr: 30 (new) / 15 (old) = 2. Therefore, for an equivalent CRI dose we should divide the amount calculated for 15 ml/hr (1000 mg) by 2 to get 500 mg in 250 ml at 30 ml/hr.

Side effects of long-term lidocaine administration include neurologic depression initially and ultimately seizures.

The table below is a guide to the preparation of a 50 µg/kg/min constant-rate infusion (CRI) of lidocaine, when the infusion is administered at 15, 30, or 60 ml/hr. It is based on using a 250-ml bag of fluids and should be used for dogs only. To use it, find the row that correlates to the dog's body weight and select the rate of infusion. The table gives both the number of mg of lidocaine to add to a 250-ml bag and the number of ml of 2% lidocaine that this represents.

WEIGHT (KG)	MG TO 250 ML @			ML OF 2% LIDOCAINE TO 250 ML		
	15 ML/HR	30 ML/HR	60 ML/HR	15 ML/HR	30 ML/HR	60 ML/HR
1	50	25	12.5	2.5	1.25	0.625
2	100	50	25	5	2.5	1.25
3	150	75	37.5	7.5	3.75	1.875
4	200	100	50	10	5	2.5
5	250	125	62.5	12.5	6.25	3.125
6	300	150	75	15	7.5	3.75
7	350	175	87.5	17.5	8.75	4.375
8	400	200	100	20	10	5
9	450	225	112.5	22.5	11.25	5.625
10	500	250	125	25	12.5	6.25
11	550	275	137.5	27.5	13.75	6.875
12	600	300	150	30	15	7.5
13	650	325	162.5	32.5	16.25	8.125
14	700	350	175	35	17.5	8.75
15	750	375	187.5	37.5	18.75	9.375
16	800	400	200	40	20	10
17	850	425	212.5	42.5	21.25	10.625
18	900	450	225	45	22.5	11.25
19	950	475	237.5	47.5	23.75	11.875
20	1000	500	250	50	25	12.5
21	1050	525	262.5	52.5	26.25	13.125
22	1100	550	275	55	27.5	13.75
23	1150	575	287.5	57.5	28.75	14.375
24	1200	600	300	60	30	15
25	1250	625	312.5	62.5	31.25	15.625
26	1300	650	325	65	32.5	16.25
27	1350	675	337.5	67.5	33.75	16.875
28	1400	700	350	70	35	17.5
29	1450	725	362.5	72.5	36.25	18.125
30	1500	750	375	75	37.5	18.75
31	1550	775	387.5	77.5	38.75	19.375
32	1600	800	400	80	40	20
33	1650	825	412.5	82.5	41.25	20.625

Table continued on next page

WEIGHT (KG)	MG TO 250 ML @			ML OF 2% LIDOCAINE TO 250 ML		
	15 ML/HR	30 ML/HR	60 ML/HR	15 ML/HR	30 ML/HR	60 ML/HR
34	1700	850	425	85	42.5	21.25
35	1750	875	437.5	87.5	43.75	21.875
36	1800	900	450	90	45	22.5
37	1850	925	462.5	92.5	46.25	23.125
38	1900	950	475	95	47.5	23.75
39	1950	975	487.5	97.5	48.75	24.375
40	2000	1000	500	100	50	25
41	2050	1025	512.5	102.5	51.25	25.625
42	2100	1050	525	105	52.5	26.25
43	2150	1075	537.5	107.5	53.75	26.875
44	2200	1100	550	110	55	27.5
45	2250	1125	562.5	112.5	56.25	28.125
46	2300	1150	575	115	57.5	28.75
47	2350	1175	587.5	117.5	58.75	29.375
48	2400	1200	600	120	60	30
49	2450	1225	612.5	122.5	61.25	30.625
50	2500	1250	625	125	62.5	31.25
51	2550	1275	637.5	127.5	63.75	31.875
52	2600	1300	650	130	65	32.5
53	2650	1325	662.5	132.5	66.25	33.125
54	2700	1350	675	135	67.5	33.75
55	2750	1375	687.5	137.5	68.75	34.375
56	2800	1400	700	140	70	35
57	2850	1425	712.5	142.5	71.25	35.625
58	2900	1450	725	145	72.5	36.25
59	2950	1475	737.5	147.5	73.75	36.875
60	3000	1500	750	150	75	37.5

12. What concurrent problems affect the required dose of lidocaine?

Reduced blood flow to the liver decreases the required dose of lidocaine and may increase side effects, including mental depression. Low cardiac output and beta-blockade decrease hepatic blood flow. Liver failure and administration of cimetidine also decrease hepatic clearance of lidocaine.

13. Digoxin is often used in the management of heart failure. Which antiarrhythmic drugs affect the pharmacokinetics of digoxin and what are their effects?

Certain class IA (quinidine and procainamide) and class IV (diltiazem) antiarrhythmics will elevate the blood levels of digoxin when these drugs are used concurrently. Careful attention should be paid to blood digoxin levels when these drugs are used concurrently and owners should be warned to be particularly vigilant in monitoring for signs of digoxin intoxication (primarily inappetance and vomiting).

BIBLIOGRAPHY

1. Lunney J, Ettinger SJ: Cardiac arrhythmias. In Ettinger SJ, Feldman EC (eds): Textbook of Veterinary Internal Medicine, 4th ed. Philadelphia, W.B. Saunders, 1995.
2. Miller MS, Tilley LP: Treatment of cardiac arrhythmias and conduction disturbances. In Miller MS, Tilley LP: Manual of Canine and Feline Cardiology, 2nd ed. Philadelphia, W.B. Saunders, 1995.
3. Tilley LP: Essentials of Canine and Feline Electrocardiography, 3rd ed. Philadelphia, Lea & Febiger, 1992.
4. Wall RE, Rush JE: Cardiac emergencies. In Murtaugh RJ, Kaplan PM (eds): Veterinary Emergency and Critical Care Medicine. St. Louis, Mosby, 1992.

16. ANTICOAGULANT AND ANTIPLATELET THERAPY

Catherine J. Baty, D.V.M., Ph.D.

1. Name some cardiovascular conditions in which anticoagulant or antiplatelet therapy may be appropriate.
• Feline cardiomyopathies—hypertrophic, dilated, and restrictive forms
• Valvular endocarditis
• Pulmonary thromboembolism
While atrial fibrillation is an indication for anticoagulation in humans, it is not in dogs, because thromboembolic complications in dogs with atrial fibrillation are rarely identified. Atrial fibrillation occurs less commonly in cats, but when it does so, it is usually a complication of myocardial disease and anticoagulation is appropriate.

2. Name the three drugs most commonly used to prevent or treat thrombosis.
• Aspirin (antiplatelet)
• Heparin (anticoagulant)
• Warfarin (anticoagulant)

3. What are some contraindications for use of anticoagulant or antiplatelet therapies?
Most contraindications are relative and would depend on the particular agent being considered, but use of these agents in a patient with a preexisting condition likely to cause active bleeding should be considered carefully. The most common side effect of heparin and warfarin therapy is hemorrhage. Risk of hemorrhage and other therapeutic complications must be weighed against the fact that no antiplatelet/anticoagulant therapy has proven efficacy for acute management or prophylaxis in those cardiovascular conditions in small animals where they are routinely used. While allergic reactions are an important contraindication in humans, they have not been described in small animals. Heparin-induced thrombocytopenia and warfarin-induced skin necrosis are important human complications; warfarin is teratogenic and should be avoided in pregnant animals. Chronic heparin therapy may contribute to osteoporosis in humans.

4. How long should anticoagulant/antiplatelet therapies be maintained?
Duration of therapy depends on many factors, especially the underlying condition requiring the therapy and the particular therapeutic agent. In principle, persistent cardiovascular risk factors would justify lifelong therapy, while acute episodes, where no risk factor is identified or it is eliminated through treatment (e.g., feline DCM associated with taurine deficiency), might be appropriately treated for 3 to 6 months.

5. What is the mechanism of action of aspirin's antiplatelet effect?
Aspirin causes a functional defect in platelets. Most of aspirin's effects on platelets are thought to be attributable to the permanent inactivation (acetylation) of prostaglandin H-synthase, a crucial enzyme in the arachadonic acid cascade. This enzyme modification results in its loss of cyclooxygenase catalytic activity and precludes the formation of thromboxane A_2, an important mediator of platelet aggregation. This effect is essentially permanent in platelets because of their limited ability to synthesize new protein due to their formation as fragments from megakaryocyte cytoplasm and lack of nuclei. The antithrombotic effect is long lasting because impaired platelets must be replaced by new platelets with cyclooxygenase activity to restore normal clotting function. Cyclooxygenase activity of endothelial cells is also impaired causing decreased formation of prostacyclin, but because endothelial cells are nucleated, de novo synthesis of

prostaglandin H-synthase blunts this effect. Prostacyclin, in contrast to thromboxane, induces vasodilation and inhibits platelet aggregation. The use of low-dose aspirin is designed to optimize aspirin's antithrombotic effect mediated by platelets while minimizing its prothrombotic effect mediated by vascular endothelial cells.

6. Is the aspirin dose used for an antithrombotic effect the same as that used for analgesic or anti-inflammatory effects?
No. Aspirin's remarkable spectrum of pharmacologic effects is apparently both dose and time dependent. Cats, with relatively impaired urinary excretion of salicylate, have longer elimination times and thus require less frequent doses than dogs. The recommended antithrombotic dose for cats is 25 mg/kg orally every 56–84 hours (usually every 72 hours for convenience), and for dogs is 0.5–10.0 mg/kg orally every 12–24 hours. Analgesic doses are 10 mg/kg orally every 48 hours for cats and 10–20 mg/kg orally every 12 hours for dogs. The highest doses are used for antiinflammatory effect: 25 mg/kg orally every 24 hours is recommended for cats and 25 mg/kg orally every 8 hours for dogs.

7. How is the intensity of aspirin therapy usually monitored?
Usually no specific monitoring is done. A complete history should reveal any concurrent medications such as nonsteroidal anti-inflammatory drugs or warfarin that would be expected to exacerbate a risk of bleeding. The owners should be carefully instructed regarding the signs and symptoms suggestive of gastrointestinal bleeding. Although low-dose aspirin can produce minor bleeding, it rarely causes clinically important bleeding except in patients with an underlying generalized coagulation defect. Such a defect may be iatrogenic if an anticoagulant such as warfarin is being administered concurrently.

8. Describe the important differences between the mechanism of action of warfarin versus heparin.
Warfarin acts to inhibit the synthesis of several clotting factors (factors II, VII, IX, and X) and anticoagulant proteins C and S; it takes several days to achieves its anticoagulant effect. Heparin's anticoagulant effect is primarily mediated through antithrombin III (AT III) and its subsequent effect on thrombin. In contrast to warfarin, this anticoagulant effect is immediate. The emergence of low molecular weight heparins has demonstrated the clinical significance of heparin's ability to inhibit activated factor X (Xa), also via AT III. Warfarin is administered orally while heparin is available only for parenteral use.

9. How is the intensity of heparin therapy monitored?
Before therapy is started, baseline data are obtained, usually including a complete blood count, chemistry panel, and coagulation panel, including a platelet count. The chemistry panel is used to evaluate for any evidence of disease that might be expected to contribute to a deficiency of AT III, such as liver disease or protein-losing disorders. The patient is evaluated for anemia, thrombocytopenia, or evidence of a preexisting coagulopathy that might complicate heparin therapy or be exacerbated by its side effects. The activated partial thromboplastin time (aPTT) is the mainstay of heparin therapy monitoring. The activated clotting time (ACT) is another potentially appropriate test, but it is less sensitive than the aPTT to the effects of conventional heparin dosages and its use is most appropriate when high plasma concentrations of heparin are sought. Guidelines for therapeutic values for heparin are extrapolated from humans and are usually considered to be 1.5–2.5 times baseline aPTT.

10. How is the intensity of warfarin therapy monitored?
The prothrombin test (PT) is the most common method used for monitoring warfarin therapy. Therapy achieving a PT range of 1.3–1.6 times normal has been recommended based on extrapolation from human data. Monitoring of warfarin therapy has been further optimized in humans through the use of the international normalized ratio (INR). There is substantial individual

variation in response to warfarin such that initially each patient must be closely monitored using PT and INR. After a stable desired dose is achieved, usually within the first 2 weeks of treatment, the frequency of monitoring can gradually be decreased until an interval of 6–8 weeks is achieved. Because of the relative difficulty of accurately manipulating the dose (the smallest tablet size of sodium coumadin is 1 mg), some cardiologists manipulate the dose given to the patient over a full week. That is, if 0.5 mg daily results in too much anticoagulation, e.g., PT 2.5 times normal, than a two-dose scheme of 0.5 mg on Monday, Wednesday, Thursday, Friday, and Sunday and 0.25 mg on Tuesday and Saturday may be considered. If the dose is close to therapeutic range, changes of 1/7 of the week's dose are recommended.

11. What is the INR and what is the basis for it?
INR is an acronym for international normalized ratio, a means of determining intensity of anticoagulation by standardizing laboratory measurement of prothrombin times (PT). The PT is measured by adding a thromboplastin reagent to citrated plasma and determining the time to clotting after the addition of calcium. However, the sensitivity of these thromboplastin reagents to the reduction of the clotting factors has been found to vary significantly. Thus, a sensitive thromboplastin reagent will result in a more prolonged PT than a PT from the same patient measured using a less sensitive reagent. The INR is the PT ratio that would have been obtained if the World Health Organization reference thromboplastin (a sensitive reagent) had been used to measure the patient's PT.
The INR is calculated in the following manner:

$$INR = (\text{patient PT/mean normal PT})^{ISI}$$

12. What is the INR of a cat if its PT is 20.0 sec, the mean normal feline PT for the laboratory is 10.0 sec, and the international sensitivity index (ISI) of the thromboplastin reagent used to determine the PT is 1.0? And if the ISI is 2.0?
The INR is 2.0 if the ISI is 1.0, and 4.0 if the ISI is 2.0. In this hypothetical example, one can see how the same level anticoagulant can be judged to be either appropriate (2.0) or too intensive (4.0) because of a difference in the thromboplastin reagent used.
Veterinarians can easily calculate the INR for a patient so long as they obtain the ISI for the thomboplastin used to determine the PT. Human laboratories routinely provide the calculated INR for patients and veterinary laboratories can be asked to do the same.

13. What is the recommended range of INR for prophylactic anticoagulant therapy in small animals?
The range of 2.0–3.0 is based on recommendations for humans. There have been no studies in small animals testing the efficacy of this range of anticoagulation.

14. Why are heparin and warfarin therapies overlapped when a patient is to be prepared for long-term warfarin prophylaxis?
Theoretically a patient on warfarin therapy alone will initially be in a hypercoagulable state because of the differences in half-lives of the critical clotting factors affected by warfarin. In humans, factors IX and X have relatively longer half-lives than others affected by warfarin, and are thought to be most important in contributing to the transient hypercoagulable state. The same imbalance of pro- and anticoagulants is assumed to occur in small animals, so cardiologists may overlap heparin and warfarin for 3–5 days to avoid this potential problem.

15. Warfarin is acknowledged to interact with many other drugs. What are the primary determinants of these interactions?
Warfarin is primarily metabolized via the cytochrome P450 pathway, and thus is subject to either enhanced or decreased rates of metabolism depending on the specific interaction. Functionally warfarin's anticoagulant effect can be enhanced by other drugs with similar (anticoagulant) or complementary (antiplatelet) effects, thus substantially increasing the risk of hemorrhage.

16. Name some drugs that might be expected to interact with warfarin.
- Cimetidine
- Phenobarbital
- Second- and third-generation cephalosporins
- Metronidazole
- Trimethoprim-sulfamethoxazole
- Prednisone
- Thyroxine
- Aspirin
- Heparin

17. Discuss several important considerations for clients who intend to treat their pets with warfarin.
- Supervision
- Watching for signs of bleeding
- Drug interactions
- Routine laboratory monitoring
- Patience

Because of the increased risk of hemorrhage in cats treated with warfarin, it is generally recommended that this therapy be restricted to cats that are well supervised, which usually means indoor cats. Owners should be specifically instructed to monitor the patient for evidence of gastrointestinal bleeding, e.g., melena, as well as more overt bleeding. In all likelihood these patients will be receiving other medications in addition to warfarin, and owners must be cautioned regarding the potential significance of what might otherwise be considered as minor changes in medications. Clients should be instructed to arrange to recheck their cat's PT/INR within a week of any medication change. Veterinarians should, of course, consider and investigate the likelihood of a drug interaction with warfarin before prescribing any new therapies for these patients. Clients should understand that their pet will require routine laboratory monitoring of PT/INR every 6–8 weeks for the duration of warfarin treatment. Veterinarians, owners, and pets may have their patience tested by the need for frequent testing and some dose manipulation until a desirable dosage is determined.

18. In a patient receiving warfarin, would you manage an episode of minor bleeding the same way as an inappropriately elevated PT/INR?

Possibly. Depending on the severity of the elevation of the PT/INR, one might choose to stop warfarin and administer vitamin K_1. In general, if the INR is above therapeutic range but less than 6.0, and the patient is not bleeding, skipping the next few doses of warfarin and starting again with a lower dose of warfarin is sufficient correction. If the INR is between 6 and 10 and the patient is not bleeding, then the next few doses of warfarin can be skipped and vitamin K_1 can be given at 1–2 mg/kg/day orally or subcutaneously for 1–3 days. When the INR returns to near therapeutic range the warfarin can be started again at a lower dose. Patients with minor bleeding and INR below 10 might be treated similarly with careful supervision. Patients with life-threatening bleeding, an INR greater than 10, or those requiring rapid reversal of anticoagulation for surgery, may require vitamin K_1 and/or transfusion with blood products. In all instances of overcoagulation with warfarin, a given patient's response to therapy must be closely monitored.

19. Why is there so much interest in the potential applications of low molecular weight heparin therapy in veterinary patients?

Low molecular weight heparins (LMWHs) offer the prospect of anticoagulation without the relatively frequent laboratory monitoring needed with warfarin. LMWHs are administered subcutaneously like standard unfractionated heparin (UFH), but there is reason to believe that they may be appropriately dosed on a once-daily basis.

The efficacy of LMWHs for both acute management and prophylaxis of thrombosis has been documented in humans for a variety of different disease conditions. The very limited need for any laboratory monitoring in humans is because LMWHs produce a predictable anticoagulation response. The smaller molecules of LMWHs have less ability to inhibit thrombin than UFH and therefore negligible effect on the aPTT. If monitoring is required to assess the intensity of anticoagulant therapy, the most appropriate test is for antifactor Xa activity. LMWHs also don't suffer from much of the nonspecific protein binding that UFH do. Preliminary clinical trials are being undertaken in small animals.

One potentially important consideration for cats at risk for thromboembolism is that LMWHs have much less inhibitory effect on collagen-induced platelet activity than UFH. If cats are indeed at a greater risk of thrombosis than other species due to their relatively hyperaggregable platelets, then antiplatelet therapy may be needed in combination with LMWHs.

BIBLIOGRAPHY

1. Fox PR: Feline cardiomyopathies. In Fox PR, Sisson D, Moise SN (eds): Textbook of Canine and Feline Cardiology: Principles and Clinical Practice. Philadelphia, WB Saunders, 1999, pp 658–678.
2. Fox PR: Myocardial diseases. In Ettinger SJ (ed): Textbook of Veterinary Internal Medicine. Philadelphia, WB Saunders, 1989, pp 1097–1131.
3. Harpster NK, Baty CJ: Warfarin therapy of the cat at risk of thromboembolism. In Bonagura JD, Kirk RW (eds): Kirk's Current Veterinary Therapy XII: Small Animal Practice. Philadelphia, W.B. Saunders, 1995, pp 868–873.
4. Hirsh J, Dalen JE, Deykin D, Poller L: Oral anticoagulants: Mechanism of action, clinical effectiveness, and optimal therapeutic range. Chest 102:312S–326S, 1992.
5. Holland M, Chastain CB: Uses and misuses of aspirin. In Bonagura JD, Kirk RW (eds): Kirk's Current Veterinary Therapy XII: Small Animal Practice. Philadelphia, W.B. Saunders, 1995, pp 70–73.
6. Kittleson MD: Thromboembolic disease. In Kittleson MD, Kienle RD: Small Animal Cardiovascular Medicine. St. Louis Mosby, 1998, pp 540–551.
7. Turpie AGG: Pharmacology of the low molecular weight heparins. Am Heart J 135:S329–S335, 1998.

17. NUTRACEUTICALS

Davin J. Borde, D.V.M., and John-Karl Goodwin, D.V.M.

1. What is a nutraceutical?

Stephen L. DeFelice, M.D., coined the term "nutraceutical" in 1976. The proposed guidelines for the U.S. Dietary Supplement Health and Education Act of 1994 defined a nutraceutical as "any nontoxic food component that has scientifically proven health benefits, including disease treatment or prevention." The association between nutrition and cardiac function has been demonstrated in several acquired disorders. In veterinary medicine, the most commonly used nutraceuticals are taurine, carnitine, and coenzyme Q10. Other nutraceuticals, such as vitamin E, B vitamins, thiamine, and omega-3 fatty acids (present in fish oils) are less well studied but are currently undergoing intense investigation both in human and veterinary medicine.

2. What is taurine?

Taurine is a sulfur-containing amino acid (2-aminoethanesulfonic acid). In animals it is largely found dissolved in the cytosol or bound to cell membranes intracellularly. The tissues with the highest taurine concentrations are retina, central nervous system, heart, and skeletal muscle. It is also found in white blood cells and platelets.

3. How does taurine affect cardiac function?

There are three major theories concerning the action of taurine on the myocardium. First, because of its small size, high charge, and osmotic activity, taurine is believed to play a role in changing cellular osmolality, which is thought to be a protective mechanism in myocardium and nervous tissue. Second, it is believed to be involved with inactivation of free radicals, which can be important in preventing apoptosis (programmed cell death). Taurine is also thought to modulate tissue calcium concentrations and calcium availability, which is important in myocardial contractility and function. Other proposed mechanisms include direct action on contractile proteins, interactions with the renin-angiotensin-aldosterone system, and N-methylation of cell membrane phospholipids.

4. Why do some animals develop taurine deficiency?

Taurine deficiency in cats has been reported to be a result of low tissue concentrations of cysteine-sulfinic acid decarboxylase (CSAD), an important enzyme in taurine biosynthesis. The inability of cats to use other amino acids, such as glycine, for bile acid conjugation (and thus rely almost exclusively on taurine even if dietary taurine is in low concentration) results in obligatory biliary taurine loss and decreased biosynthesis, resulting in taurine deficiency. One means by which taurine deficiency can be induced is through feeding a high-fat and low-protein diet, which has been shown to produce low plasma, whole blood, and tissue taurine in both dogs and cats. Bacterial overgrowth with consequent interruption of the normal enterohepatic circulation of taurine-conjugated bile acids and increased fecal taurine loss has been shown to result from this type of diet in cats.

The cause of taurine deficiency in some breeds of dogs is largely unknown. Increased urinary loss, decreased synthesis, or increased intestinal loss are proposed as possible mechanisms. Taurine is not an essential amino acid in the dog and normal dogs fed taurine-deficient diets demonstrated normal whole blood and plasma taurine concentrations. Although dogs conjugate bile acids solely with taurine (as in the cat), CSAD activity is high compared to the cat and does not explain why some dogs develop taurine deficiency.

5. What are normal taurine concentrations in animals and how should samples be obtained?

Taurine is measured from heparinized whole blood or heparinized plasma samples. Typically, samples should be stored and shipped frozen or on ice. Normal feline and canine plasma and whole blood taurine concentrations are shown in the table below. Cats with plasma values of less than 30 nmol/ml or whole blood values less than 100 nmol/ml are considered at risk. Plasma taurine concentration is very labile (especially in cats) and 24 hours of fasting can produce abnormally low plasma taurine. The laboratory performing the procedure should be consulted regarding their accepted normal ranges and procedures for sample collection.

Normal Feline and Canine Taurine Concentrations

	FELINE	CANINE
Plasma taurine (nmol/ml)	> 60	> 45
Whole blood taurine (nmol/ml)	> 200	> 250

6. What are the clinical signs and diagnostic findings in patients with taurine deficiency?

Not all dogs and cats with taurine deficiency develop myocardial failure. In one study, 25% of cats experimentally depleted of taurine over a 2-year period developed overt myocardial failure. In dogs and cats that demonstrate clinical signs associated with taurine deficiency, signs typical of dilated cardiomyopathy are seen. Dyspnea, exercise intolerance, weakness, and weight loss are typical presenting complaints. Physical examination may demonstrate a low-intensity systolic murmur (typically grade I–III/VI), an S_3 gallop rhythm, weak femoral pulses, respiratory crackles, and increased bronchovesicular sounds. Signs of right-sided congestive heart failure such as jugular venous distention and jugular pulses, ascites, and hepatomegaly may also be noted. Since taurine is essential for normal retinal function, particularly in cats, central retinal degeneration can also be seen.

Thoracic radiographs typically demonstrate signs of congestive heart failure, including generalized cardiomegaly, pulmonary edema, and pulmonary venous distention. Electrocardiography can demonstrate waveform changes consistent with chamber enlargement. Echocardiography reveals systolic dysfunction characterized by reduced left ventricular fractional shortening and dilation of the left ventricle and left atrium. Plasma and whole blood taurine concentrations will typically be reduced, although tissue determination is necessary for a definitive diagnosis.

7. Which animals are prone to taurine deficiency?

An association between cardiomyopathy, low plasma taurine concentration, and diet in cats was made in 1987. Since that time, most commercial diets have been supplemented with taurine, which has significantly reduced the prevalence of feline dilated cardiomyopathy.

More recently, taurine deficiency and a taurine-responsive cardiomyopathy have been seen in some breeds of dogs, including the American cocker spaniel, golden retriever, and Welsh corgi. Taurine deficiency associated with cystine and urate urolithiasis has also been seen in some breeds, including the Dalmatian, English bulldog, dachshund, French bulldog, and Newfoundland. Exact pathophysiologic mechanisms explaining the association between urolithiasis and taurine deficiency have not been determined; however, feeding of low-protein diets to these patients in the treatment of the uroliths is suspected to play a role.

8. Which animals with dilated cardiomyopathy should be treated with taurine and at what dosage?

Patients with evidence of dilated cardiomyopathy and congestive heart failure should be treated with conventional therapy, including diuretics, angiotensin-converting enzyme (ACE) inhibitors, and digoxin as needed. Any patient with documented plasma and/or whole blood taurine deficiency in addition to evidence of dilated cardiomyopathy should be treated with taurine supplementation. Any cat demonstrating signs of dilated cardiomyopathy with a history of being fed a noncommercial diet that might be low in taurine (such as a diet primarily consisting of fish) should have plasma and whole blood taurine concentrations checked and taurine supplementation started.

Taurine supplementation should be considered in any American cocker spaniel with dilated cardiomyopathy. It should also be considered in golden retrievers with dilated cardiomyopathy as well as any breed at risk for cystine or urate urolithiasis that develops dilated cardiomyopathy. Although studies are still underway, taurine supplementation is relatively inexpensive and, at this time, no serious side effects of supplementation have been noted.

The dosage used in cats is 250 mg taurine administered orally every 12 hours. The dosage for taurine in large dogs is 1–2 g of taurine given orally every 8–12 hours. Smaller dogs (< 25 kg) may be supplemented with 500–1000 mg every 8 hours. Taurine may be mixed with food for administration.

9. How long after supplementation will clinical improvement be noted?

Clinical improvement in taurine-responsive cardiomyopathy can be seen as early as 2 weeks following initiation of taurine supplementation. However, this can be variable, and some patients demonstrating critical systolic dysfunction and congestive heart failure may fail to be maintained on traditional cardiac medications and inotropic support long enough for the benefit of taurine therapy to be manifest. Echocardiographic improvement may be seen in 2–4 months.

10. What is the prognosis for patients with dilated cardiomyopathy and taurine deficiency?

Because research in the area of taurine supplementation is in its infancy and studies performed to date are sparse and anecdotal, it is difficult to provide a definitive prognosis. Many of the American cocker spaniels diagnosed with and treated for taurine-responsive cardiomyopathy can be weaned off traditional cardiac medications and remain on taurine as the sole treatment. The authors have also treated other breeds, such as golden retrievers, with similar results. The prognosis for these patients appears to be good. Whether this applies to other breeds remains to be seen.

11. What is levocarnitine?

L-Carnitine is a quaternary amine (β-hydroxy-γ-trimethylaminobutyric acid) synthesized from lysine and methionine. It is found in high concentrations in mammalian cardiac and skeletal muscle. It is believed to be a nonessential compound in the diet of the dog. Only the L-isomer of carnitine is biologically active in mammals and thus any reference to carnitine in this chapter assumes L-carnitine unless stated otherwise.

12. What role does carnitine play in cardiac function?

Carnitine is important in myocardial oxidation of fatty acids and also likely plays a role in glucose metabolism within the myocardium. Sixty percent of the total energy used by the heart is obtained from fatty acid metabolism. Fatty acid oxidation and subsequent energy production occurs in the mitochondria and transport of free fatty acids in the cytosol across the mitochondrial membrane is accomplished by the "carnitine shuttle." Furthermore, free carnitine in the mitochondrial matrix is believed to scavenge and transport toxic free acyl groups out of the mitochondria.

13. What are normal carnitine concentrations in dogs and how should samples be obtained?

Normal total, free, and esterified plasma and myocardial concentrations for dogs are given in the table below. Total, free, and esterified carnitine can be measured both in heparinized plasma and tissue. Myocardial tissue samples can be obtained by standard endomyocardial biopsy techniques.

Normal Canine Plasma and Myocardial Carnitine Concentrations

	PLASMA	MYOCARDIUM
Total carnitine (mmol/L)	12–38	5–13
Free carnitine (mmol/L)	8–36	4–11
Esterified carnitine (mmol/L)	0–7	0–4

14. How is carnitine deficiency diagnosed?

Carnitine deficiency can be classified as plasma carnitine deficiency (low free plasma carnitine), myopathic carnitine deficiency (low free myocardial carnitine), or systemic carnitine deficiency (low concentrations of free plasma and tissue carnitine). Unlike taurine, whose plasma concentrations usually (but not necessarily) follow tissue levels, dogs with myopathic carnitine deficiency may have plasma carnitine concentrations that are normal or even elevated; thus, if low plasma carnitine is obtained, carnitine deficiency can be suspected. However, the finding of a normal plasma carnitine concentration does not rule out myopathic carnitine deficiency. An endomyocardial biopsy is required for a definitive diagnosis.

15. In which breeds has carnitine deficiency been documented?

Carnitine deficiency was initially diagnosed in a family of boxer dogs. Significant echocardiographic improvement was noted in at least two of these dogs following diagnosis of myocardial carnitine deficiency and supplementation with carnitine. Carnitine deficiency was also found in 13 of 18 Doberman pinschers diagnosed with dilated cardiomyopathy. A significant increase in survival times was noted for the dogs demonstrating carnitine deficiency and undergoing supplementation compared to the dogs demonstrating no carnitine deficiency. Most of the dogs in these studies demonstrated low myocardial carnitine with normal plasma carnitine concentrations.

The Multicenter Spaniel Trial (MUST) study, which examined 11 American cocker spaniels with dilated cardiomyopathy, used administration of both taurine and carnitine and demonstrated improved myocardial performance with this treatment. Subsequently, however, several anecdotal reports as well as cases seen by the authors have demonstrated clinical and echocardiographic improvement in American cocker spaniels with dilated cardiomyopathy using taurine as the sole therapy. Carnitine deficiency has been associated with myocardial disease in humans, hamsters, and turkeys. To date, there has been no report of myocardial disease associated with carnitine deficiency in cats.

16. What are the clinical signs and diagnostic findings in dogs with carnitine deficiency?

The presenting clinical signs and diagnostic findings for carnitine-deficient dogs are similar to those seen in taurine-deficient dogs (see above). In addition, carnitine deficiency can also result in muscle weakness, encephalopathic signs, and recurrent infections. Like taurine deficiency, carnitine-deficient cardiomyopathy cannot be distinguished from idiopathic dilated cardiomyopathy except by endomyocardial biopsy assessment of carnitine concentration, evidence of low plasma carnitine concentration, or may be suspected based on clinical and echocardiographic improvement following carnitine supplementation.

17. Which dogs with dilated cardiomyopathy should be treated with carnitine and at what dosage?

In boxer dogs diagnosed with dilated cardiomyopathy consideration should be given to supplementation with carnitine. American cocker spaniels diagnosed with dilated cardiomyopathy should have combined taurine and carnitine considered as part of their therapeutic regimen, although if finances are limited, taurine supplementation alone may be sufficient. The dosage of carnitine has not been clearly defined, but 50–100 mg/kg of carnitine (only the l-isomer is biologically active and should be used) given orally every 8 hours has been recommended. Myopathic carnitine deficiency may require higher dosages (as much as 200 mg/kg given every 8 hours), but this may cause diarrhea.

Since most cases of carnitine deficiency appear to require endomyocardial biopsy for a definitive diagnosis, most practitioners will likely want to try carnitine supplementation without documentation of a deficiency. The major drawback to this approach is the cost of carnitine, which can be as high as $200.00 per month depending on the source, and may be prohibitive for some clients.

18. When will improvement be noted following initiation of carnitine supplementation?

As with taurine, clinical improvement may be noted in 1–2 weeks, but echocardiographic improvement may take as long as 3–4 months to become evident.

19. What is coenzyme Q10?

Coenzyme Q10 is a lipid-soluble molecule that belongs to a family of substances known as quinones. It is found on the inner surface of inner mitochondrial membranes, in the cell nucleus and cell membranes, in serum, and is present in most cells in the body. Increased tissue levels are found with stress, and levels appear to decrease with age. Coenzyme Q10 concentrations in the body are maintained by a combination of biosynthesis and dietary intake. Meats, fish, some nuts and vegetable oils are dietary sources for coenzyme Q10; however, food processing or cooking can destroy coenzyme Q10.

20. What role does coenzyme Q10 play in cardiac function?

Coenzyme Q10 plays a role in cellular production of energy through attraction and transport of electrons during oxidative phosphorylation. It can also act as an antioxidant in the cell membrane, scavenging free radicals that are produced as toxic byproducts of cellular metabolism.

21. Is there evidence for the use of coenzyme Q10 in the treatment of congestive heart failure?

Since coenzyme Q10 is important in cellular energy production, tissues that have high and continuous energy demands, such as myocardial and nervous tissue, are suspected of manifesting dysfunction when concentrations of coenzyme Q10 are inadequate. Several studies in humans have demonstrated a significant decrease in morbidity, improvement in ejection fraction, cardiac output, and increased stroke volume when coenzyme Q10 was used in the treatment of congestive heart failure, including cases of dilated cardiomyopathy. There have been no blinded, placebo-controlled trials studying the effects of coenzyme Q10 in the treatment of clinical cases of congestive heart failure or cardiomyopathy in animals.

22. In which dogs should coenzyme Q10 be used and at what dosage?

Considering the lack of significant signs of toxicity or intolerance noted in people or noted anecdotally in animals, coenzyme Q10 is considered a relatively safe nutraceutical. It can be considered as part of the therapeutic regimen in any patient with congestive heart failure, particularly in cases of dilated cardiomyopathy. The dosage has not been clearly determined in animals, but dosages of 30–90 mg/day given orally have been recommended. Coenzyme Q10 may also be added to food.

CONTROVERSY

23. What is the future role of nutraceuticals in veterinary medicine?

Much of the information regarding efficacy and use of nutraceuticals in the treatment of heart disease has been derived from anecdotal case reports and poorly controlled studies. Part of the reason for this chasm in strong scientific research has been the ingrained bias in human and veterinary medicine against "untraditional" or "alternative" therapy. Although this prejudice has more recently been tempered, it remains a persistent obstacle. As a result, those in veterinary medicine that are hopeful of finding further pharmaceuticals to use in the battle against congestive heart failure are forced to rely on these limited, weakly supported studies and imperfect extrapolations from human medicine. Furthermore, proponents of alternative therapies and companies selling these nutraceuticals may contribute to perpetuating unconfirmed claims of efficacy that may not maintain integrity under more intense scrutiny. While veterinarians should demonstrate continued enthusiasm about future promise in the field of nutraceuticals, we must avoid allowing such enthusiasm to create false hope.

BIBLIOGRAPHY

1. Costa ND, Labuc RH: Case report: Efficacy of oral carnitine therapy for dilated cardiomyopathy in boxer dogs. J Nutr 124(Suppl):S2687–S2692, 1994.
2. Fox PR, Sturman JA: Myocardial taurine concentrations in cats with cardiac disease and in healthy cats fed taurine-modified diets. Am J Vet Res 53:237–241, 1992.

3. Freeman LM, Michel KE, Brown DJ, et al: Idiopathic dilated cardiomyopathy in Dalmatians: Nine cases (1990–1995). J Am Vet Med Assoc 209:1592–1596, 1996.
4. Huxtable RJ: Physiological actions of taurine. Physiol Rev 72:101–163, 1992.
5. Keene BW, Panciera DP, Atkins CE, et al: Myocardial L-carnitine deficiency in a family of dogs with dilated cardiomyopathy. J Am Vet Med Assoc 198:647, 1991.
6. Kittleson MD, Keene B, Pion PD, et al: Results of the Multicenter Spaniel Trial (MUST): Taurine- and carnitine-responsive dilated cardiomyopathy in American cocker spaniels with decreased plasma taurine concentration. J Vet Intern Med 11:204–211, 1997.
7. Langsjoen PerH, Langsjoen PetH, Folkers K: Long-term efficacy and safety of coenzyme Q10 therapy for idiopathic dilated cardiomyopathy. Am J Cardiol 65:521–523, 1990.
8. Pion PD, Kittleson MD, Skiles ML, et al: Dilated cardiomyopathy in the cat: Response to taurine supplementation. J Am Vet Med Assoc 201:275–284, 1992.
9. Pion PD, Sanderson SL, Kittleson MD: The effectiveness of taurine and levocarnitine in dogs with heart disease. Vet Clin North Am Small Anim Pract 28:1495–1514, 1998.
10. Sanderson S, Gross KL, Osborne CA, et al: Dogs fed a high-fat diet have reduced plasma taurine concentrations [abstract]. FASEB J 10:A506, 1996.
11. Sanderson S, Osborne C, Ogburn P, et al: Canine cystinuria associated with carnitinuria and carnitine deficiency [abstract]. J Vet Intern Med 9:212, 1995.
12. Sinatra ST: Coenzyme Q10: A vital therapeutic nutrient for the heart with special application in congestive heart failure. Conn Med 61:707–711, 1997.
13. Soja AM, Mortensen SA: Treatment of congestive heart failure with coenzyme Q10 illuminated by meta-analyses of clinical trials. Mol Aspects Med 18(Suppl 1):S59–S68, 1997.

III. Examination of the Cardiovascular System

18. PHYSICAL EXAMINATION

John D. Bonagura, D.V.M, M.S.

1. What general aspects of the physical examination are especially pertinent to cardiovascular diseases?

Observe the animal walk; gait will be abnormal in thromboembolism to a limb. Observe the posture; dyspnea leads to a posture with extended neck and abducted elbows. Cats assume a position of sternal recumbency, while a dyspneic dog will refuse to lie down and will usually stand or sit. The animal may be weak if blood pressure is low, if muscle mass has been lost (e.g., dilated cardiomyopathy in dogs), or if there is hypokalemia (e.g., from diuretic treatment). Cats with muscular weakness often hang their heads (or can't lift them at all).

The overall body condition may be revealing as heart failure can cause dramatic loss of condition and body mass (cardiac cachexia). Stunting can occur with some congenital heart diseases. General hydration should be assessed (particularly in animals receiving diuretic therapy). Dependent areas should be examined for subcutaneous edema, a potential sign of right-sided cardiac failure, though this is relatively rare in small animals. The rectal temperature may be elevated in bacterial endocarditis, phlebitis, infective pericarditis, or infective myocarditis. Tachypnea, with increased work of breathing, may cause hyperthermia. Hypothermia develops with cardiogenic shock. An accurate body weight is essential for accurate drug dosage and monitoring diuretic therapy; sudden weight changes often reflect fluid retention or loss.

2. What causes the palpable femoral arterial pulse?

The pulse is related to the differences between systolic and diastolic pressures (pulse pressure). The intensity of the pulse depends on a number of additional factors including the physical characteristics of the tissue around the artery (e.g., fat), the absolute pressure, and the rate of pressure rise in early systole.

3. What is the normal pulse rate for the dog and the cat?

Normal rates are between 60–180 for the dog and 120–240 for the cat. Autonomic tone, body temperature, endocrine status, drugs, and other factors affect the pulse rate.

4. Can arterial blood pressure be determined by palpation of the femoral artery pulse?

No, the blood pressure cannot be reliably determined by palpation. Generally a systolic pressure of less than 60 mmHg will make the pulse difficult to detect. Measurement of arterial blood pressure is discussed in Chapter 25.

5. What are the clinical conditions associated with a hypokinetic (weak) arterial pulse?

Reduced stroke volume or decreased rate of rise of the arterial pressure lead to a hypokinetic pulse. This is often due to left ventricular failure, dilated cardiomyopathy, hypovolemia, or left ventricular outflow tract obstruction (e.g., aortic stenosis).

6. What are the clinical conditions associated with a hyperkinetic (water-hammer, Corrigan's) arterial pulse?

Conditions that widen the pulse pressure (systole minus diastole) and situations that increase the rate of ejection into the aorta often lead to a more prominent arterial pulse. A higher systolic pressure can be related to an increased stroke volume, as with patent ductus arteriosus (PDA) or aortic regurgitation (AR). A lower diastolic pressure develops when there is peripheral vasodilation, with arteriovenous fistulas (including PDA), and when blood leaks back into the left ventricle (as with AR). Faster ejection rates can be due to sympathetic stimulation of the heart, and this is accentuated when there is vasodilation. Examples include hyperthyroidism, anemia, and fever.

7. What are the clinical conditions associated with a variable arterial pulse?

Variable pulses typically indicate variation in stroke volume. Cardiac arrhythmias are the most common cause. In some cases the variation is subtle and quite normal, as with respiratory sinus arrhythmia in the dog. In other cases, the variation is marked, as with atrial fibrillation or ventricular tachycardia. Pronounced hyperpnea or dyspnea can lead to variable pulses probably by influencing intrathoracic pressure and venous return. Pulsus paradoxus is a special example of respiratory variation associated with cardiac tamponade; in this situation, the pulse pressure falls during inspiration.

8. What are the conditions associated with an absent arterial pulse?

Excluding severe hypotension, aortic thromboembolism is the most common cause of an absent pulse. Clinical associations include feline cardiomyopathies, bacterial endocarditis in dogs and cats, renal amyloidosis in dogs, and trauma. Rare causes include tumor invasion or compression of the distal aorta, missile (e.g., shotgun pellet) embolization, or a tumor or granuloma embolus. In the case of feline cardiomyopathy, distal aortic embolization also leads to ischemic neuropathy and severe rhabdomyolysis.

9. What causes a normal jugular pulse?

The normal jugular pulse is only observed at the thoracic inlet and no higher than the point of the shoulder in the standing dog or cat. The positive waves are related to atrial contractions and to venous return to the atrium. The negative waves are related to negative atrial pressures that occur in early systole and early diastole. Cardiac diseases can lead to changes in these pressures, producing an abnormally prominent jugular pulse that extends towards the mandible.

10. What are causes of abnormal jugular pulses?

High-pressure atrial contractions can be reflected up the jugular vein as observed with severe cases of pulmonic stenosis or pulmonary hypertension. Severe tricuspid regurgitation can elevate the right atrial pressure leading to a prominent pulse. Arrhythmias characterized by atrioventricular dissociation (complete AV block, ventricular tachycardia) are additional causes. These rhythms generate jugular "cannon" waves that indicate the right atrium is contracting on a closed tricuspid valve.

11. What causes jugular venous distention?

Elevated jugular venous pressure is generally related to increased central venous pressure. Typical causes are right-sided heart failure, cardiac tamponade, constrictive pericardial disease, hypervolemia, and high-output heart failure (anemia, hyperthyroidism, and arteriovenous fistula). Large pleural effusions can also increase jugular venous pressure.

12. What is the cranial vena cava syndrome?

This condition is caused by an obstruction of the cranial vena cava, usually from a tumor, and leads to jugular distention and intermandibular edema. Thrombosis of the vena cava due to an indwelling jugular venous catheter is another cause.

13. What is cyanosis and what are common causes?

Cyanosis is a bluish discoloration of the mucous membranes. Central cyanosis is caused by an increased concentration of desaturated hemoglobin (usually > 5 g/dl). Causes include severe respiratory dysfunction (airway obstruction, pulmonary edema, pneumonia, or atelectesis) and right-to-left cardiac shunts such as tetralogy of Fallot or cardiac septal defects with severe pulmonic stenosis or pulmonary hypertension (Eisenmenger's physiology). Peripheral cyanosis is caused by extreme reduction in blood flow to mucous membranes as might be seen with some forms of shock or an arterial occlusion. Differential cyanosis is indicated by pink cranial membranes and blue caudal membranes. This is a sign of "reversed" patent ductus arteriosus (PDA with severe pulmonary hypertension).

14. What are causes of mucous membrane pallor?

Common causes are anemia and extreme arterial vasoconstriction in response to reduced arterial blood pressure. For example, the latter condition might be observed with congestive heart failure caused by dilated cardiomyopathy.

15. What are some ocular abnormalities that may be associated with cardiovascular diseases?

Taurine deficiency in cats can lead to retinal degeneration with hyperreflective lesions in the tapetal fundus. Hypertension can cause vascular change, edema, detachment, or hemorrhage of the retina. Hyphema is also observed in some animals.

16. What are the clinical signs of right-sided congestive heart failure?

The history often indicates exercise intolerance, weakness, or syncope. There is jugular venous distention and possibly jugular pulsations that are accentuated during palpation of the liver (hepatojugular reflex). The liver is palpably enlarged and ascites is typical. There may be pleural effusion evidenced by dyspnea, ventral muffling of heart and lung sounds, and possibly a pleural fluid line detectable by percussion. There is often an auscultatory abnormality of the heart (see below).

17. What are the clinical signs of left-sided congestive heart failure?

The history indicates respiratory problems such as tachypnea, restlessness, respiratory distress, or cough. The patient has an increased respiratory rate. There may be signs of small airway disease (crackles or rales) or pleural effusion. There is often an auscultatory abnormality of the heart (see below).

18. What is the value of precordial palpation?

Cardiomegaly or hypertrophy may displace the apical impulse or render it more prominent. Loud cardiac murmurs can produce a palpable precordial vibration (thrill). The left apex is an important auscultatory landmark because the first heart sound is loudest and murmurs of mitral regurgitation are frequently heard best at this point.

19. What is the relative caudal to cranial location of the cardiac valve areas?

The mitral area is located over the left apical impulse (and slightly dorsal to that point); the aortic valve is one or two intercostal spaces craniodorsal to the mitral valve area; the pulmonic valve is one intercostal space cranioventral to the aortic valve. The tricuspid area is slightly cranial to the mitral area but is located over the right hemithorax.

20. What are the parts and functions of the stethoscope?

The chestpieces consist of a diaphragm and a bell. The diaphragm is flat, is firmly applied to the thorax, and is used for detecting higher frequency sounds and breath sounds. The bell chestpiece is applied to create an air seal, which is used to accentuate lower-pitched sounds such as gallops and some diastolic murmurs. Some stethoscopes combine these two components into a single chestpiece. The chestpieces are connected to the stethoscope tubes, which transmit sound from the chestpiece to the ears. The biaurals and earpieces are the extensions of the stethoscope tubes. These should be oriented rostrally to create a comfortable and snug fit within the examiner's ear canals.

21. What are appropriate conditions for cardiac auscultation? What artifacts must be considered?

The room must be quiet, the patient gently restrained and calm, and the examiner relaxed. It is preferable for the animal to stand in order to locate the valve areas accurately. Ventilation and purring should be controlled if possible. Synchronous ventilation can mimic cardiac murmurs. Gently holding the mouth closed, whistling, or briefly obstructing the nares are effective maneuvers for reducing ventilation artifacts. Showing a cat water in a sink, holding the cat, or gently pressing the larynx may reduce the degree of purring. Artifacts include ventilation and panting (mimics murmurs); twitching (sounds like an extra heart sounds); and friction from rubbing the chestpiece across hair (sounds like pulmonary crackles or rales). Excessive pressure on the chest can distort the thorax of small animals and create abnormal flow patterns and murmurs.

22. Describe an approach for cardiac auscultation.

One approach is to begin over the left apex beat where mitral sounds radiate and the first heart sound is best heard. Find other valve areas from this point. The aortic valve area is craniodorsal to the left apex and the second heart sound is loudest there. Once the aortic second sound is identified, the stethoscope can be moved one interspace cranial and slightly ventral (over the pulmonary valve area). The tricuspid valve is over the right hemithorax, cranial to the mitral area, and covers a relatively wide area. The pulmonary artery extends dorsally from the valve. The left ventricular outlet is in the center of the heart and aortic murmurs usually radiate well to each hemithorax. Cats should be carefully auscultated along the left and right caudal sternal borders, as the apex is more ventral and midline in this species.

23. What causes the normal heart sounds in dogs and cats?

The first sound (S_1) is associated with the closure of the atrioventricular (AV) valves at the onset of ventricular systole. The second sound (S_2) is caused by near-synchronous closure of the aortic and pulmonic valves. The period between the first and second sounds is systole. The period between the second and ensuing first sound is diastole.

24. What abnormalities in the normal heart sounds might be detected?

Pericardial or pleural effusion or myocardial failure from dilated cardiomyopathy can decrease the intensity of the first heart sound. Arrhythmias lead to variable intensity heart sounds. Both heart sounds tend to be loud in healthy animals under high sympathetic drive or those with an ectomorphic conformation. Splitting of the sounds may be detected with asynchronous ventricular activation as with ventricular ectopia or bundle branch block. Severe pulmonary hypertension increases the intensity of S_2 or leads to audible splitting of this sound when left and right ventricular ejection times become very disparate.

25. What are gallops and what is their clinical significance?

The third and fourth heart sounds are lower-frequency sounds associated with vibrations that attend the termination of rapid ventricular filling and atrial contraction, respectively. These sounds indicate ventricular diastolic dysfunction when detected in dogs or cats. A third sound is typical of a ventricle with poor compliance that is filled under high venous pressures (as with mitral regurgitation or dilated cardiomyopathy and concurrent left-sided congestive heart failure). An atrial sound is typical of impaired ventricular relaxation (as with hypertrophic cardiomyopathy or myocardial ischemia). If both sounds are present and the heart rate is rapid, the third and fourth heart sounds may be superimposed, producing a summation gallop. Gallops may be the only auscultatory abnormality of cardiomyopathy and can vary with heart rate and filling pressures.

26. What are systolic clicks and what is their significance?

Clicks are high-pitched, systolic transient sounds. Midsystolic clicks are not uncommon in dogs with mitral or tricuspid valve disease and are probably indicative of prolapse from abnormal chordae tendineae or valve redundancy. Isolated clicks suggest mild disease, though clicks are often superimposed over murmurs in dogs with advanced mitral endocardiosis. Ejection clicks are infrequently detected with valvular pulmonic stenosis.

27. What is the differential diagnosis for "extra" heart sounds?

This should include gallops (atrial and ventricular) and clicks as well as split sounds and premature beats. Atrial or ventricular premature beats often cause an "extra" first heart sound followed by a very soft or even absent second sound.

28. Are all heart diseases associated with a cardiac murmur? Explain.

No. For example, cardiac murmurs are inconsistent in a number of conditions. Tetralogy of Fallot with pulmonary artery hypoplasia and polycythemia may not lead to a murmur. With pericardial diseases one may note distant or muffled heart sounds with pericardial effusion, an early diastolic "knock" of restricted filling in constrictive pericardial disease, or (rarely) a friction rub in pericarditis. Heartworm disease or other causes of pulmonary hypertension may cause a loud, single, second heart sound, or even a split S_2 if there is cardiac failure or right bundle branch block. A murmur is variable. In systemic hypertension a gallop sound may be the major feature of hypertensive heart disease and the second sound may also be prominent. Murmurs are inconsistent findings in cardiomyopathies, though gallops and arrhythmias may be detected.

29. What are typical auscultatory features of cardiac arrhythmias?

Auscultatory findings of abnormal heart rate, irregular cadence, irregular intensity of the heart sounds, extra or absent heart sounds, or splitting of S_1 or S_2 should alert the clinician to a possible rhythm or conduction disturbance. (These findings indicate the need for an electrocardiogram.)

30. What is a cardiac murmur and what is its significance?

A cardiac murmur is a prolonged audible vibration heard during a normally silent period of the cardiac cycle. A murmur frequently indicates heart disease; however, many heart murmurs are innocent or functional (i.e., the heart is structurally normal).

31. What causes a cardiac murmur? Give examples.

Murmurs are often associated with high-velocity blood flow (typically > 1.6 m/sec) or with fluid vibrations that develop as a result of disturbed or turbulent flow. Turbulence tends to develop when the velocity of flow increases or the viscosity of blood decreases (as with anemia). Turbulence is also more likely when blood enters a large vessel or chamber.

Common clinical causes of cardiac murmurs include:
- Sympathetic stimulation as with exercise, fever, or hyperthyroidism (which can increase the velocity of ejection into the great vessels and can also lead to dynamic ventricular outflow tract obstruction)
- Anemia (which decreases viscosity of blood and is also associated with increased sympathetic drive)
- Flow into dilated vessels (especially those that abruptly change in diameter)
- Increased flow volume across otherwise normal heart valves
- Abnormal paths of blood flow from high to low pressure.

Examples of high-velocity flow across otherwise normal heart valves include atrial and ventricular septal defects (increased flow across the pulmonary valve) and complete AV block (increased flow across the aortic valve due to increased stroke volume and lower aortic diastolic pressure). Pathologic causes of increased velocity flow include stenotic valves, incompetent valves, ventricular septal defects, and aortic-to-pulmonary shunts (PDA). Heart murmurs are often detected in cats with dilated aortas related to either hypertension or degeneration (aortic redundancy). Dynamic right ventricular outflow tract obstruction has been proposed as another cause of ejection murmurs in stressed cats. Hypovolemia can also predispose to dynamic outflow tract obstruction and murmur development.

32. How are cardiac murmurs described or classified?
Cardiac murmurs should be described based on timing, intensity, point of maximal intensity, radiation, pitch and quality. The timing of the murmur is systolic, diastolic, continuous, or to-and-fro (systolic–diastolic). The intensity of the murmur is arbitrarily graded on a 1–6 scale.

33. What is an example of murmur grading?
One example is the following system:
- **Grade 1:** a very soft, localized murmur detected only in a quiet room after minutes of intense listening.
- **Grade 2:** a soft murmur, heard immediately, localized to a single valve area.
- **Grade 3:** a moderate-intensity murmur that is evident at more than one location.
- **Grade 4:** a moderate-intensity to loud murmur; radiates well; but a consistent precordial thrill is not present.
- **Grade 5:** a loud murmur accompanied by a palpable precordial thrill.
- **Grade 6:** a loud murmur with a precordial thrill, audible when the stethoscope is removed from the thorax.

34. What is the point of maximal murmur intensity?
The point of maximal intensity (PMI) is communicated by indicating the location, valve area, and intercostal space where the murmur is loudest. A murmur usually projects from the PMI in the direction of abnormal blood flow. Murmurs can also radiate through solid structures (e.g., down to the apex). The radiation of a loud cardiac murmur can be extensive.

35. What is meant by murmur "quality" or "configuration"?
The quality and configuration of a heart murmur pertains to the frequency (pitch), timing, and subjective assessment of the murmur by the examiner. Murmurs consisting of one fundamental frequency with overtones are described as "musical," whereas murmurs of mixed frequencies are typically noted to be "harsh." Most murmurs are of mixed frequency. The timing within the cardiac cycle, development, and murmur intensity create an impression of the murmur's "shape" as it might be recorded graphically by a phonocardiogram. Ejection murmurs are typically crescendo-decrescendo whereas regurgitant murmurs are generally longer (holosystolic or pansystolic) and plateau-shaped.

36. What is a functional heart murmur?
Functional murmurs are not associated with any obvious cardiac pathology. Innocent murmurs in puppies should abate by the time of the rabies vaccination. Physiologic murmurs are functional murmurs related to an altered physiologic state and include those of the athletic heart, anemia, fever, high adrenergic tone, peripheral vasodilation, hyperthyroidism, and marked bradycardia. Most physiologic murmurs are ejection in timing and detected best over the aortic and pulmonic valves and the great vessels (at the left dorsocranial cardiac base or right cranial thorax). Some functional murmurs are musical.

37. Describe the murmur of mitral regurgitation and indicate some potential causes.
Mitral regurgitation (MR) is one of the most common flow disturbances responsible for a pathologic systolic heart murmur. MR develops secondary to malfunction of any portion of the mitral apparatus. Causes include congenital mitral dysplasia, degenerative valve disease (endocardiosis or prolapse) in the dog, bacterial endocarditis, myocardial disease, redundancy or rupture of a chorda tendineae (in the dog), and causes of left ventricular dilatation or hypertrophy, such as cardiomyopathy, hyperthyroidism, systemic hypertension, and PDA. This systolic murmur is prominent over the mitral valve area and transmits prominently down to the left apex where it is often loudest (near the left sternal edge in cats). MR murmurs radiate both dorsally and to the right (usually one grade softer on the right hemithorax). The MR murmur can be decrescendo in peracute leakage (from equilibration of left ventricular and left atrial pressures) or

in mild cases (as the regurgitant orifice closes in late systole). The murmur can be very soft in hypotensive patients; alternatively, hypertension can increase the intensity. Accordingly, the intensity of the murmur in many causes of MR is not reliably correlated to the severity.

38. Describe particular aspects of mitral regurgitation murmurs associated with endocardiosis in dogs.

In addition to the points made above, there may be other auscultatory phenomena detected in mitral valve endocardiosis. The musical systolic "whoop" (murmur is musical and sounds like the word "whoop") is a striking frequency phenomenon in some dogs. Progressive increase in the intensity of the first heart sound is a unique feature of MR in dogs with endocardiosis, probably indicating cardiac dilatation with maintenance of left ventricular contractility. In endocardiosis, the intensity of the MR murmur does increase with the degree of valvular incompetency (assuming normal arterial blood pressure).

39. Describe the murmur of mitral regurgitation in cats with hypertrophic cardiomyopathy.

Cats with hypertrophic cardiomyopathy may have a labile murmur of MR related to dynamic left ventricular outflow tract obstruction and systolic anterior motion of the mitral valve. The murmur may not be holosystolic. It is typically loudest along the left apical sternal border.

40. Describe the murmur of tricuspid regurgitation and indicate some potential causes.

Tricuspid regurgitation (TR) is a common cardiac murmur and much of what was stated concerning mitral regurgitation is applicable here. Causes include valve malformation, endocardiosis, valve degeneration, right ventricular enlargement (pulmonic valve stenosis, right sided cardiomyopathy, chronic bradycardia, pulmonary hypertension), dirofilariasis, and rarely tricuspid endocarditis. The PMI of this systolic murmur is the tricuspid valve area and dorsal radiation is typical.

41. How does one distinguish a separate murmur of tricuspid regurgitation in the setting of concurrent mitral regurgitation?

The following support concurrent TR in the setting of MR: a prominent jugular pulse, right precordial thrill, different frequency murmur than that heard at the left side, or right-sided congestive heat failure.

42. Describe the murmur of the ventricular septal defect.

When the defect communicates the left ventricular outlet with the perimembranous ventricular septum or the right ventricular inlet septum, the holosystolic murmur is loudest just below the tricuspid valve, along the right sternal border. When the defect communicates the left ventricular outlet with the right ventricular outlet septum, the murmur may be most prominent over the craniodorsal left cardiac base. If the aortic valve has prolapsed into the ventricular septal defect, there may be a diastolic murmur of aortic regurgitation.

43. Describe the causes and the murmur of aortic stenosis.

Aortic stenosis (AS) is most common in dogs as a congenital, subvalvular, fibrous obstruction in the left ventricular (LV) outflow tract. The valve may be both stenotic and mildly incompetent. Other causes of LV outflow obstruction are hypertrophic cardiomyopathy or mitral valve malformation; these conditions can cause dynamic outflow obstruction. Bacterial endocarditis of the aortic valve causes aortic regurgitation before the vegetation is large enough to obstruct the valve. Cases of isolated, congenital, aortic valvular stenosis are seen sporadically. The systolic murmur of AS is flow dependent, crescendo-decrescendo in configuration, and, like most ejection murmurs, becomes louder following exercise, inotropic stimulation, a ventricular premature beat, and increases in venous return. When intense, this murmur can be loudest over the right dorsal cardiac base owing to radiation of the murmur into the ascending aorta. The murmur tends to radiate up the carotids and even to the head. A diastolic murmur of aortic regurgitation (AR) may develop, leading to a to-and-fro murmur of AS/AR.

44. Describe the causes and the murmur of pulmonic stenosis.

Pulmonic valve stenosis is a congenital malformation of the valve characterized by valve thickening, varying degrees of leaflet fusion, hypoplasia, and thickening at the valve base. Subvalvular pulmonic stenosis (PS) occurs as an isolated lesion or in association with ventricular septal defect (VSD) or tetralogy of Fallot. The systolic crescendo-decrescendo murmur is heard best over the pulmonic valve (left second or third intercostal space) and radiates prominently in a dorsal direction into the poststenotic dilatation of the main pulmonary artery. Thus, the murmur tends to be heard very well at the dorsal, left, cardiac base. Valvular PS also may be associated with an early systolic ejection click (fused valve) or a murmur of TR caused by secondary right ventricular enlargement. Following balloon catheter valvuloplasty there may be enough pulmonary insufficiency to create an audible diastolic murmur.

45. Describe the causes and the murmur of aortic regurgitation.

Aortic regurgitation is the most important diastolic cardiac murmur in dogs and cats. Causes include bacterial endocarditis, congenital aortic valve disease, prolapse of an aortic valve cusp into a subaortic ventricular septal defect, and aortic root dilatation in aged cats. This murmur is a long, diastolic, decrescendo murmur heard best over the aortic valve at the left hemithorax. The murmur is also well heard at the right cardiac base.

46. What are other causes of diastolic heart murmurs in dogs and cats?

Aside from aortic regurgitation, diastolic murmurs are rare in dogs and cats. The soft, low-pitched rumble of congenital mitral or tricuspid stenosis is difficult to detect unless one listens carefully with the bell. There is often concurrent valvular regurgitation, which may lead to a systolic murmur.

47. What is the most important cause of a continuous cardiac murmur?

A continuous murmur is one that begins in systole and continues without interruption past the second heart sound. Effort must be made to distinguish a continuous murmur from the "bellows" or "to-and-from" murmurs that can result from the presence of concurrent outflow tract obstruction and semilunar valve incompetence or a VSD complicated by aortic valve regurgitation. Patent ductus arteriosus is the most important cause of a continuous murmur and is described as "distant" and "machinery-like" (like a machine shop) in quality. The murmur must be carefully located dorsally on the cranial left base, over the main pulmonary artery. The stethoscope should be "inched" up and back to the PMI of the continuous murmur at the left base. In very small dogs, the murmur can be louder over the manubrium. In neonates, in cats, and in cases of developing pulmonary hypertension, the murmur may not sound continuous, but instead seem a very "long" systolic murmur (entering early diastole). Often in cases of PDA with left ventricular dilatation there will also be a systolic murmur of mitral regurgitation over the left apex.

48. What are other causes of continuous murmurs?

Continuous murmurs (bruits) may also be detected over congenital or acquired arteriovenous fistulas, including those associated with thyroid carcinomas, declawing operations, or limb injuries.

49. What are normal respiratory sounds?

Normal respiratory sounds include vesicular and bronchovesicular sounds, bronchial breathing, and tracheal sounds (panting). Normal sounds (and abnormal sounds) may only become evident after enforcing deeper breathing. This can be encouraged by closing the mouth and holding off one nostril or by occluding both nostrils for a brief period to encourage deep breaths or sighs.

50. What conditions lead to variations in the normal sounds?

Normal sounds may become accentuated or decreased in diseases of the thorax or in congestive heart failure. An increase in bronchial sounds is often detected as a nonspecific finding of pulmonary disease including pulmonary edema. Decreased sounds may indicate pleural fluid (ventral fluid line) or air. Displaced sounds may indicate a mass lesion or diaphragmatic hernia.

51. What are abnormal upper respiratory sounds and their clinical significance?

Abnormal upper airway sounds include: tracheal snaps, which may be heard in tracheal collapse; stertor (inspiratory snoring), typical of pharyngeal or nasopharyngeal diseases, and stridor, an inspiratory wheeze over the larynx, which is typical of upper airway obstruction. Low-pitched inspiratory noise may also indicate upper airway obstruction.

52. What are abnormal lower respiratory sounds and their clinical significance?

Abnormal lower airway (adventitious) sounds include rhonchi, wheezes, and crackles. A sonorous rhonchus is an inspiratory or expiratory noise (be sure to rule out transmission of upper respiratory stertor), which suggests the presence of fluid or exudate in larger airways, as with bronchitis or pneumonia. Wheezes (sibilant rhonchi) are high-pitched expiratory sounds typical of bronchial narrowing. The usual associations are bronchial disease (bronchitis, asthma) or attenuation of a main bronchus caused by left atrial dilation, hilar lymphadenopathy, primary bronchial collapse, or a pulmonary mass lesion. Crackles (rales) are discontinuous sounds similar to radio static or the sound of Velcro pulled apart. These sounds are caused by the explosive opening of collapsed small airways.

53. Do crackles (rales) indicate fluid in the lungs?

Though there is a tendency to relate these sounds to "fluid in the lungs," there is not a consistent correlation as crackles may be detected with pulmonary edema, pneumonia, bronchitis, or pulmonary fibrosis. The loudest crackles are typically detected in primary lung diseases. Subtle crackles are evident only after a deep breath.

BIBLIOGRAPHY

1. Constable PD, Hinchcliff KW, Olson J, Hamlin RL: Athletic heart syndrome in dogs competing in a long-distance sled race. J Appl Physiol 76:433–438, 1994.
2. Detweiler DK, Patterson DF: Abnormal heart sounds and murmurs of the dog. J Small Anim Pract 8:193–205, 1967.
3. Detweiler DK, Patterson DF: A phonograph record of heart sounds and murmurs of the dog. Ann NY Acad Sci 127:322–340, 1965.
4. Haggstrom J, Kvart C, Hansson K: Heart sounds and murmurs: Changes related to severity of chronic valvular disease in the cavalier King Charles spaniel. J Vet Intern Med 9:75–85, 1995.
5. Smetzer DL, Breznock EM: Auscultatory diagnosis of patent ductus arteriosus in the dog. J Am Vet Med Assoc 160:80, 1972.
6. Smetzer DL, Hamlin RL, Smith CR: Cardiovascular sounds. In Swenson MJ (ed): Dukes' Physiology of Domestic Animals. Ithaca, NY, Comstock, 1970, pp 159–168.

19. ELECTROCARDIOGRAPHY

Andrew W. Beardow, B.V.M.&S., MRCVS

1. What does the electrocardiogram measure?

By design, an imbalance of ion concentrations across the membrane of cardiac muscle causes the interior of the myocyte to be more negative than the exterior; this leaves the cell electrically charged, i.e., there is a potential gradient across the cell membrane. Active pumping of sodium and potassium ions maintains this "resting membrane potential. " Some fluctuations in the resting membrane potential may occur, but significant changes do not occur until a "threshold" potential is reached. If the cell is stimulated and the threshold is reached, ion channels in the membrane open, allowing rapid membrane depolarization due to the influx of sodium ions. This rapid change in membrane potential triggers the opening of other ion channels, in particular calcium channels. It is this influx of calcium that stimulates mechanical contraction. Reversal of this process due to ion diffusion and active ion pumping resets the membrane potential ready for the next depolarization. Cells in the heart are triggered to depolarize by depolarization in adjacent cardiac cells. These cells may either be "working" myocytes or myocytes that are part of the specialized conduction system that rapidly carries a wave of depolarization throughout the heart. This specialized conduction system ensures rapid, coordinated contraction of the cardiac muscle. The membrane potential of a single cell during depolarization is known as a monophasic action potential (MAP). Summation of all these MAPs generates an electrical field, whose effects radiate throughout the body. Changes in the electrical field manifest as small (mV) potential differences that can be measured by electrodes attached to the skin. These potential differences are amplified and recorded by the equipment used to record an electrocardiogram.

2. What is the diagnostic use of the electrocardiogram?

The electrocardiogram provides information regarding: (1) heart rate; (2) rhythm; (3) chamber size; (4) the cardiac conduction system; and (5) myocardial ischemia. While definitive assessment of cardiac size should be reserved for diagnostic modalities such as radiography or echocardiography, electrocardiography can give an indication of chamber enlargement. Coronary vessel disease resulting in regional myocardial hypoxia or infarction is uncommon in small animals. Therefore, in small animals, the primary use of electrocardiography is in the diagnosis of arrhythmias.

3. What is meant by the term "lead," and how many are there?

When recording an ECG, the recording electrodes are always attached in a standardized way. These electrodes may be self-adhesive pads or more typically specially prepared alligator clips. If the standards are not followed, the recorded information cannot be related to established "normal" patterns of electrical activity. A lead defines the points between which we are measuring the potential differences generated in the body by the hearts electrical field. For instance, lead II is defined as measuring the potential difference between the electrode attached to the patient's left leg (LL) and right arm (RA). The standard also defines the polarity assigned to each electrode. In lead II the LL is positive and the RA negative. By selecting different leads we are able to assess the electrical field generated by the heart from several different perspectives. This field, which changes with time, will have both strength, and when looked at in three dimensions, direction. Looking at multiple leads enables us to build a three-dimensional perspective of the changes in the electrical field. The tissues undergoing depolarization or repolarization at any one time will determine the strength and direction of the field. Therefore, the field strength may give an indication of the mass of the tissue being depolarized, and its direction will be determined by the pattern of conduction through the entire heart.

To build a three-dimensional perspective from leads comparing two points of reference, we need to assess the ECGs measured in three different planes. Most often a single plane is used and the plane that is used the most is known as the frontal plane. The frontal plane is defined by six leads, three bipolar (i.e., one electrode is defined as positive and the other as negative) and three augmented unipolar leads. Leads I, II, and III are bipolar, i.e., we define one as positive and one as negative (see table below). Leads aVR, aVL, and aVF are augmented unipolar leads, i.e., only one electrode has a defined polarity. In the case of the augmented unipolar leads the electrode in question (e.g., right arm in aVR lead) is positive and compared to an average of the other two (left arm and left leg), as shown in table below. These six leads thus allow us to look at the heart's electrical field from six different perspectives in the plane defined by their points of attachment (the frontal plane). The other planes are defined by moving the points of attachment. In veterinary patients these additional points are on the chest wall. Most electrocardiographs have an exploring electrode (C or V) that can be used to measure a unipolar lead when it is attached to defined points on the chest wall (see table below). Four unipolar chest (precordial) leads are defined for veterinary patients. A complete electrocardiogram thus consists of a total of ten leads—six frontal plane leads and four unipolar chest leads.

LEAD	ELECTRODES AND ELECTRODE PLACEMENT
I	LA (+); RA (−)
I	LL (+); RA (−)
III	LL (+); LA (−)
AVR	RA (+); average of LA and LL (left foot LF)
AVL	LA (+); average of RA and LL (LF)
AVF	LL (LF); average of RA and LA
Chest Leads	
V_1 (CV_5 RL)	V electrode at 5th right intercostal space close to sternum
V_2 (CV_6 LL)	V electrode at 6th left intercostal space close to sternum
V_4 (CV_6 LU)	V electrode at 6th left intercostal space at the costochondral junction
V_{10}	Over the dorsal spinous process of T6–T7 vertebrae

4. What is the electrophysiologic basis of heart rate?

The pacemaker cells located in the sinoatrial node determine the heart rate. Unlike the cells that make up the bulk of cardiac muscle, a pacemaker cell is able to undergo spontaneous depolarization. The process of spontaneous depolarization is a complex one and involves the movement of sodium, potassium, and possibly calcium across the cell membrane. Once threshold is reached, the pacemaker cell depolarizes, triggering depolarization of adjacent cells and thus triggering another cardiac cycle. Alteration in the rate at which threshold is reached will alter the heart rate. Autonomic influences that determine heart rate do so by altering the rate at which threshold is reached. Sympathetic stimulation will increase the rate at which threshold is reached, thus speeding heart rate, while parasympathetic stimulation will have the opposite effect of slowing heart rate. Besides the pacemaker cells in the sinoatrial (SA) node, there are a number of other cells that normally undergo spontaneous depolarization and can also act as pacemakers. Under normal circumstances they do not act as pacemakers because the pacemaker in the SA node is firing at the highest rate. However, should the rate at the SA node drop below the intrinsic rate of any of the other pacemakers, they will then become the dominant pacemaker and will drive the heart rate. These auxiliary pacemakers are located in the His bundle, the bundle branches, and Purkinje cells. Other cardiac cells can become auxiliary pacemakers if their membranes become leaky due to cell damage. This "abnormal automaticity" is one mechanism for the development of arrhythmias when the rate of depolarization of the injured cells becomes predominant.

5. What deflections are usually seen in a lead II ECG and what are their origins?

The diagram below shows a normal electrocardiogram and a schematic representation of the origins of each phase of the ECG. The arrows in the diagram represent the net direction of the wave of depolarization at that point in the electrocardiographic cycle. The amplitude of the deflection on the electrocardiogram represents the magnitude of the electrical field. The positive and negative symbols represent the orientation of the electrodes recording a lead II electrocardiogram. Waves of depolarization that move toward the positive electrode will give a positive deflection on the ECG. Waves of depolarization moving away from the positive electrode give negative deflections. A wave moving perpendicular to the line (the isopotential line) joining positive and negative electrodes will give no deflection. The electrocardiogram in each lead represents both the magnitude of the electrical field associated with depolarization and the direction of its movement relative to the lead electrodes. From the diagram we see that the P wave is associated with atrial depolarization, the Q wave with early ventricular depolarization, the R wave with the bulk of left ventricular depolarization, and the S wave with late ventricular depolarization including the bulk of right ventricular depolarization. Hence changes in the right ventricle will be manifest in changes in the S wave.

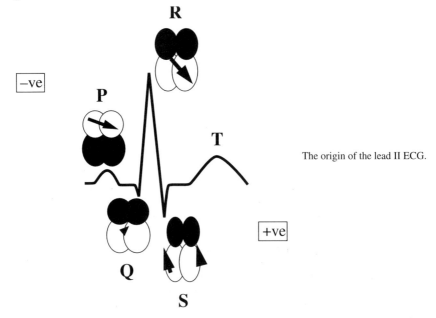

The origin of the lead II ECG.

6. We commonly measure the PR and QT intervals. What are they and what is their significance?

The diagram below illustrates the PR and QT intervals. The PR interval, measured from the beginning of the P wave to the beginning of the Q wave (or R wave if no Q wave is present), represents the time taken for the electrical impulse to travel across the atria and cross the AV node. Conduction through the AV node is deliberately slow, facilitating ventricular filling from the contracting atria before ventricular systole is initiated. PR prolongation is usually a result of excessive slowing of conduction through the AV node. An excessively long PR interval thus defines a first-degree AV block. If conduction fails intermittently, a second-degree AV block has occurred. Complete lack of AV node transmission is described as a third-degree AV block. For the AV node to fulfill its role as a gatekeeper between the atria and the ventricles, it must be the only point of contact between them. An abnormality known as ventricular pre-excitation can result from the presence of a congenital accessory conduction pathway between the atria and the ventricles. The accessory pathway does not slow conduction, the result being a decrease in the delay between atrial and ventricular depolarization and shortening of the PR interval. The presence of accessory pathways can lead to tachyarrhythmias because they form one arm of a re-entrant loop. For example, an impulse passing through the accessory pathway may depolarize the ventricle, enter the AV node in a retrograde direction, and, if the timing is correct, arrive back at the atria once they have repolarized, triggering another cycle through this loop.

The QT interval represents the time taken from the start of ventricular depolarization to the end of ventricular repolarization. The major influences on the QT interval are the heart rate and the factors that influence the rate of active chemical processes (e.g., body temperature). QT interval is inversely related to heart rate. Animals that become severely hypothermic during surgery frequently have significant prolongation of the QT interval. The repolarization phase is an active process, and therefore factors affecting active processes will be manifest here. The ST segment represents early repolarization and will thus be influenced by these factors. Elevation or depression of this segment can be an indication of changes in the electrolyte and acid-base milieu of the heart as well as regional myocardial hypoxia.

Diagram of PR and QT intervals.

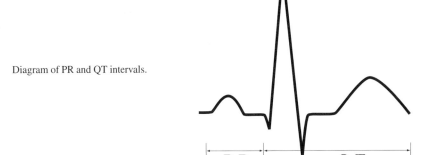

7. What is meant by the term mean electrical axis and how is it calculated?

The electrical axis describes the net direction of shift in the heart's electrical field during the cardiac cycle. It is significant because it may be affected by certain clinically important factors. For instance, a shift in the balance between the left and right ventricle due to right ventricular hypertrophy will alter the net direction of the electrical field, as will factors that affect the sequence of chamber depolarization, including bundle branch blocks that affect the pattern of action potential conduction through the heart's conduction system. The six leads of an electrocardiogram are in effect six representations of the shift in the heart's electrical field viewed from six different directions. If the net shift is toward the positive electrode of a lead, a large positive deflection will be seen. It is likely that if the net shift is positive toward one electrode of one lead, it will be less positive or even negative relative to the positive electrodes of other leads. Knowing this, and assuming that we always place the electrodes and measure the leads in the same way each time, allows us to take the information collected from each lead and calculate the mean or average direction of movement of the heart's electrical field. The figure below shows the orientation of leads I, II, and III. They can be represented as an equilateral triangle (Einthoven's triangle), illustrating their relative orientation to each other. The zero baseline for each lead is the point at which no net positive or negative deflection is seen. If we then represent the ECG deflections for two of these leads, in this case leads I and III on their respective zero baselines, we can see how these ECG tracings relate to each other. It is the same electrical field that each is seeing, but it is seeing it from a different perspective. When these perspectives are related to each other, we can calculate the net positive or negative deflection from each lead. The dashed lines represent the net deflections of each lead. The intersection of these gives us the reference point for the mean electrical axis. In theory, if we had also reflected the ECG recorded in lead II, its mean deflection would also have intersected at the same point. Therefore, if the net deflections of any two leads can be reflected in this way, the mean electrical axis can be calculated (see figure, top of next page).

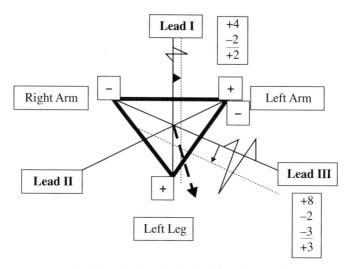

Orientation of leads I, II, and III (Einthoven's triangle).

To simplify the matter, not only is this true for leads I, II, and III, but also for the augmented unipolar leads aVR, aVL, and aVF. If the axes of all the frontal leads are superimposed over a central point of zero potential, a hexaxial reference diagram results:

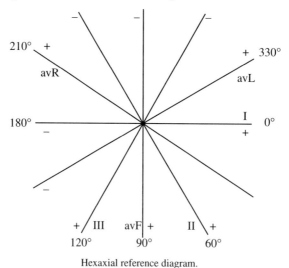

Hexaxial reference diagram.

When the six frontal leads are depicted in this fashion, the positive pole of each lead is assigned a value in degrees that relates to an arbitrary zero at the positive pole of lead I. Thus, the positive electrode of lead aVF is at the 90° position and aVL is at 330°. Note that the baseline of the augmented leads runs along the isopotential line for leads I, II, and III. In particular, leads aVF and I are perpendicular; hence these two leads are often selected when making a determination of mean electrical axis.

An exact value of MEA is not always necessary to make clinical judgements. When applying these results clinically, we often divide the results into ranges or quadrants. For instance, the left lower quadrant runs from 0–90°. MEA values falling into this quadrant are normal. An axis that lies in the right upper quadrant (180 to –90°) is indicative of a right axis deviation in canine patients. This being said, we can get an indication of the MEA by assessing the appearance of the QRS complex in any two perpendicular leads. If, for example, the net deflections of leads I and aVF are both positive, the MEA must fall in the left lower quadrant, i.e., between 0 and 90° (see figure below).

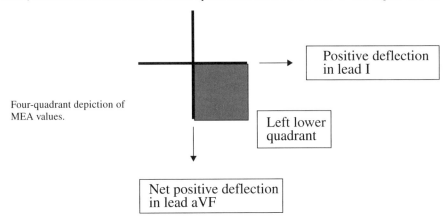

Four-quadrant depiction of MEA values.

If both leads I and aVF are positive and the magnitude of the net deflection in lead aVF exceeds that of lead I, the MEA is greater than 45° but less than 90°. In the case where the net deflection of lead I is 0, the complex is said to be isoelectric and the MEA falls along lead aVF at 90°. When using the isoelectric lead method of calculating MEA, we simply identify an isoelectric lead (one in which the net deflection is zero) and determine the magnitude of the net deflection in the perpendicular lead. If lead I is isoelectric and the net deflection of lead aVF is positive, the MEA is 90° (see figure below). To simplify further, recall that the MEA is approximated by the lead that has the largest positive deflection; if lead aVF is the "most positive," the MEA is approximately 90°.

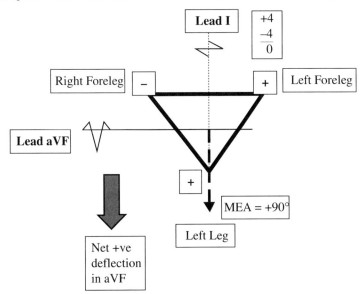

Using the isoelectric lead method of calculating MEA. Lead I is isoelectric; therefore, the MEA lies along its isopotential line. To determine the direction along the isopotential line we look at the complex seen in the lead perpendicular to it, in this case aVF. If the net deflection is positive, the MEA lies at +90°. If the net deflection is negative, the MEA lies at –90°.

8. What are the normal values for the amplitude and duration of the deflections and intervals in lead II for the dog and cat?

Normal ECG Parameters in Lead II

PARAMETER	DOG	CAT
Heart rate	70–160 adult; 60–140 giant breeds; up to 180 in toys; up to 220 in puppies	140–180; up to 240 probably normal
P wave	0.4 mV high; 0.04–0.05 seconds	0.2 mV high; 0.04 seconds
PR interval	0.06–0.13 seconds	0.04–0.09 seconds
QRS	2.5–3.0 mV high; 0.05–0.06 seconds	0.75–0.9 mV high; 0.04 seconds
MEA	40–100°	Very wide (0–180°)
QT	0.15–0.25	0.12–0.18
ST	No greater than 0.2 mV deflection	
T wave	No greater than 25% amplitude of R wave; a very variable component of limited value	0.3 mV high

The governing influence in determining ranges is usually body size.

9. Describe a systematic approach to ECG evaluation.

In evaluating an ECG it is important to develop a systematic approach to ensure that all facets of rate and rhythm are evaluated. Several systems have been developed. One such system is to always ask and answer the following questions:

1. What is the heart rate? Why? This helps to determine the presence of bradyarrhythmia or tachyarrhythmia. In order to obtain the heart rate from the ECG we can count the number of complexes that occur during a specific period of time. Remember that the x axis of the ECG represents time. When the ECG is recorded at a paper speed of 50 mm/sec, a 150-mm section represents 3 seconds. The number of complexes during that 3-second period multiplied by 20 provides the heart rate in beats per minute (bpm). Many commercial ECG papers have tick marks that are spaced at 75-mm intervals, which means that the space between alternate tick marks represents 3 seconds when the paper speed is 50 mm/sec and 6 seconds when the paper speed is 25 mm/sec. Counting the number of complexes during a 3- (or 6-) second period and multiplying by 20 (or 10) provides the heart rate during that interval. Alternatively, 60 divided by the RR interval (in seconds) determined from the ECG provides an "instantaneous" heart rate.

2. Is every QRS preceded by a P wave and is every P wave followed at a fixed distance by a QRS? Why? This determines the source of each QRS complex and determines if any P waves go unconducted. If the beat is a sinus beat, it will be preceded by a P wave and the PR interval will be relatively constant. If the QRS does not originate from the sinus node there may be no preceding P wave, or the P wave may be abnormal and the PR interval altered if the beat is supraventricular in origin.

3. Are there complexes that come early or late? Why? Is there evidence of premature beats or escape beats?

4. Do the QRS complexes from these beats look like those we have previously identified as having a sinus origin? Why? This is done to determine if the complexes are of ventricular or supraventricular origin. A supraventricular beat is one that arises from above the bifurcation of the AV bundle, while a ventricular beat arises from the ventricles. The QRS of a supraventricular beat almost always looks like those that arise from the sinus because the conduction from the AV node through the conduction pathways in the ventricle is the same, and it is this part of the electrical cycle that generates the QRS complex. The exception is a phenomenon known as aberrancy of ventricular conduction, in which very "early" premature supraventricular depolarizations, or rapid supraventricular tachycardias, result in QRS complexes that have abnormal configuration due to conduction system dysfunction. The QRS from a beat that arises in the ventricle will not

be conducted via the normal conduction pathways of the ventricle and will have a very abnormal-looking QRS complex compared to those arising from the sinus.

  5. Are the ECG parameters normal in the sinus beats? Why? Is there evidence of conduction abnormalities or chamber enlargement?

  6. Is every complex that we are calling a QRS followed by a T wave? Why? Some artifacts can look like abnormal QRS complexes. To help differentiate between them, we look for evidence of repolarization following the depolarization, i.e., the presence of a T wave.

10. What ECG changes are most indicative of left heart enlargement?

  The QRS complex represents depolarization of the ventricular myocardium. Normally left ventricular activity drives the amplitude and duration of the QRS complex because it is the dominant ventricle by virtue of its mass. An increase in the size of the left ventricle will emphasize this dominance. Left ventricular enlargement is usually characterized by an increase in the amplitude and duration of the QRS complex in lead II.

11. What is a left anterior fascicular block pattern and why is it important?

  This pattern has been most commonly described in cats. It is characterized by a net negative deflection in leads II and III with a positive deflection in lead I. This ECG abnormality has been associated with cardiac disease in cats, in particular cardiomyopathy. Its presence should rise the index of suspicion for heart disease, but is not diagnostic of it.

12. Describe the ECG changes most suggestive of a right ventricular hypertrophy.

  In the normal heart the left ventricle dominates by virtue of its mass. With right ventricular hypertrophy this dominance is diminished. This manifests in two main ways. The amplitude of the R wave may be diminished, its amplitude driven by the left ventricular electrical influences, and the S wave deepens as the thickened right ventricle pulls the mean electrical axis toward it. (see diagram below). The ECG changes most sensitive for right ventricular hypertrophy are thus a right axis deviation in the frontal plane (due to the presence of deep S waves) and deep S waves in the chest leads.

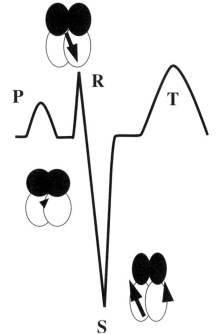

The origin of a right axis deviation in lead II. The right ventricle predominates in the latter portion of ventricular depolarization.

13. What are the common causes of artifact when recording an electrocardiogram in veterinary patients?

Artifacts are usually seen for the following reasons:

1. Lack of electrical contact between the patient's skin and the electrode. This is usually due to the animal's fur getting between the skin and the electrode or because of a lack of a suitable electrical coupling medium such as alcohol.

2. Electrical interference due to failure to insulate the patient from the table, contact between the electrode and the person restraining the patient, or electrodes on adjacent limbs coming into contact with each other. Patients should be placed on a rubber mat when recording an electrocardiogram or a thick, dry, wool blanket. Sixty-cycle (50 in Europe) interference can occur if the ECG is recorded with the patient near high-voltage sources such as x-ray machines or some overhead lights. Several different positions in the clinic may need to be tested to ensure that this type of interference is minimized.

3. Movement is perhaps the greatest source of artifact. Even respiration can cause variability in the amplitude of the complexes. Purring is another source of motion artifact. When recording an ECG the electrodes should be attached below the elbows and stifles to minimize the effects of body motion. The patient should be restrained in right lateral recumbency with the forelegs perpendicular to the body. Movement or malposition of the forelimbs is another common source of artifact. If we are unable to restrain the patient in this way due to a patient's clinical status, the ECG can be recorded with the patient sitting sternally. This may negate some of the assumptions that are based on complex size and configuration, as the standards are calculated for the patient restrained in right lateral recumbency. There should be no effect, however, on our ability to make a diagnosis of rate and rhythm.

14. What is meant by the term wandering pacemaker?

The sinoatrial node does not consist of one pacemaker cell. Rather, it is a nest of cells and the individual cell responsible for initiating nodal depolarization may change from one moment to another. Fluctuations in autonomic tone can bring different pacemaker cells to dominance and change the path taken from the SA node over the atrium. This may manifest as variations in P wave morphology and can be a normal variation. If one studies such an ECG, one can occasionally pick up a rhythm in this variability and correlate it to physiologic variables, i.e., the respiratory cycle.

15. What is the significance of small complexes in lead II?

Small complexes in lead II (less than 0.5 mV) in dogs may be indicative of pleural effusion, pericardial effusion, hypothyroidism, or obesity. However, in some breeds small complexes may be a normal variation.

BIBLIOGRAPHY

1. Kittleson MD: Electrocardiography: Basic concepts, diagnosis of chamber enlargement, and intraventricular conduction disturbances. In Kittleson MD, Kienle RD (eds): Small Animal Cardiovascular Medicine. Mosby, St. Louis, 1998, pp 72–94.
2. Miller MS, Tilley LP, Smith FWK Jr, Fox PR: Electrocardiography. In Fox PR, Sisson D, Moise NS (eds): Textbook of Canine and Feline Cardiology: Principles and Clinical Practice. W.B. Saunders, Philadelphia, 1999, pp 67–106.
3. Tilley LP: Essentials of Canine and Feline Electrocardiography: Interpretation and Treatment. 3rd ed. Philadelphia, Lea & Febiger, 1992.

20. AMBULATORY ELECTROCARDIOGRAPHY

Teresa C. DeFrancesco, D.V.M.

1. What is ambulatory electrocardiography?

Ambulatory electrocardiography is a prolonged continuous recording of the cardiac rhythm that is ideally obtained while the patient is engaged in normal daily activities. The two most common applications of ambulatory electrocardiography are a Holter monitor, a 24–48-hour continuous ECG recording, and an event recorder.

2. What is the advantage of an ambulatory electrocardiogram over an in-hospital electrocardiogram?

An ambulatory ECG provides a longer and more thorough assessment of the cardiac rhythm as opposed to a routine 3–5-minute in-hospital ECG. This allows a more complete assessment of the cardiac rhythm, particularly if an intermittent arrhythmia is documented or suspected. Ideally, the patient would wear the ambulatory ECG in the home environment to allow a more complete assessment of the heart rate and rhythm out of a stressful hospital environment and with various activities such as exercise or sleep. Typically, a diary of events and clinical signs are carefully recorded and correlated to the cardiac rhythm.

3. List the most common clinical indications for ambulatory electrocardiography.
- Syncope
- Quantification of cardiac arrhythmia
- Efficacy of antiarrhythmic therapy
- Screening for subclinical cardiomyopathy

Other less common veterinary indications are for ST segment analysis in ischemic heart disease, and an accurate assessment of heart rate control in the treatment of atrial fibrillation.

4. What is a Holter monitor?

A Holter monitor is a long-term continuous recording (usually 24 hours) of the cardiac rhythm. It is named after a physicist Norman "Jeff" Holter who first designed and adapted the technology in the early 1960s to a small portable recording unit, thus making it clinically useful. Although Holter monitoring has been used in human medicine for close to 40 years, it has only been used in veterinary medicine in the last 10 years. Currently available Holter monitors usually weigh about 0.5 kg and are applied noninvasively via adhesive ECG patches to the skin in the area of the precordium.

5. What is an event recorder?

An event recorder is a patient-activated (or client-activated in veterinary medicine) recording of a short loop of the ECG. This technology is most useful in evaluation of infrequent syncope in which an intermittent arrhythmia is suspected. The unit continually records and then erases 5 minutes of an ECG loop until the owner activates the recording button. The event recorder will then store 5 minutes of ECG, 1 minute prior and 4 minutes after the recording button was activated. The stored ECG is typically immediately transmitted by telephone to a central recording station and analyzed. The event recorder is smaller in size than a Holter monitor and these units are typically worn for longer periods of time, such as 1 week to a month.

6. What is the advantage of an event recorder over a continuous electrocardiographic recording?

The main advantage of an event recorder is in the evaluation of a collapsing patient with infrequent clinical signs and/or of small size (< 7 kg).

7. What is the technology used in ambulatory electrocardiography?

Many technological advances have been made in ambulatory electrocardiography. Traditional Holter monitoring systems use a battery-operated cassette tape electromagnetic recorder that records two or three modified precordial leads over a 24-hour period. The recorder usually has an event and calibration marker, and an internal clock. The cassette tape is then digitized and analyzed by a technician-assisted computer. Newer solid-state technologies in the form of real-time microcomputer systems are gaining popularity because of the immediate availability of data after the recording. The event recorder is a solid-state device that stores a loop of ECG when activated by the owner. The ECG recording can then be sent trans-telephonically to the base station where it is printed on a standard ECG machine or microcomputer for interpretation.

8. Can ambulatory electrocardiography be performed in cats?

Yes. There are reports in the literature of Holter monitoring in both normal cats and cats with hypertrophic cardiomyopathy. However, the technique is limited to medium to large cats with a friendly demeanor. A Holter monitor may be too big and stressful for a small cat to wear. An event recorder may be more feasible if warranted by the clinical scenario.

9. Where does one obtain the recording unit for ambulatory electrocardiography?

Common sources for both general practitioners and cardiology specialists are LabCorp, Ambulatory Holter Monitoring Division, Burlington, NC (800-289-4358) and Cardiopet, Little Falls, NJ (800-726-1212). These centers will provide the recorder, hook-up kit, detailed instructions for the hook-up and application of the recording unit to the patient, and tape analysis. In addition, most veterinary university teaching hospitals and specialty referral hospitals will offer ambulatory electrocardiography.

10. Who performs the ambulatory electrocardiographic analysis and interpretation?

If the recording unit is obtained from a commercial ambulatory electrocardiographic company, a human electrocardiographic technician will usually perform the analysis. This may be problematic if he or she is not experienced with canine electrocardiograms. However, in the author's opinion, this problem has improved with time and greater exposure to canine electrocardiograms. Upon request, LabCorp will provide oversight by a veterinary cardiologist. Cardiopet Holter monitors and event recorders are typically over-read by experienced veterinary cardiologists. The final interpretation of the recording is made by the primary clinician and should take into consideration the patient's clinical signs. A cardiology specialist should be consulted if the interpretation is not straightforward.

11. Describe a normal canine 24-hour ambulatory electrocardiogram.

A normal canine 24-hour ambulatory electrocardiogram should have a wide variation in heart rate. Normal heart rates at sleep can be as low as 30–40 per minute with periods of sinus arrest, occasional ventricular escape complexes, and second-degree AV block. Normal heart rates during extreme exercise can be very high (> 250 per minute) for brief periods of time. Sinus arrhythmia is common. There is controversy about the number of ventricular premature complexes that is considered normal. Some feel that even one ventricular premature complex is worrisome; however, two studies evaluating the cardiac rhythm in normal dogs by Holter monitoring showed that 18–50% of dogs had a low frequency of ventricular extrasystoles (usually < 50 per 24 hours).

12. Describe a normal feline 24-hour ambulatory electrocardiogram.

The normal feline 24-hour ambulatory electrocardiogram was reported recently, and average heart rates over a 24-hour period ranged from approximately 110–200 per minute. Most cats had periods of sinus arrhythmia noted during sleep. Isolated ventricular extrasystoles occurred in some of the cats, more commonly in the older ones.

13. Are there guidelines for the antiarrhythmic therapy based on 24-hour ambulatory electrocardiography?

There are no rigid guidelines for antiarrhythmic therapy based on Holter monitoring. If the patient is having clinical signs correlated to an arrhythmia, appropriate antiarrhythmic therapy is indicated. Other potential indications for therapeutic intervention include frequent triplets or paroxysms of ventricular tachycardia, especially if these arrhythmias occur at fast rates, are multiform in nature, or are very premature (R-on-T complexes).

14. How useful is ambulatory electrocardiography in determining efficacy of antiarrhythmic drug therapy?

It is extremely useful and desirable to guide antiarrhythmic therapy based on long-term ambulatory Holter monitoring. Because there is substantial spontaneous variation in the frequency of ventricular arrhythmias, standard in-hospital ECGs may over- or underestimate the efficacy of the antiarrhythmic therapy. Human studies show that a 90% decrease in ventricular tachycardia is generally believed to represent true reduction in the number of ventricular ectopics.

15. How useful is ambulatory electrocardiography in the clinical evaluation of syncope?

A recent retrospective study evaluated the clinical utility of Holter monitoring in syncopal dogs. Holter monitoring was helpful in establishing a diagnosis in 42% of cases, but no relationship was detected between the frequency of episodes occurring before Holter recording and the likelihood of a diagnostically useful Holter. An arrhythmia was ruled out in 12% of the recordings and was implicated as the cause of syncope in 30% of recordings.

16. How useful is ambulatory electrocardiography as a screen for subclinical cardiomyopathy?

In combination with echocardiography, ambulatory electrocardiography is a commonly used screening test for occult cardiomyopathy. The only longitudinal study evaluating the usefulness of Holter monitoring as a screening tool for cardiomyopathy was performed in Dobermans in the early 1990s. Calvert showed that the presence of ventricular extrasystoles is a reliable marker for Doberman cardiomyopathy and may significantly precede clinical signs of heart disease. In apparently normal Dobermans, 100% that had greater than 50 ventricular extrasystoles/24 hours went on to develop overt dilated cardiomyopathy or sudden death. Thus, if more than 100 ventricular extrasystoles or ventricular tachycardias are identified on a 24-hour Holter monitor, occult cardiomyopathy is highly suspected. Most normal dogs will have less than 50 ventricular extrasystoles and no runs of ventricular tachycardia.

BIBLIOGRAPHY

1. Calvert CA, Jacobs GJ, Smith DD, et al: Association between results of ambulatory electrocardiography and development of cardiomyopathy during long-term follow-up of Doberman pinschers. J Am Vet Med Assoc 216:34–39, 2000.
2. Calvert CA, Jacobs GJ, Pickus CW: Bradycardia-associated episodic weakness, syncope and aborted sudden death in cardiomyopathic Doberman pinschers. J Vet Intern Med 10:88–93, 1996.
3. Goodwin JK: Holter monitoring and cardiac event recording. Vet Clin North Am Small Anim Pract, 28:1391–1407, 1998
4. Goodwin JK, Lombard CW, Ginnex DD: Results of continuous ambulatory electrocardiography in a cat with hypertrophic cardiomyopathy. J Am Vet Med Assoc 200:1352–1354, 1992.
5. Hall LW, Dunn JK, Delaney M, et al: Ambulatory electrocardiography in dogs. Vet Rec 129:213–216, 1991.
6. Lemkuhl LB, Bonagura JD: Results of Holter monitoring in dogs with congenital subaortic stenosis. Proceedings, 11th Annual Forum, American College of Veterinary Internal Medicine, 1993, pp 553–556.
7. Marino DJ, Matthiesen DT, Fox PR: Ventricular arrhythmias in dogs undergoing splenectomy: A prospective study. Vet Surg 23:101–106, 1994.

8. Miller RH, Lehmkuhl LB, Bonagura JD, et al: Retrospective analysis of the clinical utility of ambulatory electrocardiographic (Holter) recordings in syncopal dogs: 44 cases (1991–1995). J Vet Intern Med 13:111–122, 1999.

9. Moise NS, DeFrancesco TC: Twenty-four-hour ambulatory electrocardiography (Holter monitoring). In Bonagura JD (ed): Kirk's Current Veterinary Therapy XII: Small Animal Practice. Philadelphia, W.B. Saunders, 1995, pp 792–799.

10. Ulloa HM, Houston BJ, Altrogge DM: Arrhythmia prevalence during ambulatory electrocardiographic monitoring of Beagles. Am J Vet Res 56:275–281, 1995.

11. Ware WA: Twenty-four-hour ambulatory electrocardiography in normal cats. J Vet Intern Med 13:175–180, 1999.

12. Ware WA: Practical use of Holter monitoring. The Compendium 20:167–177, 1998.

21. CANINE CARDIAC RADIOLOGY

Charles S. Farrow, B.Sc., D.V.M.

1. What is the use of cardiac radiology?

Radiographic studies provide an excellent assessment of global cardiac size. Because the pulmonary vessels and parenchyma can be evaluated with respect to cardiac size, it is possible to make an indirect assessment of cardiac performance. Thoracic radiography is the only noninvasive means through which one can make a diagnosis of left-sided congestive heart failure.

2. What are the limitations of cardiac radiology?

Radiographic assessment of the heart is limited to *exterior* analysis, although related *interior* abnormalities may be inferred. This limitation is illustrated by the radiographic appearance of a large pericardial effusion. When a large pericardial effusion is present, the cardiac silhouette is enlarged when the heart itself might, in fact, be small. Additionally, the size of specific cardiac chambers can only be inferred through characteristic changes in the contour of the cardiac silhouette. Because the heart is apparent radiographically as a single fluid density, it is not possible to distinguish the atrial or ventricular septae.

Unlike echocardiography, radiology cannot directly assess heart function; however, an experienced radiologist can often infer cardiac dysfunction, especially as suggested by aortic and pulmonary arterial disfigurement and altered lung circulation.

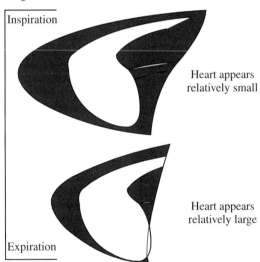

Inspiration

Heart appears relatively small

FIGURE 1. Depth of respiration related to heart size in lateral projection.

Heart appears relatively large

Expiration

3. What effect does breathing have on the radiographic appearance of the heart?

Breathing is associated with thoracic movement, which may in turn cause blurring of the heart and lungs especially when longer exposure times are used. The resultant motion unsharpness can be mistaken for lung disease.

However, even when exposure times are brief enough to assure crisp intrathoracic imagery, breathing may still influence radiographic appearances, depending on whether the exposure was made during inspiration or expiration. In an inspiratory film, the heart appears both relatively and absolutely smaller than it does during expiration. Conversely, during expiration the heart appears larger than it does during inspiration. These differences pertain to both lateral and dorsoventral projections (see Figs. 1 and 2).

Of equal importance, especially when attempting to render a judgement on heart failure, is the appearance of the lung, which appears relatively dense during expiration, often resembling pulmonary edema.

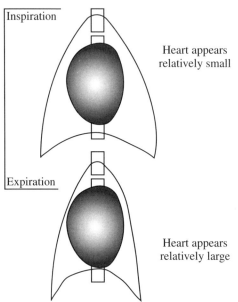

FIGURE 2.   Depth of respiration related to heart size in ventrodorsal projection.

4. What effect do systole and diastole have on the radiographic appearance of the heart?

Just as breathing influences the appearance of the heart, cardiac emptying and filling may likewise be appreciated radiographically, especially in dorsoventral thoracic projections of larger dogs with slow heart rates. To generalize: the heart appears slightly to moderately larger and rounder during maximal filling (ventricular end-diastole), while during emptying (end ventricular systole), the heart appears relatively smaller, often featuring prominent atria and tapered ventricles (Fig. 3).

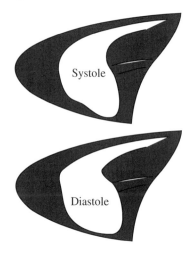

FIGURE 3.   Circulatory variability of the heart.

5. Does the shape of the heart vary with breed?

In general, the heart of a dog conforms to its thorax. Thus, an Irish setter, with its tall, laterally compressed rib cage, has a tall, narrow, upright heart, while that of a pug appears relatively short and round, reflecting its more cylindrical torso. The heart of a Labrador retriever falls somewhere in between (Fig. 4).

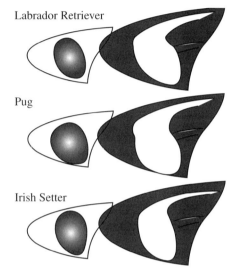

Labrador Retriever

Pug

FIGURE 4. Breed-related variability in heart shape.

Irish Setter

6. How does the radiographic appearance of the heart differ in dorsoventral versus ventrodorsal projection?

Generally, the heart appears longer and narrower when projected ventrodorsally than when projected dorsoventrally. This difference results in large part from the caudal displacement of the cardiac apex, owing to its relatively weak moorings compared to that of its base (Fig. 5). For the same reason, the heart often tips to the right or left of midline, in some instances markedly altering its silhouette. Overall, the dorsoventral projection more accurately portrays the cardiac anatomy than does the ventrodorsal view.

7. How does the radiographic appearance of the heart differ in right versus left lateral projection?

In the right lateral projection the cardiac apex appears relatively conical, and the caudal vena cava appears to blend imperceptibly with the caudal boarder of the left ventricle. In contrast, the left lateral projection features a relatively rounded cardiac apex and a distinctive caval overlap. With practice, a right lateral projection can be readily differentiated from a left lateral view (Fig. 6).

8. What is the cardiothoracic ratio?

In people, where cardiac mensuration is currently used as an adjunct in assessing heart size on a frontal view of the chest, the cardiothoracic ratio is calculated by dividing the widest transverse cardiac diameter by the widest inside thoracic diameter. In dogs, cardiac mensuration has never achieved clinical popularity, largely due to breed variation and low sensitivity. One published method is illustrated (Fig. 7).

9. What is cardiac emphasis?

Cardiac emphasis refers to the relative contributions made by the right and left halves of an enlarged heart. By determining which side of the heart is the more enlarged, right or left, the number of potential explanations becomes smaller (Fig. 8).

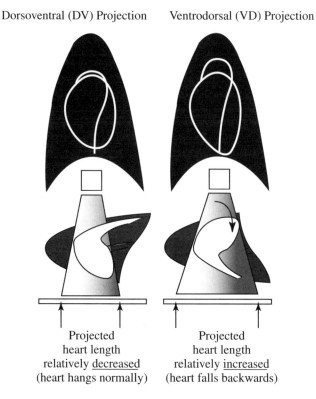

Dorsoventral (DV) Projection   Ventrodorsal (VD) Projection

Projected
heart length
relatively <u>decreased</u>
(heart hangs normally)

Projected
heart length
relatively <u>increased</u>
(heart falls backwards)

FIGURE 5.   Projectional variability of heart shape.

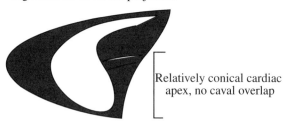

Right side down lateral projection

Relatively conical cardiac
apex, no caval overlap

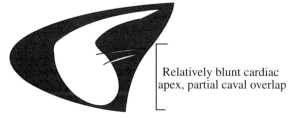

Left side down lateral projection

Relatively blunt cardiac
apex, partial caval overlap

FIGURE 6.   Influence of right- vs. left-sided lateral projections on heart size and caval overlap.

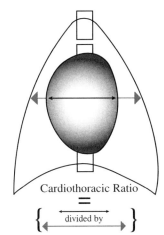

FIGURE 7.   Determination of the cardiothoracic ratio.

10. How is right atrial enlargement determined radiographically?

Medical imaging specialists readily acknowledge the difficulty in evaluating the right atrium radiographically; most advocate ultrasonography instead. The difficulty lies with the right atrium not being profiled in either of the two standard thoracic projections (Fig. 9). Right atrial enlargement has been reported to eliminate the normally tapered appearance of the cranial aspect of the heart base (referred to as "loss of cranial waist") as seen in lateral projection, but so may right ventricular enlargement.

11. How is right ventricular enlargement determined radiographically?

Right ventricular enlargement may be detected in lateral, dorsoventral, and ventrodorsal thoracic radiographs. In lateral projection, the cranial margin of the heart may bulge forward, thus increasing the length and area of the heart. In the opposite plane (dorsoventral, ventrodorsal) the right border of the heart appears abnormally convex, termed by some a reverse "D" sign (Fig. 10).

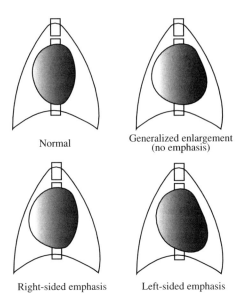

FIGURE 8.   Cardiac emphasis.

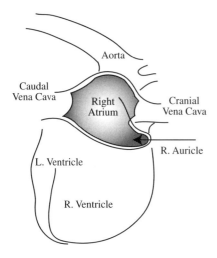

FIGURE 9. The right atrium and auricle from a right lateral perspective.

12. How is left atrial enlargement determined radiographically?

Unlike the right atrium, the left atrium is clearly profiled in a lateral thoracic radiograph. When moderately enlarged, the left atrium causes the caudal heart margin to assume a distinctive recurved appearance (Fig. 11). In the opposite plane, left atrial enlargement may be inferred by the abnormal spreading apart of the principal bronchi to the caudal lung lobes, which is best seen with a penetrated view.

13. How is left ventricular enlargement determined radiographically?

Left ventricular enlargement is best seen in a lateral thoracic radiograph as a backward bulging of the caudal heart margin (Fig. 12). It is also possible to see increased left marginal convexity in the dorsoventral or ventrodorsal views, but not as obviously as when the right ventricle is enlarged.

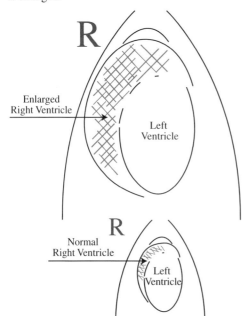

FIGURE 10. Right ventricular enlargement as determined by ventrodorsal projection.

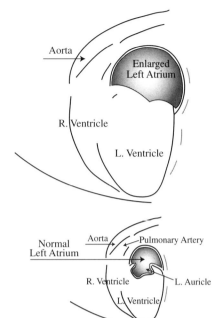

FIGURE 11. Left atrial enlargement as determined by right lateral projection.

14. How is proximal aortic enlargement determined?

The proximal aorta is identified most easily in the dorsoventral or ventrodorsal views as a sharply curving line crossing the precardiac portion of the mediastinum from right to left, immediately cranial to the edge of the heart, which gradually straightens as it passes over the length of the heart, disappearing into the abdomen. In the ventrodorsal view, especially in light films, the aorta may blend imperceptibly with the heart making it appear distorted. In a lateral projection an enlarged proximal aorta may visibly press into the cranial mediastinum and resemble a mediastinal

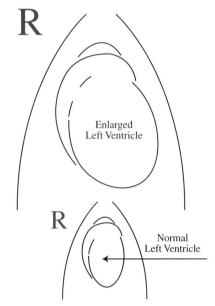

FIGURE 12. Left ventricular enlargement as determined by ventrodorsal projection.

mass. Enlargement of the proximal aorta is often a feature of severe subaortic stenosis and of persistent patency of the arterial duct.

15. How is proximal main pulmonary arterial enlargement determined?

Enlargement of the proximal part of the pulmonary artery (also known as the main pulmonary artery, or pulmonary arterial segment) results in its extension beyond the edge of the adjacent right heart margin, which profiles its lateral edge—typically just to the right and slightly below the aorta. Pulmonic stenosis and causes of pulmonary artery hypertension including heartworm disease can be associated with the development of proximal main pulmonary arterial enlargement.

16. How is generalized pulmonary vascular enlargement (pulmonary hyperemia) determined?

Pulmonary hyperemia (pulmonary overcirculation, pulmonary congestion) is characterized by increased vessel size and number. Visual assessments of this nature are notoriously inaccurate, although some authors have suggested otherwise. The most widely used method of vascular mensuration compares the diameter of a cranial lobe artery or vein to that of a nearby rib (as viewed in lateral projection).

17. What is shunt vasculature?

Shunt vasculature is a term used in the radiographic diagnosis of congenital heart disease to describe abnormal lung circulation and, inferentially, the direction of blood flow through a defective intraventricular or intra-atrial septum, or through an interarterial shunt (persistent arterial duct). A diminished pulmonary circulation is characteristic of a right-to-left shunt, while overcirculation is usually a feature of a left-to-right shunt.

18. What is cardiac remodeling?

Cardiac remodeling is the process by which a diseased heart changes in size or shape. Such changes usually are the result of abnormal increases in blood volume or chamber pressure, which in turn cause dilation and hypertrophy.

19. What is a cardiac (disease) pattern?

A cardiac pattern is a group of related cardiopulmonary abnormalities that characterize a particular disease. Experts often immediately recognize specific heart disease or disease groups by their patterns.

20. What is the cardiac pattern of shock?

A small heart, diminished lung circulation, and a relatively hyperlucent and hyperinflated lung are most characteristic of hypovolemic shock.

21. What is the cardiac pattern of congestive heart failure?

An enlarged heart with left-sided emphasis, enlarged pulmonary vessels, and an abnormally dense lung due to pulmonary edema define the radiographic appearance of left-sided congestive heart failure. The resultant lung consolidation often results in improved bronchial or alveolar visibility (air bronchograms and air alveolargrams).

22. What is the cardiac pattern of excessive intravenous fluid administration?

A normal or mildly enlarged heart, a mild to mild-moderate increase in pulmonary circulation, and occasionally interstitial edema are most characteristic of fluid overload.

23. What is the cardiac pattern of mitral regurgitation?

An enlarged heart with left-sided emphasis (due in greatest part to left atrial enlargement) is characteristic of mitral regurgitation (mitral insufficiency). The appearance of the lung and vasculature provide an indirect assessment of cardiac performance; in the setting of compensated mitral valve regurgitation, the lung is clear. Elevations in left atrial pressures may be manifest as pulmonary congestion or the development of frank edema.

24. What is the cardiac pattern of cardiomyopathy?

In the dog, dilated cardiomyopathy is the most common form of heart muscle disease and the radiographic appearance is characterized in the advanced stages by generalized heart enlargement. Often, there is left-sided emphasis; the presence of edema indicates left-sided congestive heart failure.

25. What is the cardiac pattern of pericardial disease?

Pericardial disease that results in a medium to large volume of fluid formation makes the heart appear larger and rounder than normal. Typically, the pulmonary circulation appears reduced. In some instances the individual lung vessels look miniscule and the lung is relatively hyperlucent. Such findings should prompt a search of the abdomen for free fluid, which would indicate right-sided congestive heart failure.

26. What is the cardiac pattern of patent arterial duct?

Patent ductus arteriosus (PDA) is best characterized by cardiomegaly with left-sided emphasis, enlargement of the proximal aorta, and pulmonary overcirculation. The three bulges on the right heart border, representing the aorta, left auricular appendage, and left atrium, respectively, are widely promoted as diagnostic features; however, it is rare that the three are observed together in a single case.

27. What is the cardiac pattern of aortic stenosis?

Aortic stenosis (AS) is best characterized by cardiomegaly with left-sided emphasis, enlargement of the aortic root, and a normal appearing pulmonary circulation.

28. What is the cardiac pattern of pulmonic stenosis?

Pulmonic stenosis is best characterized by cardiomegaly with right-sided emphasis, enlargement of the main pulmonary artery, and a normal or small peripheral lung circulation.

29. What is the cardiac pattern of ventricular septal defect?

Ventricular septal defects are characterized by cardiomegaly (which may be generalized), enlargement of the main pulmonary artery, and an increased pulmonary circulation.

BIBLIOGRAPHY

1. Buchanan JW, Bucheler J: Vertebral scale system to measure canine heart size in radiographs. J Am Vet Med Assoc 206:194–199, 1995.
2. Carlson E: Experimental studies of ventricular mechanics in dogs using the tantalum-labeled heart. Fed Proc 28:1324–1329, 1969.
3. Douglas SW, Williamson HD: Veterinary Radiological Interpretation. Philadelphia, Lea & Febiger, 1970, pp 186–188.
4. Farrow CS: Radiology of the Cat. St. Louis, Mosby, 1994, p 93.
5. Kealy K: Diagnostic Radiology of the Dog and Cat. Philadelphia, W.B. Saunders, 1987, p 172.
6. Miller SW: Cardiac Radiology: The Requisites. St. Louis, Mosby, 1996, p 6.
7. Ruehl WW, Thrall DE: The effect of dorsal versus ventral recumbency on the radiographic appearance of the canine thorax. Vet Radiol 22:10–16, 1981.
8. Silverman S, Suter PF: Influence of inspiration and expiration on canine thoracic radiographs. J Am Vet Med Assoc 166:502–510, 1975.
9. Ticer JW: Radiographic Technique in Veterinary Practice. Philadelphia, W.B. Saunders, 1984, pp 275–281.

22. FELINE CARDIAC RADIOLOGY

Charles S. Farrow, B.Sc., D.V.M.

1. How does the cat's thorax differ from that of the dog?

The cat's thorax appears relatively conical compared to that of the dog when viewed in lateral perspective. Seen in the ventrodorsal or dorsoventral planes, the feline chest is more tapered cranially (see figure below).

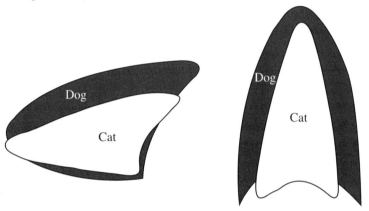

Comparative lateral (*left*) and ventrodorsal (*right*) silhouettes of the dog and cat thorax illustrate differences in both size and shape.

2. How does the cat's heart differ from that of the dog?

The cat's heart appears more tapered ventrally than that of the dog in both lateral and ventrodorsal views (see figure below). Viewed laterally, the long axis of the feline heart is inclined forward, while that of the dog is more vertically oriented.

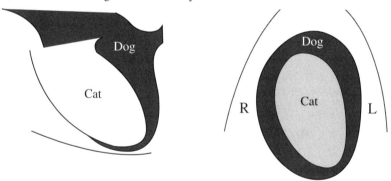

Comparative lateral (*left*) and ventrodorsal (*right*) silhouettes of the dog and cat heart illustrate differences in both size and shape.

3. Can cardiac measurement reliably predict heart enlargement in cats?

Yes. Cardiovascular measurement is an accurate means of determining heart enlargement in cats, but only provided that the standard thoracic projections used for measurement are made within close anatomic and physiologic tolerances.

4. Is the appearance of the feline heart altered by the cardiac cycle (systole/diastole)?

Yes. When the ventricles are fully filled, the heart appears larger than when partially empty—assuming one is comparing lateral thoracic images positioned identically and made during similar respiratory phases. However, in most instances the difference is comparatively small—about 5–10% depending on the heart rate. Atrial differences are harder to appreciate because of vascular and bronchial superimposition.

BIBLIOGRAPHY

1. Douglas SW, Williamson HD: Veterinary Radiological Interpretation. Philadelphia, Lea & Febiger, 1970.
2. Farrow CS: Radiology of the Cat. St. Louis, Mosby, 1994.
3. Kealy K: Diagnostic Radiology of the Dog and Cat. Philadelphia, W.B. Saunders, 1987.
4. Miller SW: Cardiac Radiology: The Requisites. St. Louis, Mosby, 1996.
5. Ticer JW: Radiographic Technique in Veterinary Practice. Philadelphia, W.B. Saunders, 1984.

23. ECHOCARDIOGRAPHY

Jonathan A. Abbott, D.V.M.

1. What is echocardiography?

Echocardiography is the medical use of ultrasound to provide information regarding cardiac structure and function. The terms echocardiography and cardiac ultrasound are synonymous.

2. What is sound? What characteristics of sound are important in diagnostic imaging?

Sound is a disturbance of a physical medium. Sound is propagated as a wave that actually represents local oscillations in air pressure. Because sound is a disturbance of a physical medium it differs from electromagnetic waves such as light in that it cannot travel through a vacuum. It is conceptually useful to portray sound as a sine wave (Fig.1). As with other waveforms, sound has a number of interrelated physical characteristics:

1. Energy
2. Frequency—the number of oscillations per unit of time; frequency is measured in cycles per second or hertz (Hz)
3. Wavelength—the distance between successive troughs or peaks in a wave
4. Velocity—the rate at which the wave travels through the medium
5. Amplitude—magnitude of the pressure changes

Sound that has a frequency between 20 and 20,000 cycles per second (Hz) is audible. Sound that has a frequency that exceeds 20,000 Hz is outside of the range of human hearing and is known as ultrasound. Diagnostic ultrasound uses sound with frequencies greater than 1,000,000 Hz (megahertz or MHz).

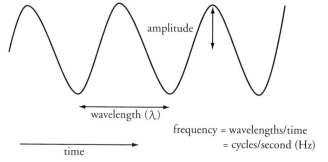

FIGURE 1. For illustration purposes, the local pressure changes that make up sound can be depicted as a sine wave. The amplitude of the wave is the magnitude of pressure chagne. The wavelength is the distance between similar points on the wave and frequency is the number of wavelengths or cycles in a given period of time. The base unit of frequency is the hertz (Hz); a single Hz is a cycle/second. The velocity of the wave is the third clinically relevant feature of sound.

3. How does ultrasound provide images of cardiac structure?

When sound strikes a boundary between media of differing density, known as acoustic interface, some of the sound is reflected and some is transmitted. It is the reflected sound, or echoes, that are used to generate image information. Because the velocity of sound in body tissues is relatively constant, the time that elapses between emission of the sound and return of the echo indicates the distance between the sound source and the echo source.

In diagnostic ultrasound, pulses of ultrasound are transmitted into the body and the returning echoes are displayed using a grayscale on a television monitor. On the resulting display, strong or high amplitude echoes are white and lower amplitude signals are various shades of gray. Fluids, such as blood, that do not reflect ultrasound are black.

4. What is a transducer?

A transducer is a device that changes one form of energy to another. In the case of echocardiography, the transducer is a piezoelectric (from the Greek *piezo* = pressure) crystal that is constructed from quartz. When the transducer is excited by electricity, it vibrates, which changes the pressure in the immediate area and therefore produces sound. When reflected sound waves strike the transducer, it again vibrates and this mechanical energy is converted to an electrical signal that is used in the production of the ultrasound image. The term transducer is often used to refer to the probe that houses the piezoelectric crystal.

5. What are the commonly used echocardiographic modalities? What distinguishes these types or modalities of echocardiography?

M-mode echocardiography is the most technologically primitive form of echocardiography. The M-mode transducer emits pulses of ultrasound within a single line. The result is a unidimensional image of the heart, sometimes known as an "icepick" view. The echoes that arise from the single line of ultrasound are presented on an oscilloscope; the information from successive ultrasound pulses is displayed before the preceding lines have decayed and the result is an image in which the x axis is time and the y axis is distance from the transducer.

Two-dimensional (2-D) echocardiography is a more recent technologic advance. The echoes that return from multiple lines of ultrasound are combined in order to create an image that has both depth (distance from the transducer) and a perpendicular, or lateral, dimension. Thus, the image is a tomographic "slice" of the region of interest. Rapid, repetitive interrogation by the transducer results in the appearance of "real-time" motion. The lines of ultrasound used to create the image can be parallel, as is the case in linear transducers, or the lines of ultrasound can be emitted in an arc producing a pie-shaped sector. Both linear and sector transducers are used in abdominal sonography while only sector transducers are employed for echocardiographic studies.

When a propagating wave is reflected from a moving object, a shift in frequency results. This frequency shift is related in a mathematical manner to the velocity of the moving object. This is known as the Doppler principle and **Doppler echocardiography** utilizes this relationship in order to determine the velocity of red blood cells. Doppler echocardiography provides information regarding the velocity, direction, and character of blood flow.

6. What are standard echocardiographic images?

With some variations, comparative studies of cardiac anatomy demonstrate great consistency; that is, with the exception of predictable differences in size, the feline heart is similar to the canine heart which is similar to the human heart. This consistency of form lends itself to the standardization of echocardiographic image planes. The standard echocardiographic images obtained in dogs and cats are derived from the images that are obtained in people. The use of standard echocardiographic images is advantageous because it provides a means of consistent and quantitative cardiac assessment.

7. What are the standard M-mode echocardiographic images?

Currently, M-mode studies are obtained by 2-D echocardiographic guidance. The three standard M-mode echocardiographic images are obtained by placing an electronic cursor through the 2-D image.

Left ventricle. This image is in a plane that is parallel to the minor axis of the left ventricle. Generally, the line of ultrasound is directed immediately ventral to the mitral valve leaflets and between the left ventricular papillary muscles. The result is an "icepick" view of the left ventricular lumen. Closest to the transducer is the right ventricle and at successively greater distances are the interventricular septum, the left ventricular lumen, and the parietal wall of the left ventricle (Fig. 2A).

Mitral valve. When the M-mode ultrasound line is directed through the center of the anterior mitral valve leaflet, a record of mitral valve motion results. In patients who are in sinus

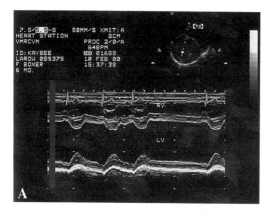

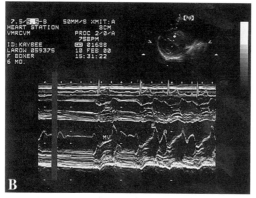

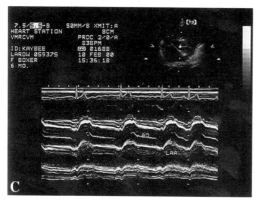

FIGURE 2. Standard M-mode echocardiographic images of a normal canine heart. *A,* M-mode echocardiogram obtained at the left ventricular level. A simultaneously recorded electrocardiogram provides a time scale. The two-dimensional image from which this M-mode was derived is shown in the inset. The echocardiographic cursor passes through the right ventricle (RV), the interventricular septum, the left ventricle (LV), and finally through the posterior or free wall of the left ventricle. The bright line adjacent to the LV posterior wall represents the pericardium. The movement of these structures during the course of the cardiac cycle is evident; the interventricular septum and left ventricular free wall move toward each other immediately following each QRS. Note that mechanical systole is typically bounded by the R and the end of the T wave of the electrocardiogram. *B,* M-mode echocardiogram obtained at the level of the mitral valve. The two-dimensional image from which this M-mode was derived is shown in the inset. The anterior mitral valve leaflet traces an M-shape. During early diastole (E) the leaflet moves toward the interventricular septum. The A-point (A) is the result of atrial contraction. *C,* M-mode echocardiogram obtained at the aortic level. The aorta (Ao) and the left atrial appendage (LAA) are labeled. The two-dimensional image from which this M-mode was derived is shown in the inset.

rhythm the anterior leaflet traces an M shape that demonstrates the biphasic motion of the normal mitral leaflets. In early diastole, during rapid ventricular filling, the anterior leaflet moves toward the septum. During diastasis, the atrioventricular pressure difference lessens and the leaflet returns to a partially open configuration. Atrial contraction in late diastole is responsible for the second peak of mitral valve motion. Generally, the posterior mitral valve leaflet is visualized less well than the anterior leaflet but its motion mirrors that of the anterior leaflet (Fig. 2B).

Aortic root. The third standard M-mode image is obtained when the line of ultrasound passes through the aortic root and then through the left atrial appendage (Fig. 2C).

FIGURE 3. Standard 2-D echocardiographic images obtained from the right parasternal transducer position (long axis views). RA, right atrium; RV, right ventricle; LA, left atrium; LV, left ventricle; TV, tricuspid valve; MV, mitral valve; LVW, left ventricular wall; PM, papillary muscle; CH, chorda tenidnea; VS, interventricular septum; LC, left coronary aortic cusp. (From Thomas WP, Gaber CE, Jacobs GJ: Recommendations for standards in transthoracic two-dimensional echocardiography in the dog and cat: Echocardiography Committee of the Specialty of Cardiology, American College of Veterinary Internal Medicine. J Vet Intern Med 7:247–252, 1993, with permission.)

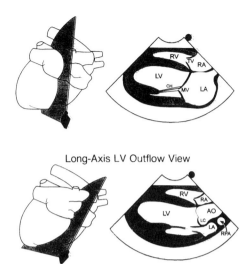

Long-Axis LV Outflow View

8. What are the standard 2-D echocardiographic images?

The standard 2-D echocardiographic images are obtained using both left and right parasternal transducer positions (Figs. 3 and 4). From the right parasternal transducer position, the heart is imaged in both the short (or cross-sectional) axis and the longitudinal, or long, axis. Thus, as an example, an image could be described as a right parasternal short axis image at the level of the heart base. The apical images and cranial images of the aorta, pulmonary artery, and right atrium are obtained using the left parasternal transducer position.

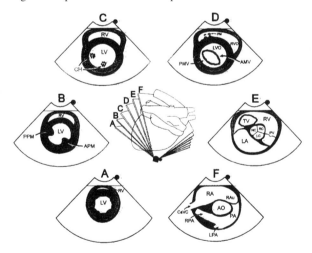

FIGURE 4. Standard 2-D echocardiographic images obtained from the right parasternal transducer position (short axis views). RA, right atrium; RAu, right auricle; RV, right ventricle; RVO, right ventricular outflow; LA, left atrium; LV, left ventricle; TV, tricuspid valve; AMV, anterior mitral valve cusp; PMV, posterior mitral valve cusp; LVW, left ventricular wall; PPM, posterior papillary muscle; APM, anterior papillary muscle; CH, chorda tendinea; VS, interventricular septum; LC, left coronary aortic cusp; NC, noncoronary aortic cusp; RC, right coronary aortic cusp; LPA, left pulmonary artery; RPA, right pulmonary artery. (From Thomas WP, Gaber CE, Jacobs GJ: Recommendations for standards in transthoracic two-dimensional echocardiography in the dog and cat: Echocardiography Committee of the Specialty of Cardiology, American College of Veterinary Internal Medicine. J Vet Intern Med 7:247–252, 1993, with permission.)

9. How is Doppler information displayed?

The Doppler echocardiograph determines the velocity and direction of red blood cells. In the case of spectral Doppler, this velocity information is displayed graphically; the horizontal axis is time and the vertical is velocity. By convention, blood flow toward the transducer is shown above an operator-determined baseline; blood flow away from the transducer is assigned a negative velocity and is below the baseline. Doppler velocity information can also be encoded as color pixels superimposed upon a 2-D or M-mode echocardiographic image. Color-flow Doppler provides a noninvasive angiogram of sorts; it is a visual representation of blood flow in relation to the structural 2-D image. The BART convention—blue away, red toward relative to the transducer—is in nearly universal use. Shades of red or blue indicate progressively higher velocities and make up what is known as a color map.

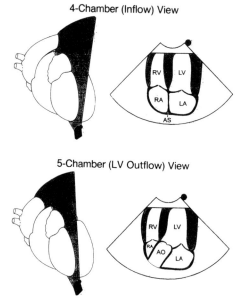

FIGURE 5. Standard 2-D echocardiographic images obtained from the left caudal parasternal transducer position. AS, atrial septum; RA, right atrium; RV, right ventricle; LA, left atrium; LV, left ventricle; AO, aorta. (From Thomas WP, Gaber CE, Jacobs GJ: Recommendations for standards in transthoracic two-dimensional echocardiography in the dog and cat: Echocardiography Committee of the Specialty of Cardiology, American College of Veterinary Internal Medicine. J Vet Intern Med 7:247–252, 1993, with permission.)

10. What is spectral Doppler?

Doppler velocity data is contained in the frequency shift that results when ultrasound is reflected from moving red cells. A computer algorithm known as the fast Fourier transform (FFT) is used to separate the components of the complex sound wave that returns to the transducer. The use of FFT for this purpose is a form of spectral analysis and it is the basis of the spectral Doppler techniques—pulsed- and continuous-wave Doppler. The velocity information provided by spectral Doppler is displayed graphically.

The pulsed-wave Doppler technique employs a single piezoelectric crystal that emits and receives ultrasound. The instrument emits ultrasound in pulses; analysis of the frequency-shifted echo is performed before the next pulse is emitted. Because the speed of sound within the body is roughly constant, the time required for the echo to return to the transducer is determined by the depth of the reflecting red cells. Control of the delay between pulse emission echo analyses specifies the anatomic location of the echo source. This ability to localize red cell movement to specific anatomic regions is referred to as range-gate specificity. Pulsed-wave Doppler therefore provides velocity information from within a distinct anatomic region; this anatomic region is known as the sample volume. The sample volume is displayed as a circle or bar on an electronic cursor and the cursor can be manipulated by the operator using a roller ball or toggle stick. Movement of the sample volume determines the time period the instrument waits before analyzing returning echoes.

Continuous-wave Doppler employs two piezoelectric crystals; one of them continuously transits ultrasound while the other receives the returning echoes. Continuous-wave Doppler lacks the property of range-gate specificity; it provides a display of the maximum Doppler shift or velocity that occurs within the linear domain of the ultrasound beam (Fig. 6).

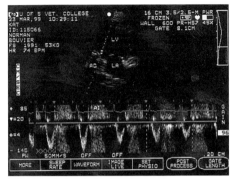 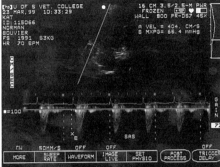

FIGURE 6. Pulsed-wave Doppler study of the left ventricular outflow tract of a dog with subvalvular aortic stenosis. As can be seen in the 2-D image *(left)*, the pulsed-wave sample volume, indicated by the two heavy lines on the cursor, is beneath the aortic valve. In systole, there is an "envelope" below the baseline indicating flow away from the transducer and into the aorta. The peak velocity of the systolic jet is close to 145 cm/s (the scale is shown on the ordinate). During diastole, a broad spectral signal indicates aortic valve incompetence (AI); because the velocity of the AI jet exceeds the Nyquist velocity of the instrument, directional ambiguity (aliasing) results. *Right,* "Mapping" of the aorta with pulsed-wave Doppler demonstrated an increase in systolic flow velocity just beneath the aortic valve; the velocity exceeded the Nyquist limit and aliasing was evident. A continuous-wave Doppler study of the left ventricular outflow revealed a peak systolic flow velocity of about 400 cm/s. Continuous-wave Doppler lacks range-gate specificity, so the anatomic site of the peak velocity cannot be determined from this image alone; however, the continuous-wave study does correctly ascertain the direction of the high-velocity jet. As it happens, the peak systolic aortic velocity was not obtained in the same plane as the AI jet and the aortic valve incompetence is not evident from the continuous-wave image.

11. What is aliasing?

Aliasing is a phenomenon of directional ambiguity that complicates the interpretation of pulsed Doppler studies; it results when the frequency of a periodic motion exceeds one-half the sampling rate. Aliasing is most easily understood through the use of an analogy.

Cinematic film is actually a series of separate, consecutively recorded photographs. When cinematic film is viewed through a projector, rapid display of the individual photographs provides the illusion of uninterrupted motion. In the case of cinefilm, the frame rate of the film, or the rate at which moving objects are photographed, is the sampling rate. If the clockwise rotation of a wheel, say on a bus or wagon, is viewed using cinefilm, the wheel appears to move backward if the frame rate of the film is less than twice the frequency of revolution of the wheel. This is because the wheel moves through greater than one half of a revolution between frames; in that time, a point at 12 o'clock on the wheel might make it to the 10-o'clock position. The point is unconsciously assumed to have taken the most direct route possible and consequently the direction of rotation is perceived to be counterclockwise.

Pulsed Doppler technologies, which include both spectral pulsed-wave Doppler and color-flow Doppler, are both subject to aliasing. The sampling rate of the pulsed Doppler instrument is known as the pulse repetition frequency, which is determined by the design of the transducer and the depth of interrogation. When the Doppler frequency shift is greater than one half the pulse repetition frequency, aliasing results. In spectral Doppler, the signal "wraps around" the graphic display and the displayed direction of flow is incorrect (see figure above). The same kind of directional ambiguity results when color-flow Doppler is used to evaluate high-velocity flow.

12. Are both pulsed-wave and continuous-wave Doppler necessary?

Pulsed-wave and continuous-wave Doppler provide information that is distinct but complementary. Pulsed-wave studies have the advantage of providing anatomic localization of flow; blood flow velocities can be determined from specific regions within the heart or vascular system. However, pulsed-wave instruments are subject to aliasing. In contrast, aliasing does not occur with the use of continuous-wave Doppler, but this modality lacks range-gate specificity. The freedom from aliasing is important because the velocity of pathologic blood flow is commonly supraphysiologic and beyond the range of pulsed-wave instruments. Typically, pulsed-wave Doppler or color-flow Doppler (which is a pulsed-wave technology) are used to localize flow disturbances; for example, the disturbed flow immediately distal to an aortic stenosis lesion. Although precise diagnostic criteria are lacking, most believe that anatomic aortic stenosis is defined by velocities that exceed 2 m/s and this velocity is greater than the Nyquist limit, or velocity at which aliasing occurs, of most pulsed-wave instruments. Thus, continuous-wave Doppler is then required to determine the peak velocity of the jet.

13. What is the role of quantitative 2-D or M-mode echocardiography?

The use of conventional, or standard, echocardiographic images lends itself to the quantitative assessment of cardiac chamber size and cardiac performance. In dogs, measurements of cardiac chamber size are for the most part related to body weight or body surface area. Most cats are about the same size and there is little correlation between echocardiographic variables and body weight in this species. Clinically important cardiac disease usually results in enlargement of one or more of the cardiac chambers. Thus, the assessment of cardiac size is the one of the primary uses of echocardiography.

The imposition of mechanical overload results in myocardial hypertrophy, or an increase in muscle mass. Volume overloads resulting from valvular incompetence or shunts cause dilation and hypertrophy; this is known as eccentric hypertrophy. In contrast, a pressure overload such as that which results from outflow tract stenosis causes hypertrophy without appreciable dilation or concentric hypertrophy. Thus, the echocardiographic appearance of concentric hypertrophy is characterized by an increase in diastolic ventricular wall thickness that can be demonstrated quantitatively. In contrast, eccentric hypertrophy results in enlargement of the diastolic chamber dimension, which is accompanied by a roughly proportional increase in wall thickness.

14. How is M-mode or 2-D echocardiography used to assess systolic myocardial function?

Most properly, systolic myocardial *function* or contractility is a load-independent quantity that is practically impossible to measure in the living animal. However, echocardiographic parameters of systolic *performance* provide clinically useful indices of contractility.

Most of the echocardiographic measures of systolic performance are ejection phase indices; they quantify the extent or rate of ventricular shortening. The difference between the end-systolic and end-diastolic ventricular volume expressed as a percentage of the end-diastolic volume is known as the ejection fraction (EF). The calculation of EF requires the echocardiographic estimation of ventricular volumes. Numerous formulas, all of which are imperfect, have been proposed for this purpose. Other means of assessing systolic ventricular performance include the fractional shortening, the velocity of circumferential shortening, fractional systolic thickening of the ventricular septum or posterior wall, and systolic time intervals such as ejection time and pre-ejection period.

15. What is the fractional shortening?

In veterinary echocardiography, the fractional shortening (FS) is the most widely used index of systolic function. It is calculated using the following equation:

$$FS = LVED - LVES/LVED$$

where LVED is the end-diastolic minor dimension of the left ventricle and LVES is the end-systolic minor dimension of the left ventricle. Most often, the left ventricular FS is obtained using M-mode echocardiography, although it can also be obtained by freezing the 2-D image at end-diastole and then at end-systole. For M-mode studies, it is convention that the end-diastolic dimension is obtained at the time the R wave is inscribed on a simultaneously recorded electrocardiogram; end-systole is taken as the time of maximal septal excursion.

The FS is similar to the EF; however, because it is derived from linear measurements it is free of the geometric assumptions that underlie the echocardiographic estimation of cardiac volumes. The FS in healthy dogs is usually about 30% (with a range of 27–45%). The FS in most healthy cats is somewhat higher, often closer to 50% (with a range of 32–65%).

16. What are the limitations of FS in evaluating systolic function?

Correct interpretation of the FS requires an understanding of its limitations. These limitations relate to both methodology and difficulties that are inherent in the use of ejection phase indices of systolic function. With regards to the latter, fractional shortening is highly dependent on afterload. This means that fractional shortening tends to be low when afterload is high. However, the effect of reduced afterload is probably of greater clinical importance. In patients with substantial mitral valve regurgitation (MR), afterload is low in relation to ventricular size. In effect, it is "easy" to eject blood into the low-impedance reservoir provided by the left atrium. In consequence, the FS is typically high in patients that have MR and normal systolic function. The finding of a low or even a normal SF in patients with MR suggests diminished contractility. Ejection phase indices are also affected by changes in preload although this tends to be of lesser clinical importance than the effect of afterload as described above.

Consideration must also be given to the method used to derive the SF. Most often, the SF is calculated from measurements obtained from M-mode images. It must be recognized that the M-mode image is a unidimensional view; therefore, a diminished SF does not necessarily reflect global cardiac performance and may result from regional wall motion abnormalities.

17. What about diastolic function?

The role played by diastolic function in cardiac performance is less easily understood than the role of systolic function. The ability of the ventricles to fill at low diastolic pressures depends on both the active, energy-requiring process of myocardial relaxation and on a mechanical property of the heart known as compliance. Diastolic function is very difficult to quantify. Analysis of the pulsed-wave Doppler mitral valve inflow signal can provide potentially useful information regarding diastolic ventricular performance. When the heart rate is less than about 150 bpm, ventricular filling is biphasic. In early diastole blood enters the ventricle, which results in the Doppler "E" wave. Flow through the atrioventricular valve slows until atrial contraction results in the "A" wave. Doppler-derived measurement of the duration of the isovolumic relaxation time, the deceleration rate of early diastolic filling, and the ratio of E and A wave velocities are all means by which to evaluate diastolic performance. Unfortunately, the use of these velocities and intervals are limited by a dependence on heart rate and cardiac loading conditions.

Echocardiographic imaging studies can provide a rough but clinically useful index of diastolic function. When diastolic dysfunction is present, diastolic ventricular pressures are high when ventricular volume is normal or small. This high diastolic pressure is reflected upon the left atrium, potentially resulting in atrial enlargement. In the absence of systolic dysfunction, atrial enlargement that is disproportionate to ventricular volume implies a decrease in ventricular compliance. For example, patients with severe hypertrophic cardiomyopathy typically have a normal or small left ventricular lumen, normal or hyperdynamic systolic performance, and left atrial dilation.

18. Do Doppler studies also provide quantitative information?

Doppler echocardiography provides precise determinations of flow velocity. In addition to measures of systolic and diastolic performance, this information can be used to quantify both flow and pressure differences within the circulation. The estimation of pressure differences, or gradients, across obstructive lesions is one of the most important applications of Doppler echocardiography. When a cardiac inflow or outflow tract is abnormally narrow, high pressures must be generated in order to maintain flow through the resistive orifice. In aortic stenosis, for example, it is necessary for the left ventricle to generate abnormally high pressures during systole in order to maintain normal systemic perfusion and pressure. As a result, there is a pressure gradient across the outflow tract and this gradient is a clinically useful measure of stenosis severity.

Pressure gradients across short-segment stenoses are related to poststenotic flow velocities by the Bernoulli equation. This complex expression accounts for factors that include convective acceleration and viscous friction. Fortunately, for clinical purposes the Bernoulli equation can be simplified to:

$$\Delta P = 4v^2$$

where ΔP is the pressure gradient and v is the postobstructive velocity. The velocity is measured by Doppler and the gradient is estimated using the modified Bernoulli equation above. In outflow tract stenosis, gradients less than 40 mmHg are generally considered to be mild, those between 40 and 80 moderate, and those greater than 80 or 100 mmHg severe. The estimation of pressure gradients is one of the most important applications of Doppler echocardiography and this use of the technology is one of the main reasons that noninvasive echocardiographic study has nearly replaced cardiac catheterization in the evaluation of patients with congenital heart disease.

19. How is a diagnosis of stenosis made by Doppler?

Flow velocities within the heart and great vessels of normal dogs have been published. Flow velocities in cats are comparable, but usually somewhat lower. When stenosis is present, flow velocity increases at the narrowed orifice. Therefore, flow velocities that are higher than normal suggest the presence of obstruction. However, it must be recognized that high flow through a normal vessel such as that which occurs in shunts or high cardiac-output states will also result in high flow-velocities. For example, right ventricular stroke volume is large when a clinically important atrial septal defect is present and, as a result, pulmonary artery flow velocities are high in the absence of pulmonic stenosis. Therefore, the diagnosis of stenosis requires documentation of abnormally high velocities and a discrete velocity increase at the level of the stenosis.

20. How is flow quantified by Doppler echocardiography?

The spectral Doppler display is a graph that relates flow velocity to time. The integral of the velocity-time curve generated during a single cardiac cycle provides a measure known as stroke distance. Multiplication of the stroke distance by the area of the vessel from which the stroke distance was obtained gives a measure of the stroke volume. The accuracy of flow quantification is limited by the accuracy of the vessel area measurement and the technique of volumetric flow quantification is not in common clinical use.

21. What is the utility of the imaging echocardiographic modalities?

The imaging modalities such as 2-D echocardiography and M-mode echocardiography provide a pictorial representation of cardiac structure; specifically, the appearance of the cardiac chambers, the valvular apparatus, and the pericardial space can be evaluated. The information provided by the imaging modalities allows inferences to be made regarding cardiac function. Systolic ventricular performance can be quantified using indices such as shortening fraction. Diastolic performance of the heart is difficult to quantify, but the finding of atrial enlargement that is disproportionate to diastolic ventricular size suggests diastolic dysfunction.

When compared to plain radiography, the echocardiographic imaging modalities have some obvious advantages. The cardiac silhouette seen radiographically is simply that, a silhouette; it is not possible to accurately distinguish the individual cardiac chambers. In contrast, the cardiac septae and the pericardial space are clearly visible using 2-D echocardiography and they can be measured with an accuracy that is not possible using plain radiographic studies. It should, however, be recognized that thoracic radiographs can provide information regarding the appearance of the lung, airways, and pulmonary vessels that cannot be obtained by echocardiographic study. The information provided by echocardiography and radiography is therefore distinct but complementary.

22. What is the utility of color-flow Doppler?

The primary use of color-flow Doppler is the detection of flow disturbances. When nearby cells move in different directions at high and disparate velocities, the juxtaposition of multiple, differently colored pixels results in a color-flow "mosaic" and this mosaic indicates the presence of disturbed ("turbulent") flow. Because turbulence has an exact mathematical definition, some prefer the use of "disturbed flow" to describe nonlaminar blood flow. The use of variance color-flow maps provides an alternative means to detect disturbed flow; however, the algorithms used to assign a "turbulent color," which is usually green, are not without limitations.

Again, the detection of pathologic flow disturbances is the primary clinical use of color-flow Doppler. For example, the appearance of a color-flow mosaic within the left atrium during systole indicates mitral valve regurgitation. Other examples of flow disturbances include the detection of high-velocity shunt flow across a ventricular septal defect or the detection of a diastolic flow disturbance beneath the aortic valve, indicating aortic valve regurgitation.

23. What is transesophageal echocardiography?

Transesophageal echocardiography (TEE) is a relatively new echocardiographic technique that employs a transducer that is incorporated into a flexible endoscope. The instrument is manipulated within the esophagus in order to provide echocardiographic images and Doppler data. The esophagus and stomach are closely associated with the heart and consequently there is little attenuation of sound energy. Thus, high-frequency transducers can be employed and the resolution of TEE is excellent. TEE has seen relatively little use in veterinary medicine in part due to the expense of the endoscopic probes and the need for general anesthesia prior to examination.

BIBLIOGRAPHY

1. Brown DJ, Knight DH, King RR: Pulsed-wave Doppler echocardiography to determine aortic and pulmonary velocities and flow variables in clinically normal dogs. Am J Vet Res 52:543–550, 1991.
2. DeMadron E, Bonagura JD, Herring DS: Two-dimensional echocardiography in the normal cat. Vet Radiol 26:149–158, 1985.
3. Feigenbaum H: Echocardiography, 5th ed. Philadelphia, Lea & Febiger, 1994.
4. Goldberg SJ, Allen HD, Marx GR, Donnerstein RL: Doppler Echocardiography, 2nd ed. Philadelphia, Lea & Febiger, 1988.
5. Jacobs G, Knight DH: Change in M-mode echocardiographic values in cats given ketamine. Am J Vet Res 46:1712–1713, 1985.
6. Lombard CW: Normal values of the canine M-mode echocardiogram. Am J Vet Res 45:2015–2018, 1984.
7. Moise NS, Fox PR: Echocardiography and Doppler imaging. In Fox PR, Sisson D, Moise NS (eds): Textbook of Canine and Feline Cardiology: Principles and Clinical Practice, 2nd ed. Philadelphia, W.B. Saunders, 1999, pp 130–172.
8. Moise NS: Echocardiography: Therapeutic implications. In Kirk RW (ed): Current Veterinary Therapy X: Small Animal Practice. Philadelphia, W.B. Saunders, 1989.
9. O'Grady MR: Quantitative cross-sectional echocardiography in the normal dog. Vet Radiol 27:34–49, 1986.
10. Thomas WP: Two-dimensional real-time echocardiography in the dog: Technique and anatomic validation. Vet Radiol 25:50–64, 1984.
11. Thomas WP, Gaber CE, Jacobs GJ: Recommendations for standards in transthoracic two-dimensional echocardiography in the dog and cat: Echocardiography Committee of the Specialty of Cardiology, American College of Veterinary Internal Medicine. J Vet Intern Med 7:247–252, 1993.
12. Weyman AE (ed): Principles and Practice of Echocardiography, 2nd ed. Philadelphia, Lea & Febiger, 1994.

24. CARDIAC CATHETERIZATION

Carl D. Sammarco, B.V.Sc., MRCVS

1. Why is cardiac catheterization done?

Cardiac catheterization fulfills both a diagnostic and therapeutic role. Although the advent of echocardiography has decreased the need for diagnostic catheterization, cardiac catheterization remains important in the definition of several cardiovascular diseases. The invasive nature of catheterization is a disadvantage of this procedure.

Diagnostic uses of cardiac catheterization include selective angiography, pressure studies, selective blood gases, oximetry and measurement of cardiac output. In dogs, congenital heart disease and left-to-right shunts may be better documented with angiography and selective blood gases or oximetry than with echocardiography. Catheterization may add useful information to a presurgical work-up prior to cardiopulmonary bypass and cardiac surgery. Although the information gleaned is not vital for every patient with cardiac disease, it can be useful in certain patients for diagnosis and guiding therapy. Therapeutic cardiac catheterization procedures include patent ductus arteriosus (PDA) closure, balloon valvuloplasty, and temporary and permanent cardiac pacing.

2. How is cardiac catheterization done?

Arterial and venous catheterization can be performed percutaneously or via a cut-down over the vessels. The carotid artery, femoral artery, jugular vein, and femoral vein are commonly used for catheter access. The jugular vein, femoral artery, and femoral vein are accessible by percutaneous approach, while the carotid artery requires surgical cut-down for catheter placement.

Percutaneous catheterization can be performed under local anesthesia, with or without light sedation. The area is surgically prepared, and access to the vessel is achieved using a modification of the Seldinger technique. This requires a needle and guide wire. The needle is placed percutaneously into the vessel. The wire is then advanced into the vessel through the needle. The needle is removed and a catheter or a commercially available introducer/sheath system can be fed over the wire and into the blood vessel. Most vascular sheath/introducers are large French (4–16), and have a hemostatic valve on them. This allows a catheter to be fed through the vessel sheath, which prevents bleeding around the catheter when multiple catheters are used and also reduces trauma to the vessel. At the end of the procedure the sheath can be removed and pressure applied to the vessel, allowing preservation of the vessel. Introducer/sheath systems can also be used if a cut-down is performed, in order to facilitate multiple catheterizations.

The right heart is catheterized via the femoral vein or jugular vein. From the jugular vein, the catheter is passed down the cranial vena cava into the right atrium. The catheter can be advanced through the tricuspid valve into the right ventricle and out into the pulmonary artery. Use of balloon-tipped catheters along with guide wires facilitates passing catheters out into the pulmonary artery, especially if cardiac disease is present. Low cardiac output, tricuspid regurgitation, right ventricular hypertrophy, and pulmonic and tricuspid stenosis could obstruct to advancement of the catheter. The right jugular vein is more commonly used to avoid problems associated with the presence of a persistent left cranial vena cava. If using the left jugular and a left cranial vena cava is present, it may be difficult to advance the catheter across the tricuspid valve because embryology dictates that a left cranial vena cava empties into the coronary venous drainage and not directly into the right atrium. Persistent left cranial vena cava is rare in dogs, but is seen with a higher frequency in dogs with other congenital cardiac anomalies. If the right heart is catheterized from the femoral vein, the catheter is fed up the caudal vena cava and into the right atrium. From here on the procedure is similar to the one described above.

The left heart is catheterized from the common carotid or the femoral artery. In either approach, the catheter is fed into the aorta and across the aortic valve into the left ventricle.

Advancing the catheter into the left atrium from the ventricle is difficult and not often attempted. In human patients, catheterization of the left atrium or mitral valve is achieved via a right heart approach, and a special catheter is then used to cross the atrial septum from the right atrium into the left atrium.

3. What is the difference between selective and nonselective angiography?

A selective angiogram is performed to highlight a specific area of interest. For example, if subaortic stenosis is suspected or needs to be evaluated, an injection of contrast is made with the catheter placed just below the aortic valve or in the left ventricular outflow tract.

A nonselective angiogram is performed by injecting contrast agent in a peripheral vein. It has the advantages of being less invasive, quicker, and less expensive. Anesthesia is not typically required, and no special equipment is needed. Nonselective studies can be performed using static radiographs, although fluoroscopy with video capability is useful. The disadvantages of nonselective studies are superimposition of contrast in several chambers and vessels and decreased visualization of the left side of the heart. Contrast agent injected into a vein will eventually reach the pulmonary veins, left atrium, left ventricle, and aorta (known as the levophase). Dilution of the contrast occurs at this phase, decreasing opacification and the ability to identify structures and defects on the left side of the heart. Placing a catheter into the pulmonary artery and performing the injection in a distal pulmonary artery branch can minimize the dilution effect. This selective, distal pulmonary artery angiogram can sometimes save the need to perform a left heart catheterization.

Selective angiography requires special long catheters (70–150 cm) and usually a high-pressure injector in order to get good results. Fluoroscopy is useful for proper placement of catheters. Typically, the catheter tip is placed just proximal to the area of interest. Many different catheter types are available depending on the study. For instance, subaortic stenosis could be evaluated by placing a pigtail catheter (see figure below) into the aorta and across the valve into the left ventricle. The approach can be from the femoral or the carotid artery. Pulmonic stenosis can be evaluated by placing an angiographic catheter via the jugular or femoral vein, through the right atrium and into the right ventricle. A very dense contrast agent is commonly used in order to achieve good opacification. Available contrast agents include Hypaque-76 (370 mg/ml of organically bound iodine, 66% diatrizoate meglumine, 10% diatrizoate sodium, distributed by Nycomed, Princeton, NJ) and Oxilan-350 (350 mg/ml of organically bound iodine, 73% ioxilan, distributed by Cook Imaging Corporation, Bloomington, IN).

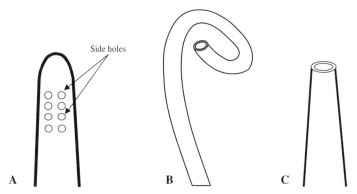

A, Angiographic catheter; *B,* pigtail catheter; *C,* End-hole catheter.

4. What type of case is a good candidate for angiography?

Angiography is especially useful for evaluating dogs with congenital heart disease. If complicated malformations are present or if left-to-right shunting (atrial septal defect [ASD] or ventricular septal defect [VSD]) is suspected, angiography may add information where echocardiography is limited. Small VSDs and ASDs that are shunting left to right may be difficult to demonstrate with echocardiography. Dogs with pulmonic stenosis need angiography as part of their evaluation prior to balloon valvuloplasty. The angiogram further delineates the extent of disease, and can be used as a means of determining the appropriate balloon size.

Angiography is essential prior to coil embolization in dogs with patent ductus arteriosus. Angiography is used to measure the size and position of the duct. This information is vital for determining the coil size and for deploying the coil in the appropriate area of the duct.

Angiography is an important part of the presurgical work-up for corrective congenital heart surgery. Inflow occlusion technique and cardiopulmonary bypass are currently performed at several veterinary centers. Corrective surgery for severe pulmonic stenosis, double-outlet right ventricle, subaortic stenosis, tetralogy of Fallot, large ASD, and VSDs are successfully completed at these centers.

5. How is trans-catheter patent ductus arteriosus occlusion done?

PDA closure is achieved by placing a catheter in the PDA from either the right or left side and deploying an occlusion device. The device used currently is an embolization coil. The coil is made of stainless steel with attached synthetic fibers. The fibers are thrombogenic and result in clot formation within the duct. The coil is packaged in a thin metal tube that allows it to be passed into a catheter. An angiogram just prior to deployment outlines the anatomy of the duct and assists in determining appropriate coil size. Several techniques have been described; in one of them, the coil is fed through a thin-walled catheter using a soft straight wire (see figure below). The duct can be approached from either the pulmonary artery or the aorta. The catheter is placed in the duct with fluoroscopic guidance. After deployment of the coil, clot formation will occur within 10–15 minutes. A repeat angiogram is performed to rule out any residual shunting. If significant shunting is present, additional coils can be placed.

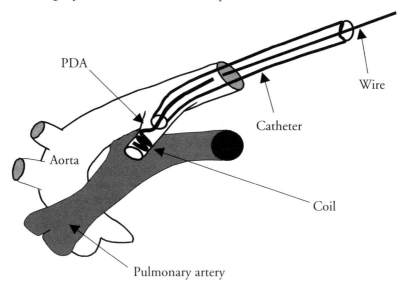

Technique of feeding a coil through a thin-walled catheter using a soft straight wire.

6. How is balloon valvuloplasty performed?

In patients with stenotic valves, a balloon can be placed across the valve and expanded in an attempt to open or relieve the obstruction. Valves with fused leaflets appear to be more amenable to valvuloplasty than hypoplastic orifices or obstruction due to a fibrous ring. In many pulmonic stenosis patients, the stenosis is purely valvular and balloon dilation is often rewarding. Work is currently in progress to test the efficacy of this procedure for relief of subaortic stenosis. Mitral and tricuspid stenosis are amenable to valvuloplasty, but these defects are very rare. Since valvuloplasty for pulmonic stenosis is the most common procedure performed, it will be described as an example.

The procedure is performed under general anesthesia. The pressure gradient across the valve is determined with an end-hole catheter. The pressure is first measured in the pulmonary artery, then the catheter is pulled back into the right ventricle to establish the right ventricular pressure. The gradient across the valve is calculated. An angiogram is rendered to determine the balloon size required to dilate the stenotic lesion. Pulmonic valvuloplasty can be accomplished by feeding a balloon from a peripheral vein (jugular or femoral), through the right atrium and ventricle, into the right outflow tract and pulmonary artery. Typically, balloon catheters are less flexible and need the help of a guide wire to pass them into the right ventricle.

Initially, an end-hole catheter is fed into a distal pulmonary artery using fluoroscopic guidance. A long guide wire is then fed down the end-hole catheter into the pulmonary artery. The distal end of the wire is left in the pulmonary artery and the pressure catheter is removed in exchange for the valvuloplasty catheter. The balloon is situated at the site of the stenosis and rapidly filled with diluted contrast material in order to tear the pulmonic valve. The balloon first has an "hourglass" appearance on fluoroscopy, and as the obstruction is torn open by pressure from the balloon, the balloon inflates fully (see figure below).

Following valvuloplasty, the pressure gradient is measured again to determine the physiologic effectiveness of the procedure. The pressure gradient can decrease due to myocardial depression from anesthesia and from hypoxia during the inflation of the balloon. Therefore, more accurate evaluation of the reduction in pressure will be determined 4–6 weeks postoperatively, when full recovery from the procedure has occurred. This is typically evaluated by echocardiogram. Dogs with hypoplastic pulmonary arteries and dysplastic-thickened valves may not benefit from valvuloplasty over the long term because return of the gradient following balloon procedure commonly occurs. Restenosis and ineffective dilation are possible reasons for the return of the gradient.

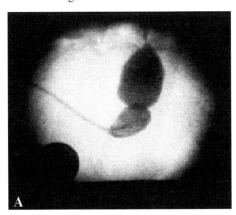 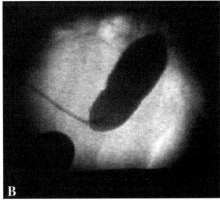

Fluoroscopy images during balloon valvulopasty. *A,* The balloon with diluted contrast agent is being inflated at the pulmonic valve. The stenotic valve causes the waist in the balloon. Note hourglass appearance. *B,* The balloon has popped to full dimension after further filling under pressure. A tiny waist still appears.

7. How are temporary and permanent pacemaker leads placed?

A temporary pacemaker lead is a special catheter with electrodes on the tip that is placed into the right ventricle. Typically, the right side is approached using a percutaneous introducer in the jugular or the femoral vein. The temporary pacing lead is fed into the right ventricle using fluoroscopic guidance. An ECG can also be used to detect the correct advancement of the pacing lead, but the fluoroscopic technique tends to be quicker. Once the lead is in the right ventricle, a pacing device is hooked onto the external end of the catheter to allow electronic stimulation and pacing. Temporary pacing is commonly established in the awake patient prior to placement of a permanent pacemaker in patients that are at risk for asystole under anesthesia (sick sinus syndrome, AV block). Since a temporary pacemaker can be placed in an awake animal with minimal sedation, there is less risk for anesthesia-induced asystole. Permanent pacing lead placement requires surgical sterility and this may be difficult to maintain in patients that are awake.

Permanent transvenous pacing leads are usually placed under general anesthesia. A cutdown over the jugular vein is performed after surgical preparation of the skin. The lead is fed down the jugular and through the right atrium into the right ventricle. There are several different types of lead tips available to assure fixation of the lead in the ventricle. Screw-tip leads and tined leads (barbed like a grappling hook) are the more common types. The external end of the lead is then hooked into a small implantable pulse generator, which is placed into a pocket surgically created under the neck muscles. Alternatively, the lead can be fed subcutaneously over the shoulder and placed under the cutaneous trunci muscles on the thorax or under the external oblique muscles on the flank. Occasionally, a second lead is fed down the same vein and placed in the right atrium. The second lead allows for dual chamber pacing and can be useful for young, active dogs. This requires a pacemaker that can take two leads and perform dual chamber pacing.

8. What are the normal pressures in the cardiovascular system?
The ranges are shown in the table below. Diagram of the heart (see figure below) shows easier to remember average systolic, diastolic, and mean (in parentheses) numbers.

LOCATION	SYSTOLIC/DIASTOLIC (MEAN)
Aorta	95–150/70–100 (80–110)
Left ventricle (LV)	120/< 10
Left atrium	5–12/< 8 (< 10)
Pulmonary artery	15–30/5–15 (8–20)
Right ventricle (RV)	15–30/< 5
Right atrium (RA)	4–6/< 4 (2–5)

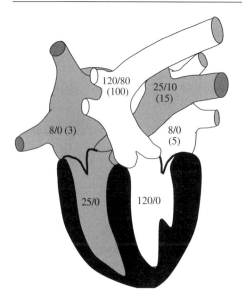

Diagram of the heart showing average systolic, diastolic, and mean (in parentheses) normal pressures in the cardiovascular system.

9. When is cardiac catheterization for pressure studies indicated?

Cardiac catheterization for measuring pressures can be useful in several case scenarios. Pressure catheters are typically 70–150 cm in length and can have single or multiple lumens. The simplest catheters will have a single lumen with the opening at the distal tip of the catheter. Many of these will have a balloon at the tip to help guide a catheter through the venous system. An inflated balloon helps a catheter "float downstream." Right heart catheterization can be performed to evaluate right-sided pressures and pulmonary wedge pressure.

Pulmonary wedge pressure is obtained by feeding a balloon-tipped pressure catheter via a peripheral vein, through the right atrium and ventricle, out into the pulmonary artery, and further out to a peripheral pulmonary artery branch. The balloon is inflated and "wedged" to eliminate proximal pressures. The open end of the catheter tip now communicates via a static column of blood with the pulmonary veins and left atrium (see figure below). The pulmonary wedge pressure is a clinically useful estimate of left atrial pressure. An elevated pulmonary wedge pressure would support a diagnosis of congestive heart failure. Once left atrial pressure is known using a pulmonary artery catheter, the wedge pressure can be monitored for effectiveness of therapy. Patients with chronic valve disease or dilated cardiomyopathy will have elevated left atrial pressures with active congestive heart failure.

Right heart catheters can be effective tools in monitoring the critically ill patient. Monitoring cardiac output, oxygen delivery, oxygen extraction, and pulmonary wedge pressures can help determine the effectiveness of therapy in patients with shock or cardiovascular compromise. Pulmonary artery catheters can be used to measure the oxygen saturation in the blood, either directly, using expensive oximetry tipped catheters, or by taking periodic blood gas samples from the catheter while the tip is in the pulmonary artery. Cardiac output can be measured with special catheters with thermistors (temperature-sensitive probes) that will derive the cardiac output using a modification of the Fick principle when a bolus of saline is given through the catheter. The cardiac output and arterial blood gas can be used to calculate oxygen delivery and extraction. In a patient with poor perfusion, the tissues will have to remove a greater amount of oxygen. Therefore, patients with poor perfusion have a greater oxygen extraction. Therapy can be chosen based on the information gained and the effectiveness of the therapy can be monitored. The use of these catheters is obviously reserved for the critical care setting.

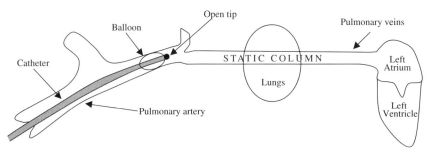

Diagram of pulmonary wedge pressure being performed. The balloon is inflated and "wedged" in the pulmonary artery. The balloon "cuts off" backward pressure creating a static column of blood from the catheter tip to the pulmonary vein. The column transmits the pulmonary vein and left atrial pressure to the catheter.

10. Why does it seem that we do less cardiac catheterization and angiograms than 10–15 years ago?

The decrease in use of cardiac catheterization is probably due to the usefulness of cardiac ultrasound. The echocardiogram has become a very important diagnostic tool in evaluating cardiac disease and its severity. Many cardiac catheterizations require anesthesia and they are invasive, so the tendency is to avoid these procedures in patients with heart disease. Accurate information can be obtained with an echocardiogram in unanesthetized patients, leaving catheter procedures for more specific diagnostic procedures and invasive therapies.

BIBLIOGRAPHY

1. Baim DS, Grossman W: Cardiac Catheterization, Angiography and Intervention, 5th ed. Baltimore, Williams & Wilkins, 1995.
2. Kienle RD: Cardiac catheterization. In Kittleson MD, Kienle RD (eds): Small Animal Cardiovascular Medicine. St. Louis, Mosby, 1998, pp 118–132.

25. MEASUREMENT OF SYSTEMIC BLOOD PRESSURE

Nigel A. Caulkett, D.V.M., M.V.Sc.

1. What factors determine blood pressure?

Blood pressure is the lateral force exerted per unit area of vascular wall. Clinically, pressure is measured in millimeters of mercury (mmHg). Intravascular pressure is referenced to the heart by adding or subtracting hydrostatic pressure. Systemic blood pressure oscillates around mean pressure. The maximum value is called "systolic pressure," and the minimum is "diastolic pressure." "Mean pressure" is the mean pressure throughout the cycle. The difference between systolic and diastolic pressure is called the "pulse pressure."

Systolic blood pressure is determined by left ventricular stroke volume, arterial compliance, and peak rate of ventricular ejection. Normal systolic pressures in dogs and cats range from 110–180 mmHg. Diastolic blood pressure is determined by peripheral vascular resistance, blood volume, duration of diastole, and the pressure at the end of systole. Diastolic pressures normally range from 70–110 mmHg. It should be recognized that blood pressure in awake animals is influenced by factors that can include patient anxiety and measurement methodology in addition to the hemodynamic variables noted previously.

Mean blood pressure is the major determinant of organ perfusion; it can be expressed as cardiac output × systemic vascular resistance. Normal mean pressures in dogs range from 85–120 mmHg. Generally it is accepted that a mean pressure of > 60 mmHg is required to perfuse all tissue beds. Mean blood pressure (BP) can be approximated by the following formula:

$$\text{Mean BP} = \text{diastolic BP} + [(\text{systolic BP} - \text{diastolic BP}) / 3]$$

This is only an approximation of mean blood pressure. It can be measured directly using the oscillometric technique, or can be more accurately calculated from a tracing of the pulse waveform.

2. What methods can be used to measure systemic pressure in dogs and cats?

Three methods are commonly used to measure systemic blood pressure in dogs and cats. Direct arterial pressure measurement is the most accurate of the three techniques, but is also the most technically demanding. Doppler and cuff and the oscillometric technique are indirect techniques; they are simple to perform and will provide good information concerning trends. Indirect techniques are good for most clinical situations, but tend to fail with severe hypotension. Photoplethysmography (see question 9) has been investigated in cats and small dogs, but is not used commonly in clinical practice.

3. How does the Doppler and cuff technique work?

There are two types of Doppler pulse-detection systems available. Doppler kinetoarteriography estimates blood pressure via the analysis of ultrasound waves reflected back from the arterial wall. The more commonly used method is the Doppler ultrasonic flowmeter. The Doppler flowmeter emits an ultrasound signal towards moving red blood cells. The frequency shift of the reflected return signal is encoded as an auditory signal by the unit. A blood pressure cuff is placed proximal to the Doppler flow probe. The cuff is inflated until the signal disappears. The cuff is gradually deflated until the signal reappears. The pressure at which the signal returns is taken as systolic pressure. The Doppler flow probe is typically placed over the common digital branch of the radial artery. Prior to placement the hair must be clipped from the palmar surface of the forelimb, and aqueous gel must be applied between the crystal and the skin.

4. How accurate is the Doppler and cuff technique?

The Doppler technique has been reported to underestimate systolic pressure in cats. A correction factor of Doppler systolic pressure + 14 mmHg was suggested to equal femoral arterial pressure. A study comparing the accuracy of Doppler, oscillometric, and photoplethysmographic devices demonstrated that the Doppler produced the most accurate prediction of systolic blood pressure in cats. This study also demonstrated that the Doppler was the most efficient of the three devices at obtaining readings.

The Doppler and cuff technique has also been shown to provide an accurate prediction of mean arterial pressure in cats. Correlation is good between Doppler systolic measurement and direct systolic measurement. This suggests that the Doppler and cuff technique is a useful tool for detecting trends, i.e., detects increases and decreases in pressure over time.

5. What factors should be considered to maximize the accuracy of the Doppler and cuff technique?

Cuff size is important in obtaining an accurate pressure measurement. A cuff width/limb circumference ratio of 0.4 has been suggested to be the most accurate. If the cuff is too small it will overestimate blood pressure; if it is too large, blood pressure will be underestimated. Movement and shivering can obscure Doppler sounds. This technique is very useful in anesthetized patients, but can be difficult to perform in awake patients.

6. What is the oscillometric technique?

The oscillometric technique senses variations in the pressure within a blood pressure cuff during deflation. The cuff is pressurized until no oscillations are seen, then it is gradually allowed to deflate until fluctuations are noted on a pressure gauge; this is taken as systolic pressure. The pressure is then allowed to fall further until maximum oscillations are reached and begin to decrease. This has been shown to be near the mean arterial pressure. The major advantages of the oscillometric technique are that it is automated, and it displays systolic, mean, and diastolic arterial pressure. The cuff is typically placed on the forelimb proximal to the metatarsal pad. It has also been evaluated on the tail. A cuff width/limb circumference ratio of 0.4 has been advocated.

7. What is the accuracy of the oscillometric technique?

The oscillometric technique has been shown to underestimate systolic pressure in cats, and tends to be less accurate than the Doppler and cuff method. The technique is relatively accurate in dogs over 7 kg, with most values for systolic and diastolic pressure falling within 10 mmHg of direct determinations. Another potential problem with the device is prolonged cycling time; it may take several minutes to obtain readings.

8. What factors will interfere with oscillometric measurement?

Sources of error include movement of the limb, inaccurate cuff size, not keeping the cuff at heart level, and inadequate pulse pressure waves due to shock or vascular compromise proximal to the cuff.

9. What is photoplethysmography?

The photoplethysmograph measures arterial volume by attenuation of infrared radiation. Arterial volume is maintained at a constant value by a microcomputer-based servosystem, so cuff pressure equals intra-arterial pressure at all times. A rapidly responding solenoid inflates and deflates the cuff, keeping the volume of the finger constant as pulsatile flow increases or decreases. In cats the cuff has been placed below the hock or on the tail.

In the previously cited study, the accuracy of photoplethysmography was comparable to Doppler. The unit overestimated at low pressures and underestimated at high pressures. An advantage of the unit is that it does illustrate rapid changes in blood pressure; it is also less prone to motion artifact than the other techniques. The unit tends to fail in darkly pigmented or calico cats. In dogs, 86% of indirectly derived mean arterial pressure measurements obtained by photoplethysmograph fall within 15 mmHg of the direct pressure measurements.

10. How is direct measurement of blood pressure performed?

Direct pressure measurement requires the placement of an indwelling catheter into a peripheral artery. The dorsal pedal artery is commonly used in dogs and the femoral artery is commonly used in cats. The femoral artery can also be used in dogs; in anesthetized dogs, systemic blood pressure measurements can be obtained from the lingual artery. The catheter is connected via noncompliant fluid-filled tubing to a pressure transducer. This transducer is in turn connected to a physiologic monitor. Most monitors will display a pressure tracing, systolic, diastolic, and mean blood pressure. Heart rate is also calculated from the pressure tracing. This technique is often performed in anesthetized animals, but can also be performed in awake dogs, following subcutaneous infiltration with lidocaine. This technique will provide the most accurate measurement of blood pressure and is useful for critically ill patients and in anesthetized patients when major fluctuations in blood pressure are anticipated.

Direct measurement of blood pressure is the most technically demanding of the techniques. The heart is used as the zero reference, and the transducer must be calibrated and zero referenced at the level of the heart to obtain accurate readings. The transducer is generally leveled at the sternum in laterally recumbent animals, and at the point of the shoulder when animals are in sternal recumbency. The length of connecting tubing should be kept to a minimum, and only noncompliant tubing should be used to decrease damping. Air bubbles should be purged from the system as they can lead to measurement error.

BIBLIOGRAPHY

1. Binns SH, Sisson DD, Buosico DA, Schaeffer DJ: Doppler ultrasonographic, oscillometric sphygmomanometric, and photoplethysmographic techniques for noninvasive blood pressure measurement in anesthetized cats. J Vet Intern Med 9:405–411, 1995.
2. Blitt CD, Hines RL (eds): Monitoring in Anesthesia and Critical Care Medicine, 3rd ed. New York, Churchill Livingstone, 1995, pp 95–130.
3. Caulkett NA, Cantwell SL, Houston DM: A comparison of indirect blood pressure monitoring techniques in the anesthetized cat. Vet Surg 27:370–377, 1998.
4. Chalifoux A, Dallaire A, Blais D, et al: Evaluation of the arterial blood pressure of dogs by two different noninvasive methods. Can J Comp Med 49:419–423, 1985.
5. Grandy JL, Dunlop CI, Hodgson DS, et al: Evaluation of the Doppler ultrasonic method of measuring systolic arterial blood pressure in cats. Am J Vet Res 53:1166–1169, 1992.
6. Goodenough DA, Muir WW 3rd: Blood pressure monitoring. Vet Med 93:48–59, 1998.

IV. Cardiovascular Diseases and Syndromes: Recognition and Management

26. ANESTHESIA AND SEDATION OF THE CARDIOVASCULAR PATIENT

Nigel Caulkett, D.V.M., M.V.Sc.

1. What are the cardiovascular effects of commonly used anesthetics and adjuncts to anesthesia?

Anesthesia of the patient with cardiac disease can be a challenge. It is important to be aware of the cardiovascular effects of anesthetic agents in order to choose an appropriate protocol for the patient. The following is a list of commonly used agents and their potential effects on the cardiovascular system. See the table in question 2 for a summary of the drugs and dosage ranges.

1. **Narcotics.** Opioids and opiates can be extremely valuable agents in the patient with cardiovascular disease. Opioids have little direct effect on cardiac contractility, but can cause decreased cardiac output via bradycardia from increased vagal tone. Potent opioids such as sufentanil or fentanyl can be used as part of a balanced technique to decrease volatile anesthetic requirements. Bradycardia can be prevented or treated with anticholinergics, if they are not contraindicated. Oxymorphone and hydromorphone are also useful in cardiac patients; both of these drugs can be used intravenously, as part of an induction regimen, or used to decrease volatile agent requirements intraoperatively. Morphine and meperidine are less useful because they produce little reduction in volatile anesthetic requirements at clinical dosages and IV administration can produce significant hypotension due to histamine release. It is important to note that potent narcotics can produce significant respiratory depression and intermittent positive pressure ventilation may be required.

2. **Benzodiazepines.** Benzodiazepine drugs have minimal cardiovascular effects and can be useful, when combined with narcotics, for sedation or induction of anesthesia. Potentiation of gamma aminobutyric acid (GABA) results in synergistic activity with ultrashort-acting barbiturates and propofol. Dose requirements for induction of anesthesia can be greatly decreased by prior or concurrent administration of a benzodiazepine agent. These agents can also be combined with ketamine to offset the increased muscle tone observed during ketamine-induced sedation or anesthesia. Midazolam and diazepam are the most useful agents for veterinary anesthesia.

3. **Phenothiazines.** Acepromazine can be a useful drug in the cardiac patient. The major advantages of acepromazine are tranquilization, antiemesis, and an antiarrhythmic effect during barbiturate or halothane anesthesia. The major side effect that can complicate anesthesia in the cardiac patient is alpha-1 blockade resulting in decreased systemic vascular resistance (SVR). This drug should be used at low doses or avoided in conditions that may be complicated by decreased SVR. For example, decreased SVR can increase the shunt fraction in conditions with a right-to-left shunt, and can increase dynamic obstruction of the left ventricular outflow tract in cats with hypertrophic cardiomyopathy.

4. **Alpha-2 agonists.** Alpha-2 agonist agents such as xylazine and medetomidine should be used cautiously in patients with cardiac disease. The major adverse effects of these drugs are bradycardia, decreased cardiac output, and increased systemic vascular resistance. Administration of an anticholinergic agent can be used to increase the heart rate, but increased rate in the

face of increased peripheral vascular resistance leads to increased cardiac work and oxygen consumption. This could be particularly detrimental in patients with ischemic heart disease. Low doses of these agents may be potentially useful in the cardiac patient, if they are used cautiously.

5. **Barbiturates.** Ultrashort-acting barbiturates should be used cautiously in patients with cardiac disease, and should be avoided in animals with heart failure. Thiopental is a potent myocardial depressant that dilates capacitance vessels, lowering venous return to the heart and decreasing cardiac output. In animals with hypovolemia or with cardiac tamponade this response may be exaggerated, leading to rapid decompensation.

6. **Propofol.** The cardiovascular effects of propofol are similar to those of thiopental. Propofol produces dose-dependent myocardial depression and venodilation. Precautions are similar to those for thiopental.

7. **Ketamine.** Ketamine has a direct myocardial depressant effect and an indirect sympathomimetic effect. Ketamine's indirect effects tend to predominate, characterized by increased heart rate, blood pressure, and myocardial oxygen demand. Ketamine can be a useful drug in patients with hypovolemia or ventricular dysfunction. Since ketamine maintains heart rate and systemic vascular resistance, it can also be helpful in animals with tamponade. Ketamine should be avoided in animals with hypertrophic cardiomyopathy because increases in heart rate and contractility are not well tolerated. Ketamine should be used cautiously in patients with outflow obstruction, because increased heart rate, intraventricular pressure, and myocardial oxygen consumption may lead to ischemia in patients with pulmonic stenosis, subaortic stenosis, or the obstructive form of hypertrophic cardiomyopathy.

8. **Etomidate.** Etomidate is a useful drug in the cardiac patient because it does not produce myocardial depression or vasodilation. It generally increases systemic blood pressure and does not change or increase cardiac output. Etomidate is better tolerated than propofol or thiopental in patients that are hypovolemic or have ventricular dysfunction.

9. **Halothane.** Halothane can be a useful drug in some patients with cardiac disease. The major cardiovascular side effects of halothane are dose-dependent myocardial depression and sensitization to catecholamine-induced ventricular dysrhythmias. Halothane decreases cardiac output and is not well tolerated in patients with ventricular dysfunction. Halothane should be used cautiously or avoided in patients that have preexisting ventricular arrhythmias, e.g., traumatic myocarditis or gastric dilatation/volvulus. Halothane may have a role in patients that tolerate decreases in SVR poorly, such as those with hypertrophic cardiomyopathy or tetralogy of Fallot. Halothane is generally well tolerated in patients with mitral regurgitation, provided that they are not in heart failure.

10. **Isoflurane.** Isoflurane is less arrhythmogenic than halothane and produces less myocardial depression. Isoflurane is a more potent vasodilator than halothane and produces more hypotension at an equivalent maximum allowable concentration (MAC) value. Isoflurane is a better choice than halothane in patients with ventricular dysfunction or preexisting arrhythmias. Isoflurane is better tolerated than halothane in patients with decompensated mitral regurgitation. Isoflurane is a potent vasodilator and must be used cautiously in patients that do not tolerate drops in systemic vascular resistance; this includes patients with hypertrophic cardiomyopathy or patients with right-to-left shunting lesions. Since the side effects of volatile agents are dose dependent it is beneficial to use a "balanced" anesthetic technique. Administration of narcotics and benzodiazepine agents can be used to significantly reduce volatile anesthetic requirements, resulting in fewer cardiovascular side effects.

11. **Sevoflurane.** Cardiovascular effects of sevoflurane are similar to those of isoflurane. Cardiac output tends to be preserved at clinically useful concentrations. As with isoflurane, blood pressure can decrease from vasodilation and, like isoflurane, myocardial sensitization is not a severe problem.

12. **Nitrous oxide.** Nitrous oxide will reduce the MAC of volatile anesthetics by up to 30%. It has minimal effects on the cardiovascular system and can be a useful adjunct to anesthesia in the cardiac patient. Concurrent administration of nitrous oxide can shorten induction and recovery times from volatile anesthesia. The major disadvantage of nitrous oxide in the cardiac patient

is that its use necessitates a decrease in fractional inspired oxygen concentration (FiO_2) of up to 66% (FiO_2 of 33% when a 2:1 ratio of nitrous:oxygen is used). A decrease in FiO_2 of this magnitude would not be well tolerated in patients with increased pulmonary venous admixture and the drug should be avoided in patients with pulmonary edema or right-to-left shunting lesions.

2. What are the most commonly used drugs in anesthesia or sedation of canine cardiac patients?

Drugs Used for Anesthesia or Sedation of Canine Cardiac Patients

Premedication	Oxymorphone	0.1–0.15 mg/kg IM
	Hydromorphone	0.1–0.2 mg/kg IM
	Midazolam	0.2–0.4 mg/kg IM
	Acepromazine	0.03 mg/kg IM
	Butorphanol	0.2–0.4 mg/kg IM
	Glycopyrrolate	0.01 mg/kg IM
IV Sedation/ Induction	Oxymorphone 0.1–0.15 mg/kg followed by diazepam 0.2–0.5 mg/kg	
	Hydromorphone 0.15–0.2 mg/kg followed by diazepam 0.2–0.5 mg/kg	
	Oxymorphone or hydromorphone as above, plus acepromazine 0.03 mg/kg	
	(Above protocols are often suitable for induction; if not, complete induction with volatile anesthesia or use one of the techniques described below.)	
Induction	Oxymorphone 0.1 mg/kg, followed by diazepam 0.2 mg/kg, followed by ketamine 2–4 mg/kg (to effect)	
	Oxymorphone 0.1 mg/kg, followed by diazepam 0.2 mg/kg, followed by propofol 2–3 mg/kg (to effect)	
	(Hydromorphone can be used instead of oxy at 0.15 mg/kg; midazolam can be used instead of diazepam at 0.1–0.2 mg/kg)	
	Thiopental 2 mg/kg, followed by diazepam 0.2 mg/kg, followed by thiopental 6 mg/kg (to effect)	
	Propofol 2 mg/kg, followed by diazepam 0.2 mg/kg, followed by propofol 4 mg/kg (to effect)	
	Etomidate 0.5–1 mg/kg (following premedication)	
	Fentanyl 6–8 µg/kg, followed by diazepam 0.5 mg/kg or midazolam 0.2 mg/kg	
	Sufentanil 2 µg/kg, followed by diazepam 0.5 mg/kg or midazolam 0.2 mg/kg	
Maintenance	Isoflurane 1.2–2%	
	Sevoflurane 2.5–4%	
	Halothane 0.9–1.5%	
	Dose requirements of the above can be decreased by approximately 30% with the addition of 60% nitrous oxide.	
	Dose requirements for volatile agents can be decreased with intermittent IV boluses of oxymorphone 0.05 mg/kg or hydromorphone 0.05–0.1 mg/kg as required (every 45–60 min).	
	Dose requirements for volatile anesthetics can be decreased with continuous infusions of either fentanyl 0.5–0.7 µg/kg/min or sufentanil 0.05–0.07 µg/kg/min. If extreme MAC reduction is required, a midazolam infusion can be administered in combination with one of the above narcotic infusions at a dose of 15 µg/kg/min. This will decrease volatile requirements by 60–80%. (These infusions should be initiated immediately postinduction with sufentanil-midazolam or fentanyl-midazolam.)	

3. How should the cardiac patient be monitored during anesthesia?

Continuous monitoring is important in the cardiac patient. Complications can occur suddenly in unstable patients and must be treated promptly. Ideally it would be valuable to continuously measure cardiac output, particularly in patients with severe ventricular dysfunction; unfortunately, this is currently not practical in veterinary medicine.

Systemic blood pressure can be readily measured in the veterinary patient by indirect techniques, such as the Doppler and cuff or oscillometric method. More accurate blood pressure measurement can be performed with direct techniques. Mean arterial pressure is the product of cardiac output and systemic vascular resistance. Decreases in cardiac output will usually result in some decrease in blood pressure. Most anesthetic techniques will result in some degree of hypotension. In general, systolic pressure should be maintained above 90 mmHg and mean arterial pressure above 60 mmHg.

Pulse oximetry is valuable in the cardiac patient, particularly in patients with pulmonary edema or right-to-left shunts. Pulse oximeters should be used in patients receiving nitrous oxide, as the risk of hypoxemia is increased due to the lower FiO_2. Hypoxemia is not uncommon in the cardiac patient, and pulse oximetry is the best tool to rapidly detect hypoxemia during anesthesia.

Arrhythmias are frequently encountered in the cardiac patient during anesthesia. *Continuous ECG monitoring* is important to rapidly characterize arrhythmias and to gauge the response to any antiarrhythmic therapy that may be administered.

Fluid overload is poorly tolerated by many patients with heart disease and can be catastrophic in patients with overt heart failure. General anesthesia often results in hypotension and increased loss of body fluids. *Continuous measurement of central venous pressure* (CVP) is useful in patients with right-sided heart disease to avoid excessive fluid administration. Ideally CVP should be maintained in the range of 1–7 cmH$_2$O. Left atrial pressure or pulmonary wedge pressure can be monitored to avoid fluid overload in the patient with left-sided heart disease. However, techniques to monitor these parameters are not practical in most veterinary hospitals.

It is important to stress that close monitoring of the cardiac patient is extremely important due to the increased risk of complications during anesthesia.

4. What are general concerns related to the sedation and anesthesia of patients with mitral regurgitation?

Patients without heart failure are generally not considered a high risk. The risk of complications will increase if heart failure is present. Patients with pulmonary edema are very high risk and should only be anesthetized if they have acute life-threatening conditions. In general, pulmonary edema should be treated prior to anesthesia or sedation.

Preanesthetic examination should include a complete blood count and total body chemistry panel. This is because anemia is not well tolerated in patients with heart failure, and these patients are usually geriatric and may have concurrent renal or hepatic disease. Electrolyte abnormalities may be present and should be corrected prior to anesthesia. Blood urea and creatinine levels should be interpreted in conjunction with urine specific gravity to determine if dehydration is present.

Fluid deficits should be carefully corrected prior to anesthesia, as hypovolemia will exacerbate decreases in cardiac output and hypotension during anesthesia. Echocardiography is useful to characterize the degree of ventricular dysfunction and regurgitant fraction prior to anesthesia. The lung fields should be carefully auscultated prior to anesthesia to detect pulmonary edema, and thoracic radiographs are indicated in any patient with abnormal lung sounds or a history of heart failure. If arrhythmias are encountered during physical examination they should be characterized with electrocardiography prior to anesthesia.

Patients with mitral regurgitation do not tolerate bradycardia or increased systemic vascular resistance. Both of these complications will lead to increased left ventricular volume and increased regurgitant fraction. Heart rate should be maintained at the resting rate or slightly elevated. Anticholinergics can be used prior to anesthesia or sedation to prevent bradycardia. Glycopyrrolate is preferable to atropine as it produces less tachycardia. If glycopyrrolate is used intramuscularly it should be administered at least 40 minutes prior to the administration of sedatives or anesthetics. Narcotics are very useful in these patients; pretreatment with an anticholinergic is indicated to prevent bradycardia.

Benzodiazepine agents are generally well tolerated. Alpha-2 agonist drugs can increase systemic vascular resistance and produce bradycardia; they should be avoided or used cautiously at a low dose. Ketamine-diazepam or etomidate can be used if they are titrated carefully to effect. Thiopental or propofol may be used in stable patients with mild disease, but should be avoided in patients with heart failure. Halothane, isoflurane, or sevoflurane can be used in stable patients. Halothane should be avoided in patients with heart failure.

5. What is a suitable IV sedative technique for a dog with mitral regurgitation?

Narcotic-benzodiazepine combinations are a good choice in these patients. The patient should be pretreated with an anticholinergic to prevent bradycardia. The narcotic should be administered first. Oxymorphone (0.1–0.15 mg/kg IV) or hydromorphone (0.15–2 mg/kg IV) are both good choices. Once the animal is sedated, diazepam is administered at 0.2–0.5 mg/kg. The patient should be monitored closely for bradycardia or respiratory depression, and supplemental oxygen should be administered by face mask. Animals sedated with these combinations are sensitive to sound and ambient noise should be kept to a minimum. In patients without heart failure a low dose of acepromazine (0.03–0.05 mg/kg) may be used instead of diazepam. If sedation is not adequate a low dose of ketamine (2–4 mg/kg) may be titrated in addition to the above.

If rapid recovery is required, the sedative effects of the narcotic may be antagonized with naloxone (0.04 mg/kg IM) or with butorphanol (0.2 mg/kg IV).

6. What is a suitable anesthetic protocol for a dog with mitral regurgitation?

Choice of anesthetic agent in these patients will depend on the severity of mitral valve regurgitation. Patients that have mild disease without heart failure or concurrent disease are generally not considered to be high-risk patients. These patients can be premedicated with either a low dose of acepromazine (0.03 mg/kg IM) or midazolam (0.2 mg/kg IM) combined with a narcotic (oxymorphone, hydromorphone, or morphine). Glycopyrrolate can be administered (0.01 mg/kg IM) to prevent bradycardia. Suitable induction agents include thiopental, propofol, or ketamine-diazepam combinations. Halothane, isoflurane, or sevoflurane can be used for maintenance.

Patients with severe mitral valve regurgitation and heart failure are high risk and efforts must be made to avoid bradycardia, myocardial depression, and increased systemic vascular resistance. Anesthesia should be avoided in patients with pulmonary edema unless they are in a life-threatening condition. Glycopyrrolate can be administered at the above dose to prevent bradycardia. Neuroleptanalgesic induction is usually well tolerated in these patients. Oxymorphone is administered IV at a dose of 0.1–0.2 mg/kg or hydromorphone at 0.15–0.2 mg/kg. Once the animal is sedated, diazepam is administered at 0.2–0.5 mg/kg IV. Many animals can be intubated following this combination.

If conditions are not suitable for intubation, ketamine can be administered in addition to the above at a dose of 2–3 mg/kg; alternatively, induction may be completed by administration of a suitable volatile anesthetic via face mask. Alternative choices for induction include IM premedication with a narcotic plus midazolam and careful IV titration of ketamine-diazepam or etomidate.

Isoflurane or sevoflurane can be used for maintenance of anesthesia. Nitrous oxide (50–70%) may be used to decrease volatile anesthetic requirements. It is advisable to monitor percent hemoglobin saturation.

Balanced electrolyte solution, such as lactated Ringer's solution (LRS), should be administered during anesthesia to replace fluid losses. Care must be taken to avoid overhydration. If fluids are required to treat hypotension, colloids such as dextran-70 or hydroxyethyl starch are more suitable than high-dose crystalloids.

Dobutamine can be carefully titrated at a dose of 2–5 µg/kg/min to improve myocardial contractility and cardiac output. Pressor agents such as phenylephrine, norepinephrine, or high-dose dopamine should usually be avoided.

These patients should be carefully monitored during anesthesia. Monitoring should include pressure measurement, ECG, and pulse oximetry. The development of rales on auscultation of the lung fields and/or hemoglobin desaturation during anesthesia may herald the development of pulmonary edema. These animals should be maintained on supplemental oxygen during recovery and monitored carefully for the development of pulmonary edema or arrhythmias.

7. How should anesthesia be managed in cats with hypertrophic cardiomyopathy?

Major concerns with hypertrophic cardiomyopathy include impaired diastolic filling, dynamic obstruction of the left ventricular outflow tract by the anterior motion of the mitral valve leaflets in some patients, mitral regurgitation, and the potential for arrhythmias and myocardial ischemia. The development of atrial fibrillation can increase risk by further decreasing ventricular filling and cardiac output. Cats that present with dyspnea or pulmonary edema are very high risk and should be stabilized prior to anesthesia.

A major concern during anesthesia includes maintaining adequate intravascular volume while avoiding fluid overload. LRS at 5 ml/kg/hr with or without dextran-70 at 2–3 ml/kg/hr can help to offset anesthetic-induced vasodilation and avoid hypotension. Hypovolemia, vasodilation, tachycardia, and increased ventricular contractility can produce dynamic obstruction of the left ventricular outflow tract. High-dose acepromazine can produce vasodilation and should be avoided. High-dose ketamine should be avoided as it can increase heart rate and contractility. Anticholinergics and beta-1 agonist drugs should be avoided as they increase heart rate. Halothane is a good choice for maintenance of anesthesia as it can decrease heart rate and contractility, and may therefore improve diastolic function. Isoflurane may be preferable over halothane, if arrhythmias are present.

Arrhythmias and pulmonary edema should be treated prior to anesthesia. Anemia is not well tolerated during anesthesia and PCV should be corrected to at least 30% prior to anesthesia. It is important to avoid stress during induction as this can produce catecholamine release, which will result in tachycardia and increased contractility.

Cats can be premedicated with oxymorphone 0.1 mg/kg plus midazolam 0.2 mg/kg IM. These drugs have minimal effects on contractility and the vagomimetic effect of oxymorphone may be beneficial in that it can decrease heart rate. Intravenous induction with etomidate (0.5–1 mg/kg) or etomidate (0.25 mg/kg), followed by diazepam (0.2 mg/kg), followed by etomidate (0.25–0.5 mg/kg) given to effect. Alternatively, 2 mg/kg of thiopental, followed by 0.2 mg/kg of diazepam, followed by 2–6 mg/kg of thiopental to effect may be used. Thiopental should be used cautiously as it can produce a transient tachycardia. An alternative technique is to mask-induce with halothane, isoflurane, or sevoflurane if the patient is adequately premedicated.

Maintenance can be accomplished with halothane, isoflurane, or sevoflurane. Monitoring equipment should include pulse oximetry, ECG, and blood pressure. Ideally direct blood pressure should be monitored although indirect blood pressure measurement should be adequate for most situations.

8. How should anesthesia be managed in the canine patient with dilated cardiomyopathy?

Patients with dilated cardiomyopathy have decreased myocardial contractility with ventricular and atrial enlargement. Ventricular enlargement is associated with mitral regurgitation. Atrial enlargement can be associated with atrial fibrillation. Risk of complications from anesthesia will be increased if the patient has pulmonary edema.

Anesthetic management should be aimed at maintaining myocardial contractility, avoiding excessive increases in heart rate (which will increase myocardial oxygen demand), and avoiding fluid overload. Bradycardia is not well tolerated in these patients since they do not have a good ability to increase stroke volume and bradycardia will reduce cardiac output. Glycopyrrolate can be administered at a dose of 0.01 mg/kg IM; this will reduce the chance of a severe bradycardia developing following the administration of potent opioids. Oxymorphone at a dose of 0.1–0.15 mg/kg IV or hydromorphone at 0.15 mg/kg followed by diazepam at a dose of 0.5 mg/kg IV will often produce conditions suitable for intubation. This combination can be followed by IV administration of 2–4 mg/kg of ketamine to increase the depth of anesthesia and facilitate intubation. Halothane should be avoided in these patients. Isoflurane is a good choice for maintenance of anesthesia at low concentrations.

Supplemental narcotics (oxymorphone 0.05 mg/kg IV) are often required intraoperatively to maintain a low concentration of isoflurane. Nitrous oxide may also be beneficial to decrease the requirement for isoflurane and maintain contractility and blood pressure. It is important to monitor hemoglobin saturation if nitrous oxide is administered. Dobutamine at 2–5 µg/kg/min is often useful to help improve myocardial contractility in these patients.

Care should be taken to avoid volume overload. Crystalloids such as LRS or normal saline can be administered at 5 ml/kg/hr. Colloidal fluids such as dextran-70 can also be administered at a dose of 2–10 ml/kg if volume exansion is required.

Central venous pressure should also be monitored during anesthesia. Hypotension is often observed in anesthetized patients with dilated cardiomyopathy; initial therapy should be aimed at decreasing the inspired concentration of the volatile anesthetic and improving contractility with dobutamine. Monitoring equipment should include pulse oximetry, accurate blood pressure measurement, and ECG.

9. What are general considerations for patients with subvalvular aortic stenosis or with pulmonic stenosis?

As with other conditions, the risk of complications will increase if the animal is in heart failure. These patients develop myocardial hypertrophy, which increases myocardial oxygen demand and the risk of ischemia. Hypotension is poorly tolerated; a reflex increase in heart rate can occur, which will decrease diastolic filling and increase myocardial oxygen consumption. Hypertension is also poorly tolerated, particularly in combination with tachycardia. Anesthetic management should be aimed at avoiding tachycardia and hyper- or hypotension, and at maintaining a normal or slightly decreased sinus rhythm. Sympathetic stimulation should be avoided. Induction should be stress-free to avoid catecholamine release. Hypoxemia and hypercarbia should also be avoided as catecholamine release can occur with these conditions. Hypoxemia can further complicate pulmonic stenosis, as it can lead to hypoxic pulmonary vasoconstriction that will increase downstream resistance and may lead to increased myocardial work.

Ketamine and tiletamine should be avoided as they trigger catecholamine release and can produce tachycardia and hypertension. Nitrous oxide should be used cautiously as it produces some sympathetic stimulation. Anticholinergics should be avoided unless heart rate becomes dangerously low. Glycopyrrolate is the anticholinergic of choice, if required. Dogs can be premedicated with either 0.05 mg/kg of oxymorphone or 0.1 mg/kg of of hydromorphone. This is followed by IV administration of 0.1 mg/kg of either oxymorphone or hydromorphone, followed by 0.2–0.5 mg/kg of diazepam. Isoflurane or sevoflurane can be used for maintenance. High doses of volatile anesthetics are to be avoided as they produce myocardial depression and vasodilation.

These patients should be monitored with pulse oximetry, ECG, and blood pressure monitoring. Fluids should be administered to maintain preload. Monitoring of central venous pressure is valuable in patients with pulmonic stenosis.

10. What are general considerations for patients with shunting lesions?

Anesthesia for patients with small ventricular or atrial septal defects is usually low risk. Patients with large left-to-right shunts and heart failure are at increased risk of complications. Patients with right-to-left shunting conditions such as tetralogy of Fallot or Eisenmenger's complex are high-risk patients that require very careful management during anesthesia. In general, management of the patient with a left-to-right shunt is aimed at avoiding volume overload, which can lead to the development of congestive signs. Precautions should also be taken to avoid factors that will increase systemic vascular resistance. Increased systemic vascular resistance will increase left-to-right flow across the shunt. Sympathetic stimulants such as ketamine and tiletamine should be used cautiously in these patients, stress should be avoided on induction and recovery, and alpha-1 and alpha-2 agonist drugs should be used cautiously. These patients can benefit from a slight decrease in systemic vascular resistance.

Isoflurane or sevoflurane is good for maintenance of anesthesia, and a low dose of acepromazine may be useful. Right-to-left shunting will be more severe if increased pulmonary vascular resistance occurs. The major causes of increased pulmonary vascular resistance are hypoxemia, acidosis, hypercapnia, and increased sympathetic tone. Hyperventilation with 100% oxygen can help to decrease pulmonary vascular resistance. Systemic vasodilation also worsens right-to-left shunting and should be avoided. Careful titration of phenylephrine may be used to increase systemic vascular resistance. Nitrous oxide should be avoided in these patients, and halothane may be more suitable than isoflurane or sevoflurane for maintenance.

11. What is a suitable technique for ligation of a patent ductus arteriosus (PDA) in a 6-month-old puppy?

Anesthesia for the patient with PDA is usually not complicated. The risk will increase if the patient has heart failure, severe pulmonary edema, or reversal of the flow across the PDA. General principles for left-to-right shunting lesions should be followed. These patients also have large pulse pressures and low diastolic pressures due to increased diastolic runoff. Patients may be in poor body condition and care should be taken to avoid hypothermia. In a small patient mask induction is not difficult and the patient can be mask-induced with sevoflurane or isoflurane, following premedication. In theory induction can be slower in patients with left-to-right shunts as increased pulmonary blood flow will slow the rate of rise of volatile anesthetics in the alveolus. Clinically this is not usually a significant effect, particularly with highly insoluble agents like isoflurane or sevoflurane.

Premedication with 0.1 mg/kg of oxymorphone plus 0.2 mg/kg of midazolam will calm the patient to facilitate induction. Acepromazine is best avoided in PDA as it could potentially lower diastolic pressure. Larger patients can be induced with etomidate, or with thiopental-diazepam or propofol-diazepam combinations. Blood pressure should be monitored and mean arterial pressure should be maintained at 50–60 mmHg. Careful administration of colloids such as dextran 70 can be used to increase diastolic pressure; 5–10 mmHg is often adequate.

Ligation of the PDA will result in increased systemic vascular resistance, which is often accompanied by a sudden drop in heart rate and pronounced increase in diastolic pressure. Heart rate will usually recover quickly. If it remains dangerously low (< 40 beats/min), administration of atropine or glycopyrrolate should be considered. Intercostal blocks, with bupivacaine, can be used to produce intra- and postoperative analgesia in these patients.

BIBLIOGRAPHY

1. Bednarski RM: Anesthetic concerns for patients with cardiomyopathy. Vet Clin North Am Small Anim Pract 22:466–465, 1992.
2. Evans AT: Anesthesia for severe mitral and tricuspid regurgitation. Vet Clin North Am Small Anim Pract 22:466–467, 1992.
3. Hensley FA, Martin DE (eds): The Practice of Cardiac Anesthesia. Boston, Little, Brown, 1990.
4. Ilkiw JE: Anesthesia and disease. In Hall LW, Taylor PM (eds): Anaesthesia of the Cat. London, Bailliere Tindall, 1994, pp 224–248.
5. Morgan EG, Mikhail MS (eds): Clinical Anesthesiology. E. Norwalk, CT, Appleton & Lange, 1992.
6. Steffey EP: Inhalation anesthesia. In Thurmon JC, Tranquilli WJ, Benson GJ (eds): Lumb and Jones's Veterinary Anesthesia. Baltimore, Williams & Wilkins, 1996, pp 297–329.

27. EMERGENCY MANAGEMENT OF CONGESTIVE HEART FAILURE

Jonathan A. Abbott, D.V.M.

1. What is heart failure?

Heart failure is a state in which cardiac output is inadequate to meet the body's metabolic demands despite adequate preload. This definition excludes extracardiac causes of reduced output such as hypovolemia. For example, a patient that suffers from hemorrhagic shock has inadequate cardiac output; however, heart failure is not present, because the failure of the circulatory system to sustain normal metabolic function is not the result of primary cardiac dysfunction. The qualifying statement regarding preload related to filling pressures localizes the cause of circulatory dysfunction to the heart; heart failure can be alternatively defined as a sustained and consequential decrease in cardiac output that results from cardiac dysfunction.

It is important to recognize that heart *failure* results from heart *disease* and that practically any heart disease can result in heart failure. In veterinary medicine, heart failure is most often manifest as congestive heart failure (CHF). The clinical signs are primarily due to the development of abnormally high systemic or, more often, pulmonary venous pressures. Left-sided CHF is typically characterized by the presence of pulmonary congestion and edema, although some feline patients develop pleural effusion as a consequence of disease that primarily affects the left ventricle. Right-sided CHF is manifest as body cavity effusions or peripheral edema.

2. What is low-output heart failure?

Most diseases that result in heart failure are chronic. Compensatory mechanisms including the renin-angiotensin-aldosterone system result in intravascular volume expansion and, ultimately, clinical signs due to venous congestion. Heart failure in which signs of reduced cardiac output such as hypothermia, weakness, and prerenal azotemia predominate is known as low-output or forward heart failure. Often, low-output and congestive failure coexist. Signs of low-output failure seem to be more common in the cat than in the dog; cats with heart failure due to myocardial disease are sometimes hypothermic, depressed, and occasionally bradycardic.

3. What is the difference between systolic and diastolic failure? How is this distinction important in case management?

Systolic cardiac performance is a global measure of the heart's pumping ability. Systolic performance is affected by myocardial function (contractility), but also by afterload, preload, and valvular competence. In this chapter, systolic failure refers to CHF that results from some deficit of pumping performance. Mitral valve regurgitation and dilated cardiomyopathy are the most common causes of systolic failure.

Diastolic cardiac performance refers to the ability of the ventricle to fill at low pressures. Pathologic ventricular hypertrophy and endomyocardial fibrosis can impair diastolic performance; restrictive myocardial diseases and hypertrophic cardiomyopathy are examples of disorders that can result in diastolic failure.

Impaired systolic and diastolic performance can coexist in a single patient. However, the therapeutic approach to patients that fall into these two somewhat artificial designations differ and for that reason the distinction is conceptually useful.

4. What cardiac diseases are most likely to cause an emergent presentation of CHF?

Most heart diseases in dogs and cats are chronic; despite this, it is common for clinical signs to develop suddenly. The reasons for this are varied. Pets are largely sedentary, and consequently subclinical heart disease can progress until a minimum of stress or exertion provokes signs of cardiac dysfunction. Additionally, subtle changes in respiratory rate and character are difficult for owners to recognize. Regardless, it is common for chronic disorders such as mitral valve endocardiosis, canine dilated cardiomyopathy, and feline myocardial disease to result in clinical signs that are apparently sudden in onset and necessitate emergent management.

In addition, there are a few examples of truly acute CHF in dogs and cats. Rupture of a first-order mitral valve chorda tendinea can result in sudden elevations of left atrial pressure and acute, left-sided CHF. Similarly, destruction of the aortic or mitral valve by an aggressive infective lesion can also cause acute heart failure. Regardless of the precise pathogenesis, the sudden development of cough or dyspnea related to heart failure is an important veterinary emergency.

5. What historical findings are associated with acute or decompensated CHF?

Respiratory distress related to pulmonary edema or pleural effusion is the most consistent historical finding in severe CHF. Heart disease in cats rarely results in cough, although this sign is observed commonly in affected dogs. Syncope, lack of appetite, and depression may also be part of the patient history. With the exception of cardiac tamponade which is discussed elsewhere, the onset of right-sided CHF is in general more insidious and less often prompts urgent veterinary evaluation.

6. What physical findings are expected?

The physical examination reflects the effects of diminished cardiac performance and attendant increases in ventricular filling pressures. Often, the disease that has resulted in heart failure is also apparent on physical examination. In dogs, tachycardia is a relatively consistent finding. It is important to recognize that the respiratory arrhythmia that is common in healthy dogs results partly from vagal influence. Vagal discharge is inhibited in heart failure and, as a result, the finding of a respiratory-related arrhythmia is virtually incompatible with a diagnosis of overt CHF. In contrast, tachycardia is a much less consistent finding in cats with heart failure. The heart rates of healthy cats differ little from the heart rates of cats in heart failure and, in fact, some cats with severe heart failure develop bradycardia.

On physical examination, elevated ventricular filling pressures are manifest as dyspnea due to pulmonary edema or pleural effusion. Crackles are often audible when pulmonary edema is present, while a large pleural effusion may muffle heart and lung sounds.

Auscultatory findings may reflect the disease that is responsible for the heart failure state. Dogs with CHF due to mitral valve endocardiosis invariably have a systolic murmur of mitral valve regurgitation; most often, the murmur is loud. Dogs with dilated cardiomyopathy may have more subtle physical findings, although careful auscultation often reveals a soft murmur of functional mitral incompetence and/or a gallop rhythm. Many cats with CHF due to hypertrophic cardiomyopathy have cardiac murmurs although this finding is certainly not consistent; similarly, the restrictive myocardial diseases may cause a murmur or, perhaps more often, a gallop rhythm.

7. How is a diagnosis of left-sided CHF made?

The clinical signs of left-sided heart failure and primary respiratory tract disease are superficially similar. Since interventions such as aggressive diuretic therapy can be lifesaving in CHF but harmful in the setting of respiratory tract disease, an accurate diagnosis is essential. A noninvasive diagnosis of left-sided CHF can be made radiographically; left atrial enlargement in the presence of pulmonary opacities compatible with edema is diagnostic. Sometimes, the fragile clinical status of the patient is an impediment to careful radiographic studies and the risk-benefit ratio is in favor of empirical therapy. In these cases, a careful assessment of the history and physical findings is essential. Prior to empirical therapy, it is important to determine that a diagnosis of acute CHF is at least plausible.

With respect to the patient history, patients with CHF are unlikely to survive for more than a few months without treatment, and so a long history of cough and dyspnea suggests that primary respiratory tract disease is at least partly responsible for the clinical signs. Again, cats with cardiac disease seldom cough; in contrast, small-breed dogs with CHF due to mitral valve disease typically have a history of cough that precedes the development of dyspnea.

Heart failure results from heart disease; therefore, it is important to consider whether or not it is likely that the patient has a cardiac disorder that could reasonably result in heart failure. The most common acquired heart diseases that result in left-sided CHF in dogs are dilated cardiomyopathy and degenerative mitral valve disease; the former most commonly affects middle aged, large breed dogs while the latter affects elderly, small breed dogs. Elderly small-breed dogs that develop CHF due to mitral valve disease have cardiac murmurs; when mitral valve disease is severe enough to cause CHF, the murmur is usually loud. Conversely, it is extremely unlikely for an elderly small-breed dog to develop CHF in the absence of a murmur; in these cases, signs such as cough and dyspnea are probably related to respiratory tract disease. Dogs with dilated cardiomyopathy may have relatively subtle auscultatory findings; a soft murmur or a gallop rhythm, however, may have great clinical importance. Myocardial diseases are the most common cause of CHF in cats; idiopathic hypertrophic cardiomyopathy is quite common, restrictive myocardial diseases somewhat less so. Feline patients with myocardial disease often have cardiac murmurs and/or a gallop, although this is not invariably true.

8. What diagnostic studies are indicated when fulminant CHF is suspected?

Thoracic radiographs can provide a noninvasive diagnosis of left-sided CHF. When restraint for radiographic studies can be tolerated by the patient, thoracic radiographs guide the therapeutic approach. When available, echocardiography can provide useful information in the setting of fulminant CHF. Echocardiography cannot provide a diagnosis of CHF; however, echocardiography can be used to determine the cause of heart failure. Sometimes, a cursory echocardiographic examination can be performed using minimal restraint and this can be used to determine if the diagnosis of CHF is at least plausible.

9. What are the therapeutic goals in the management of acute or decompensated CHF?

The primary goals in the management of severe CHF are the restoration of normal ventilatory function and, when possible, augmentation of cardiac performance. Ancillary therapies such as narcotics and oxygen supplementation are important; however, these goals are achieved largely through manipulation of the primary determinants of cardiac output: heart rate, preload, afterload, and contractility.

10. How do these goals differ from those in the management of chronic CHF?

The therapy of acute CHF is different from the therapy of chronic CHF in terms of method and intent. Current evidence suggests that activation of compensatory neurohumoral mechanisms such as the adrenergic nervous system and the renin-angiotensin-aldosterone system play an important role in the progression of CHF; pharmacologic blunting of these mechanisms has been shown to improve long-term prognosis. For example, drug efficacy studies performed in people indicate that the long-term use of beta-blockers has a "cardioprotective" effect despite the fact these drugs, at least acutely, can have a negative effect on cardiac performance. In contrast, the hemodynamic effect of therapy is foremost in the management of acute CHF and specific therapeutic interventions can be classified based upon their effect on the four primary determinants of cardiac output : preload, afterload, contractility, and heart rate.

11. How is preload manipulated in acute or decompensated CHF?

Preload is the force that distends the ventricle at end-diastole. It is approximated in the living animal by end-diastolic ventricular pressure or volume. Although end-diastolic left ventricular pressure can be estimated through the measurement of the pulmonary capillary wedge pressure, this quantity is not routinely measured in small animal patients. However, the concept of preload and its pharmacologic manipulation is theoretically useful.

Cardiogenic pulmonary edema results when elevated diastolic ventricular pressures are communicated back to the pulmonary veins and capillaries. Diuretics cause patients to produce large volumes of urine; the administration of a powerful diuretic agent such as furosemide rapidly decreases intravascular volume and, therefore, preload. The consequent decrease in left atrial pressure alters the Starling forces at the level of the pulmonary capillary and facilitates the reabsorption of edema fluid.

Furosemide is a high-ceiling loop diuretic appropriate for use in the setting of fulminant CHF. Published furosemide doses vary widely and to a large extent the dose and dosing interval are dictated by clinical circumstances. Intravenous doses in the range of 2–7 mg/kg in dogs or 1–4 mg/kg in cats are reasonable when faced with patients suffering from fulminant CHF. The intravenous route is generally preferred when it can be obtained without imposing undue stress on the patient. Other diuretics such as the thiazides, spironolactone, and amiloride may have a role in the management of patients with chronic CHF; however, they have a weaker diuretic effect than does furosemide and see little use in the treatment of fulminant CHF.

12. Do nitrates have a role in the management of acute or decompensated CHF?

Nitrates such as nitroglycerin (NG) may have beneficial effects in severe CHF. These drugs cause dilation of capacitance veins and specific arterial beds through the release of nitric oxide. The clinical efficacy of NG in small animals is uncertain; however, based on what is known of its pharmacology, the administration of NG would be expected to decrease thoracic blood volume and therefore preload, limiting the accumulation of pulmonary edema.

The transdermal formulation of NG is utilized most often. Transdermal NG is available as a cream and as a controlled-dose adhesive patch. The former allows somewhat greater flexibility of dosing; in cats, 1/8–1/4 inch of the cream is applied to an area of hairless skin. In dogs, the dose is adjusted based on body weight; smaller dogs may receive 1/4 inch of NG and large dogs as much as 1 inch. NG is commonly applied to the interior of the pinnae although more central sites such as the inguinal area might lead to more rapid and reliable absorption.

13. How else can excessive preload be reduced?

While it is seldom used, phlebotomy is an alternative means of rapidly decreasing preload. It has the obvious disadvantage that it results not only in the loss of intravascular fluid, but also in a loss of blood cells and proteins.

14. How does preload reduction affect cardiac performance?

Preload is related to cardiac performance through the Frank-Starling law of the heart; a decrease in preload diminishes the force of ventricular contraction and therefore decreases stroke volume. As a result, preload reduction generally results in a decrease in cardiac output. However, a few factors likely mitigate this effect in some cases.

Patients with systolic heart failure due, for example, to mitral valve regurgitation or dilated cardiomyopathy have large ventricles and, potentially, a "flat" Frank-Starling relationship. Thus preload can be reduced until pulmonary vein pressures are low enough to prevent edema formation with little effect on stroke volume. When mitral valve regurgitation is the main factor that limits stroke volume, a reduction in preload can decrease mitral annular dilation, reduce valvular regurgitation, and conceivably increase stroke volume.

In general, preload reduction can be expected to have a negative effect on cardiac performance but this effect is buffered by a large ventricular volume. Patients with diastolic dysfunction, such as those with hypertrophic cardiomyopathy or restrictive myocardial disease, develop signs of CHF when ventricular volumes are normal or small. In these cases, aggressive preload reduction can result in a precipitous decline in stroke volume. Similarly, patients that develop dyspnea due to respiratory disease are likely to have normal or decreased ventricular filling pressures and therefore tolerate aggressive diuresis poorly.

15. Is preload reduction indicated in diastolic failure?

Hypertrophic and restrictive myocardial diseases are the most common causes of diastolic failure in small animals. The use of furosemide is indicated when cardiogenic pulmonary edema is present and this is true irrespective of the nature of the heart disease that is responsible for congestive signs. Again however, patients with diastolic failure develop pulmonary edema when ventricular volumes are normal or small, and as a result aggressive diuresis tends to be poorly tolerated. Diuretic use is indicated in order to reduce pulmonary vein pressures; however, high diuretic doses can dangerously limit stroke volume.

16. How is afterload manipulated in systolic failure?

Afterload is the sum of forces that oppose myocardial shortening; it has an inverse relationship with cardiac performance such that an increase in afterload decreases stroke volume. Afterload is related not only to blood pressure but also to ventricular geometry. When CHF results from systolic myocardial dysfunction, afterload is inappropriately high, and as a result contractility and afterload are mismatched. When mitral valve regurgitation is the cause of CHF, elevated systemic vascular resistance is a primary factor that limits stroke volume.

It is useful to consider the relationship that exists among perfusion pressure, vascular resistance, and cardiac output. By analogy to Ohm's law, $BP = SVR \times Q$ where Q represents cardiac output, BP is blood pressure, and SVR is systemic vascular resistance. Systemic vascular resistance, which can be decreased through pharmacologic dilation of arterioles, is an important determinant of afterload. In the setting of systolic failure, judicious vasodilation reduces vascular resistance and, potentially, afterload, allowing stroke volume to increase. Because of the relationship described by Ohm's law, a reduction in resistance need not translate into clinically evident hypotension provided the drop in vascular resistance is accompanied by an increase in stroke volume. Vasodilators are not indicated in systolic failure because affected patients have abnormally high blood pressure; they are indicated because vascular resistance is abnormally high. Vasodilation alters hemodynamics in such a way as to increase stroke volume.

17. What parenteral agent can be used to reduce afterload or vascular resistance in systolic failure?

Nitroprusside is a balanced vasodilator that has a pronounced effect on the systemic arterioles. Metabolism of nitroprusside is rapid and results in the release of cyanide and nitric oxide. It is the nitrate metabolite that possesses vasodilatory properties. The agent is infused intravenously at a rate of 1–10 µg/kg per minute. Nitroprusside is a potent vasodilator and should be used only in carefully controlled circumstances. Measurement of systemic blood pressure is recommended and the dose should be titrated based upon serial blood pressure measurements and indices of peripheral perfusion. Cyanide toxicosis is a potential adverse effect associated with the use of this drug and it is suggested that the use of nitroprusside be limited to periods of less than 48 hours.

18. Are oral vasodilators useful in acute or decompensated CHF?

ACE inhibitors are the oral vasodilators used most commonly in the management of CHF. However, the efficacy of these drugs has been demonstrated in chronic heart failure, not in the setting of acute cardiac decompensation. In fact, the ACE inhibitors are not potent vasodilators and it is possible that many of the benefits of ACE inhibition are realized only after long-term use; further, these benefits are likely to result as much from reduced neurohumoral activation as from the mechanical effect of vasodilation. In contrast, hydralazine is a potent vasodilator. While the neurohumoral activation that is associated with hydralazine administration is probably of lesser concern in fulminant CHF, the potency of hydralazine may represent a liability as this drug can cause clinically important hypotension.

The use of all oral vasodilators is problematic in that it can be difficult to titrate an oral drug according to effect and gastrointestinal absorption in the critically ill may be unpredictable. Vasodilators must always be administered with caution in patients with fulminant CHF. In general, the ACE inhibitors are well tolerated and may be beneficial. Hydralazine may have a role although the risk of clinically important hypotension is greater than that associated with the use of ACE inhibitors.

19. Is afterload reduction indicated in diastolic failure?

Hypertrophic cardiomyopathy (HCM) is the most common cause of diastolic failure in animals. In this disease, systolic performance is usually normal and clinical signs are related to increases in diastolic ventricular pressure that result from impaired myocardial relaxation or reduced ventricular compliance. Many patients with HCM have hyperdynamic systolic performance, meaning that the end-systolic chamber size is small. When this is the case, there is no "systolic reserve"—stroke volume cannot increase substantially in response to vasodilation and systemic hypotension can result. There may be benefits to the use of vasodilators such as ACE inhibitors in the long-term management of diastolic failure but, in general, afterload reduction is not indicated in the management of acute or decompensated CHF that results primarily from diastolic dysfunction.

20. Are inotropic drugs indicated in fulminant CHF?

Pharmacologic inotropic support is indicated in patients with fulminant CHF due to impaired systolic myocardial function. Thus, short-term inotropic support is considered in patients with CHF due to dilated cardiomyopathy.

21. Compare and contrast the available positive inotropes.

Positive inotropes act by increasing the availability of calcium within the sarcomere or by increasing the calcium sensitivity of the contractile apparatus. The positive inotropes that are used in the management of acute CHF fall into one of three pharmacologic categories. The digitalis glycosides include digoxin and digitoxin. The phosphodiesterase inhibitors that are used as positive inotropes are the bipyridine derivatives amrinone and milrinone. The other clinically useful inotropes are catecholamines or synthetic analogues of these hormones. Dopamine, dobutamine, and epinephrine fit in this category.

Digoxin can be administered intravenously or orally. The cardiac glycosides bind to and inhibit the Na/K pump of the cardiomyocyte. The resulting change in cellular tonicity increases intracellular calcium concentration which, in turn, increases the inotropic state. The digitalis glycosides also have autonomic effects that are likely favorable in the setting of CHF. However, the glycosides are relatively weak inotropes and the therapeutic index of these agents is low. They are indicated in the chronic therapy of CHF but have a limited role in the critical care setting.

Amrinone and milrinone are potent positive inotropes that also exert a vasodilatory effect. The action of these agents is mediated through inhibition of phosphodiesterase, an enzyme that catalyzes the breakdown of cAMP, an intracellular second messenger that has many effects, including elevation of the intracellular calcium concentration. Inhibition of phosphodiesterase results in an increase in cAMP. Clinical trials in people have not shown inotropes, other than possibly digitalis, to have a beneficial effect when given for extended periods. Consequently, these drugs are not available for oral administration and they must be administered by intravenous infusion. The increase in intracellular calcium concentration is potentially arrhythmogenic and electrocardiographic monitoring is recommended during administration.

Dobutamine and other catecholamine derivatives or analogues stimulate adrenergic receptors. Adrenergic receptors are coupled by G-proteins to adenylate cyclase, an enzyme that catalyzes the release of cAMP. Increases in cAMP levels result in increased intracellular calcium concentration. These drugs must be administered by intravenous infusion. Dobutamine is a relatively selective agonist of beta-adrenergic receptors. In contrast, dopamine is referred to as a "flexible molecule" and can stimulate beta adrenergic receptors, dopaminergic receptors, and alpha-adrenergic receptors. It should be noted that all catecholamine analogues lose receptor specificity at higher doses. Consequently, it is possible to increase peripheral vascular resistance to the patient's detriment using these drugs. The administration of dobutamine results in greater increases in stroke volume relative to increase in heart rate and for this and other reasons is superior to dopamine. Electrocardiographic monitoring is recommended during infusion of adrenergic agonists.

22. How is heart rate manipulated in severe CHF?

Tachycardia develops in most canine patients with severe CHF. Partly, this results from the compensatory adrenergic nervous system activation that is a feature of the heart failure state. However, anxiety associated with the uncomfortable sensation of breathlessness likely contributes to the development of tachycardia and resolution of pulmonary edema is usually accompanied by a return of the heart rate to normal or near normal. Pharmacologic control of physiologic tachycardia is rarely indicated; the management of pathologic tachyarrhythmias is discussed elsewhere.

23. What can be done to improve diastolic function?

Attempts are made to improve diastolic function using drugs that slow heart rate and/or speed myocardial relaxation. The calcium channel antagonist diltiazem is widely used in the management of congestive heart failure due to HCM. This drug has a modest slowing effect on the sinoatrial node and is believed to increase the rate of myocardial relaxation. The beta blockers effectively slow heart rate and indirectly improve diastolic function when ventricular filling is impaired by high heart rates.

In general, the use of these agents is reserved for chronic therapy; the emergent management of diastolic failure is based primarily upon the use of furosemide, sometimes nitroglycerin, and general measures such as cage rest, supplementary oxygen administration, and pleurocentesis when indicated.

24. What is the role of oxygen supplementation?

The administration of supplemental oxygen is indicated when CHF is the cause of dyspnea. Patients with CHF are fragile and every effort should be made to limit stress and anxiety. An oxygen cage is a convenient method by which to increase the fraction of inspired oxygen; when tolerated, alternative methods include the use of a nasal cannula or face mask.

25. Should anxious animals with CHF be sedated?

Anxiety may increase respiratory rate and unnecessarily increase the work of breathing. Cautious sedation should therefore be considered for anxious patients with CHF. Morphine has an established role in the management of severe CHF in people and dogs. This drug reduces anxiety and as a favorable ancillary effect it results in venodilation; the latter serves to reduce pulmonary vein pressures facilitating the reabsorption of edema fluid. Morphine should be used cautiously because high doses result in central respiratory depression and can therefore worsen hypoxemia. In cats, narcotics must be used cautiously, and these drugs are not generally used in the management of feline CHF.

26. What role does pleurocentesis play in the management of fulminant CHF?

Pleural effusion in the absence of ascites is a fairly common manifestion of CHF in cats; in this species, pleural effusion can be associated with cardiac diseases that primarily affect the left ventricle. In dogs, cardiogenic pleural effusion is usually a manifestation of right-sided cardiac disease and it is generally observed in patients that also have ascites. When radiographic or physical findings suggest that pleural effusion is the cause of dyspnea, pleurocentesis is indicated. The procedure can be performed with manual restraint following aseptic preparation of the lateral thorax. A butterfly or over-the-needle catheter is introduced into the pleural space and then connected to a fluid administration set and syringe for removal and diagnostic evaluation. The seventh or eighth right intercostal space is used commonly, although it may be necessary to attempt pleurocentesis from both sides of the chest.

The temptation to delay pleurocentesis in hopes that diuretic therapy will adequately remove a large pleural effusion should be resisted. Diuretics mobilize body cavity effusions less effectively than they eliminate excess tissue fluid; aggressive diuresis in patients with large pleural effusions can result in hypovolemia and reduced stroke volume that precedes any useful reduction in the volume of effusate.

27. What about fluid therapy?

Except when a vehicle is required for the administration of medications, intravenous (IV) fluids should not be administered to patients suffering from overt, left-sided CHF. In other, noncardiac causes of circulatory failure, the administration of IV fluids expands intravascular volume, increases preload, and, through the Frank-Starling law of the heart, improves cardiac performance. However, patients develop cardiogenic pulmonary edema *because* of elevations in venous pressures; in a sense, preload is maximal and excessive. Therefore, when cardiogenic pulmonary edema is present, the administration of IV fluid is certain to worsen congestive signs; it will not provide the beneficial effects of increased cardiac output and renal blood flow that are expected in noncardiac disease. The cautious administration of IV or subcutaneous fluids can be considered for anorexic or dehydrated patients that have recovered from a bout of cardiogenic edema.

28. Does empirical therapy have a role? What response is expected when CHF is the cause of dyspnea?

In some patients with severe dyspnea, the risk associated with restraint for diagnostic evaluation cannot be justified and empiric therapy is reasonable. When physical and historical findings suggest a diagnosis of fulminant CHF, furosemide is administered with careful monitoring of clinical response. The concurrent use of bronchodilators and nitroglycerin might be beneficial and can also be considered. In cats, allergic bronchitis can be difficult to distinguish from acute CHF based only on physical and historical findings. While the indiscriminate use of corticosteroids is obviously to be avoided, a single dose of prednisone is usually tolerated and can be justified if diagnostic evaluation is pursued following resolution of respiratory distress.

When cardiogenic pulmonary edema is the cause of dyspnea the response to brisk diuresis is usually prompt and dramatic. Failure to respond to one or two doses of furosemide suggests that the presumptive diagnosis of CHF is incorrect, or possibly that the patient is refractory to conservative medical management. When patient response is poor, the risk-benefit ratio associated with diagnostic evaluation may shift so that restraint for diagnostic procedures can be justified. Prolonged and aggressive diuretic therapy can result in clinical deterioration in cases in which respiratory disease is in fact responsible for clinical signs.

29. Suggest a protocol for the management of severe systolic failure.

- Supplemental oxygen
- Cage rest
- Morphine for anxious patients
- Furosemide (± nitroglycerin) administered based on clinical status and response

Many if not most animals that are destined to survive an episode of acute, severe CHF are likely to do so with conservative therapy of this sort. In cases in which a definitive diagnosis of the disease responsible for CHF has been established, ancillary therapy might include:

- Nitroprusside titrated based on blood pressure and indices of peripheral perfusion for patients with mitral valve endocardiosis
- Dobutamine used together with nitroprusside for patients with severe CHF due to dilated cardiomyopathy

The following table includes doses of drugs that may be of use in the medical management of acute or decompensated systolic failure. The most common causes of systolic failure in small animals are dilated cardiomyopathy and mitral valve regurgitation due to endocardiosis; thus, the doses listed apply to the dog only.

Drugs Used in the Management of Acute or Decompensated Systolic Failure
Due to Canine Dilated Cardiomyopathy/Mitral Valve Regurgitation

DRUG	PRIMARY MECHANISM OF ACTION	DOSE	ADDITIONAL NOTES
Furosemide	Decreases preload through diuretic effect	1–8 mg/kg IV, IM, PO q1–12h	Wide dose range; dosage and interval determined by clinical status and response Parenteral administration preferred in the critical care setting
Nitoglycerin	Decreases preload through vasodilation	2% transdermal ointment 0.5–1.5 in topically q12h	Used most often in combination with diuretics
Morphine	Decreases anxiety	0.05–0.1 mg/kg IV, 0.1–0.5 mg/kg IM, SC	Morphine may have favorable hemo-dynamic effects in the setting of fulminant congestive failure
Nitroprusside	Balanced vasodilator that potentially re-duces afterload and preload	Administered only as a constant rate infusion at 1–10 µg/kg/min	Potent arteriolar dilator; monitoring of systemic blood pressure is advisable
Dobutamine	Catecholamine used as positive inotrope	Administered only as a constant rate infusion at 2.5–20 µg/kg/min	Used only in the short-term management of fulminant congestive failure due to dilated cardiomyopathy EKG monitoring is advisable Dobutamine has less effect on heart rate than dopamine when administered at equipotent doses
Dopamine	Catecholamine used as positive inotrope	Administered only as a constant rate infusion at 2.5–15 µg/kg/min	Used only in the short-term management of fulminant congestive failure due to dilated cardiomyopathy EKG monitoring is advisable
Amrinone	Phosphodiesterase inhibitor used as positive inotrope	1–3 mg/kg loading dose IV followed by constant rate infusion at 10–100 µg/kg/min	Used only in the short-term management of fulminant congestive failure due to dilated cardiomyopathy EKG monitoring is advisable

IV, intravenously; IM, intramuscularly; PO, orally; EKG, electrocardiogram.

30. Suggest a protocol for the management of severe diastolic failure.
  • Cage rest.
  • Oxygen supplementation.
  • Furosemide administered based upon clinical status and response. Feline patients with di-astolic dysfunction are intolerant of overly aggressive diuresis. Monitoring of the blood urea nitrogen, hematocrit. and total protein can be used to guide therapy.
  • Specific interventions such as diltiazem are usually reserved for chronic management of patients following echocardiographic evaluation.
  The following table includes doses of drugs that may be of use in the medical management of acute or decompensated failure resulting from diastolic dysfunction. The most common causes of diastolic failure in small animals are feline hypertrophic and restrictive cardiomyopathies; thus, the doses listed apply to the cat only. Note that pleural effusion is a relatively common man-ifestation of congestive failure in the cat; pleural effusions resulting in dyspnea are most appro-priately treated by centesis.

Drugs Used in the Management of Acute or Decompensated Diastolic Failure
Due to Feline Myocardial Disease

DRUG	PRIMARY MECHANISM OF ACTION	DOSE	NOTES
Furosemide	Decreases preload through diuretic effect	1–4 mg/kg IV, IM	Wide dose range; dosage and interval determined by clinical status and response Parenteral administration preferred in the setting of fulminant congestive failure
Nitroglycerin	Decreases preload through veno-dilation	2% nitroglycerin ointment 1/8–1/4 in topically	Used most often in combination with diuretics
Diltiazem	Positive lusitrope	7.5 mg/cat PO q8h	Commonly used in the chronic management of feline patients with hypertrophic cardiomyopathy Role in the management of fulminant failure uncertain

IV, intravenously; IM, intramuscularly; PO, orally.

31. What monitoring is appropriate for a patient with acute or severe CHF?

Patients with CHF are fragile and the relative risk-benefit ratio of manipulation for diagnostic procedures must be carefully considered. Invasive monitoring including the placement of a Swan-Ganz catheter and an arterial cannula provides nearly complete hemodynamic information that can be used to modify therapy. However, complete instrumentation such as this requires intensive nursing care, is difficult to maintain, and is expensive.

The use of indirect blood pressure measurement devices can provide useful information if the limitations of these techniques are recognized. Systemic blood pressure is a valuable measure because it is known that a mean perfusion pressure of about 60 mmHg is necessary to maintain the viability of vital capillary beds in the brain and kidney. However, blood pressure is not a measure of flow and it is possible for blood pressure to be maintained at the expense of cardiac output. The measurement of central venous pressure (CVP) can provide useful information and the technique is relatively easy. However, CVP is a measure of right ventricular filling pressure; it does not provide information about pulmonary venous pressure in the setting of left ventricular dysfunction.

Despite the availability of numerous relatively elaborate monitoring techniques, most patients with severe CHF can be managed with careful attention to the vital signs. Monitoring of heart rate, respiratory rate and character, assessment of femoral arterial pulse, and observation of the mucous membranes provide invaluable information regarding response to therapy and short-term prognosis.

32. What is a Swan-Ganz catheter? What information can it provide?

A Swan-Ganz catheter is a multilumen catheter that is "flow-directed" by a small balloon located near the catheter tip. The catheter is introduced into the jugular or femoral vein and, following balloon inflation, is passed into the pulmonary artery under fluoroscopic guidance or through observation of the distinctive pressure contours of the cardiac chambers and pulmonary artery. The catheter is connected to a fluid-filled manometer system and can provide simultaneous central venous pressure and pulmonary artery pressure. Inflation of the balloon when the catheter is positioned in a peripheral pulmonary artery provides the pulmonary capillary wedge pressure, which is an estimate of left atrial pressure. In addition, the catheters are equipped with a thermosistor device that can provide measurements of cardiac output when used with a compatible cardiac-output computer.

A Swan-Ganz catheter can provide estimates of left and right ventricular filling pressures, measurement of pulmonary artery pressure, and a measure of cardiac output. If this information is supplemented by knowledge of the systemic blood pressure, the vascular resistance can be calculated. The use of the Swan-Ganz catheter as a monitoring tool in veterinary medicine is generally restricted to larger referral centers. However, the knowledge that their use provides can be invaluable in the management of critically ill patients with CHF; it allows therapeutic decisions to be made based upon knowledge of hemodynamics.

33. What is the prognosis?
Ultimately, the prognosis of patients with CHF is poor; unless the cause of heart failure can be identified and remedied, CHF is terminal and survival of 4–8 months is typical even with palliative medical therapy.

BIBLIOGRAPHY

1. Braunwald E, Colucci WS. Pathophysiology of heart failure. In Braunwald E (ed): Heart Disease: A Textbook of Cardiovascular Medicine, 4th ed. Philadelphia, W.B. Saunders, 1997, pp 394–420.
2. The COVE Study Group. Controlled clinical evaluation of enalapril in dogs with heart failure: Results of the Cooperative Veterinary Enalapril Study Group. J Vet Intern Med 9:243–252, 1995.
3. Hamlin RL: Pathophysiology of the failing heart. In Fox PR, Sisson D, Moise NS (eds): Textbook of Canine and Feline Cardiology: Principles and Clinical Practice, 2nd ed. Philadelphia, W.B. Saunders, 1999, pp 205–215.
4. Keene BW, Rush JE: Therapy of heart failure. In Ettinger SJ, Feldman EC (eds) : Textbook of Veterinary Internal Medicine, 4th ed. Philadelphia, W.B. Saunders, 1993, pp 867–892.
5. Kittleson MD: Management of heart failure. In Kittelson MD, Kienle RD (eds): Small Animal Cardiovascular Medicine. St. Louis, Mosby, 1998, pp 149–194.
6. Kittleson MD: Pathophysiology of heart failure. In Small Animal Cardiovascular Medicine. St. Louis, Mosby, 1998, pp 136–148.
7. Knight DH: Efficacy of inotropic support of the failing heart. Vet Clin North Am Small Anim Pract 21:879–904, 1991.
8. Packer M, Bristow MR, Coth JN, et al: The effect of carvedilol on mobidity and mortality in patients with chronic heart failure. N Engl J Med 334:1349–1355, 1996.
9. Sisson D, Kittleson MD: Management of heart failure: Principles of treatment, therapeutic strategies and pharmacology. In Fox PR, Sisson D, Moise NS (eds): Textbook of Canine and Feline Cardiology: Principles and Clinical Practice, 2nd ed. Philadelphia, W.B. Saunders, 1999, pp 216–250.

28. MANAGEMENT OF CHRONIC CONGESTIVE HEART FAILURE

Jonathan A. Abbott, D.V.M.

1. What is heart failure?

Heart failure is present when cardiac output is inadequate to meet the body's metabolic demands despite adequate preload. This definition excludes extracardiac causes of reduced cardiac output, such as hypovolemia. For example, a patient that suffers from hemorrhagic shock has inadequate cardiac output; however, the patient does not have heart failure, because the failure of the circulatory system to sustain normal metabolic function is not the result of primary cardiac dysfunction. The qualifying statement related to preload localizes the cause of circulatory dysfunction to the heart; heart failure can be alternatively defined as a sustained and consequential decrease in cardiac output that results from cardiac dysfunction.

It is important to recognize that heart *failure* results from heart *disease* and that practically any heart disease can result in heart failure. In veterinary medicine, heart failure is most often manifest as congestive heart failure (CHF). The clinical signs are due primarily to the development of abnormally high systemic or, more often, pulmonary venous pressures. Left-sided CHF is characterized by pulmonary congestion and edema while right-sided CHF is manifest as body cavity effusions or peripheral edema.

2. What is chronic CHF?

The diseases that cause CHF in small animals are typically chronic and progressive; despite this, however, the onset of CHF is apparently sudden in many affected animals. Unfortunately, the improvement in clinical status that accompanies the elimination of pulmonary edema does not herald recovery from CHF. The complex neuroendocrine responses that comprise the syndrome of CHF persist despite resolution of clinical signs. The term *overt CHF* is used to refer to patients that have clinical signs such as dyspnea or cough resulting from pulmonary edema. Patients with *chronic heart failure* have persistent cardiac dysfunction that has at some time resulted in signs of pulmonary or systemic congestion.

3. What is meant by neuroendocrine activation?

The compensatory response to diminished cardiac performance involves the activation of the adrenergic, or sympathetic, nervous system and the release of renin from the kidney. The former serves to provide inotropic and chronotropic support to the failing heart. Additionally, elevations in adrenergic tone result in vasoconstriction; this increases systemic vascular resistance, which allows maintenance of normal systemic blood pressure when cardiac output is low. Through an enzymatic cascade, the release of renin results in the elaboration of angiotensin II. Angiotensin II is not only a potent vasoconstrictor but it also induces the release of aldosterone and antidiuretic hormone and potentiates the activity of the adrenergic nervous system. Together, these effects result in vasoconstriction and contribute to the renal retention of salt and water. The compensatory responses observed in patients with cardiac dysfunction represent neuroendocrine activation. The results of clinical trials using people and animals suggest that the renin-angiotensin-aldosterone system (RAAS) and the adrenergic nervous system (ANS) contribute to the progressive nature of CHF; from this has evolved the concept of CHF as a neuroendocrine or neurohumoral syndrome.

4. How does the management of chronic heart failure differ from the management of acute or decompensated CHF?

Current evidence suggests that the activation of compensatory mechanisms such as the adrenergic nervous system and the renin-angiotensin-aldosterone system (RAAS) play an important role in the progression of CHF; tempering these responses with drug therapy has been shown to improve long-term prognosis. In fact, drug efficacy studies performed in people demonstrate that long-term use of beta blockers has a "cardioprotective" effect despite the fact that these drugs can have a negative effect on cardiac performance in the short term. Thus, the treatment of patients with chronic CHF is aimed not only at the elimination of clinical signs but also at modifying the maladaptive compensatory responses associated with chronic cardiac dysfunction. In contrast, the therapeutic objectives in the management of acute CHF are simpler and perhaps more intuitive; in acute CHF, interventions are directed toward improving oxygenation through the elimination of pulmonary edema and, when possible, toward increasing cardiac performance.

5. What is the difference between systolic and diastolic failure? How is this distinction important in case management?

Systolic cardiac performance is a global measure of pumping performance; it is affected by myocardial function or contractility, and also by afterload, preload, and valvular competence. In this chapter, systolic failure refers to CHF that results from some deficit of pumping performance. Mitral valve regurgitation and dilated cardiomyopathy are the most common causes of systolic failure.

Diastolic cardiac performance refers to the ability of the ventricle to fill at low diastolic pressures. Pathologic hypertrophy and endomyocardial fibrosis can impair diastolic performance; restrictive myocardial diseases and hypertrophic cardiomyopathy are examples of disorders that can result in diastolic failure.

Impaired systolic and diastolic performance can coexist in a single patient. However, the therapeutic approach to patients that fall into one of the two somewhat artificial designations differ and for that reason the distinction is conceptually useful.

6. Why are vasodilators effective in the management of chronic systolic failure?

Resistance is the quantity that determines the amount of blood that flows through a vascular bed when it is subject to a given pressure. In a sense, resistance is a measure of how difficult it is to force blood through the vessels. Resistance is dependent on a number of factors but the most important of these is vessel diameter, because this factor is subject to physiologic influences and manipulation by vasodilating drugs.

Vascular resistance is an important determinant of blood pressure and therefore afterload. However, afterload is best approximated by wall stress, which is related not only to blood pressure but also to ventricular diameter and wall thickness. If ventricular dilation is not offset by hypertrophy, afterload is increased even if blood pressure is normal. This is the case in patients with dilated cardiomyopathy; the dilated, thin-walled ventricle functions at a mechanical disadvantage because afterload is high even if blood pressure is normal.

In CHF, increases in adrenergic tone and vasoactive hormones such as angiotensin II result in vasoconstriction. In the short term, this has the favorable effect that systemic blood pressure can be maintained when cardiac output is low. However, in patients with dilated, thin-walled ventricles, systolic wall stress (afterload) is elevated and this increase in afterload comes at the price of an increase in myocardial oxygen demand. When systolic myocardial failure is present, there is a mismatch between contractility and afterload. Judicious vasodilation reduces afterload, which permits an increase in stroke volume. When mitral valve regurgitation is the cause of CHF, there is an analogous mismatch between vascular resistance and the resistance imposed by the regurgitant orifice; the compensatory increase in vascular resistance is the factor that limits stroke volume.

Vasodilators are not indicated in systolic failure because systemic hypertension is present; rather, they are effective because they decrease vascular resistance and allow stroke volume to increase. The favorable effect of vasodilation is one of degree; excessive vasodilation results in hypotension in animals with systolic failure as it does in normal individuals.

7. Are vasodilators effective in chronic diastolic failure?

Hypertrophic cardiomyopathy (HCM) is probably the most common cause of diastolic failure in animals. Usually, systolic performance is normal and clinical signs are related to increases in diastolic ventricular pressure that result from impaired myocardial relaxation or reduced ventricular compliance. Although the neuroendocrine status of patients with heart failure due to feline HCM is not well described, it is reasonable to believe that both the adrenergic nervous system and RAAS are activated. Vascular resistance may therefore be high as a compensatory measure to maintain blood pressure when stroke volume is diminished. However, unless the patient has substantial mitral valve regurgitation, it is unlikely that a decrease in vascular resistance will result in an increase in stroke volume. Many patients with HCM have hyperdynamic systolic performance, that is, the end-systolic chamber size is small. When this is the case, there is little "systolic reserve"; stroke volume cannot increase substantially and vasodilation could conceivably result in systemic hypotension. It should be recognized, however, that many patients with HCM do have mitral valve regurgitation and that the ancillary effects of vasodilators such as ACE inhibitors might have a favorable effect.

8. Why is the renin-angiotensin-aldosterone system (RAAS) important in the management of chronic systolic failure?

The RAAS is activated when cardiac performance declines. Ultimately its endocrine products result in vasoconstriction and the renal retention of salt and water. In systolic failure, pharmacologic interference with this system through the use of angiotensin converting enzyme (ACE) inhibitors results in vasodilation and a favorable decrease in afterload. The ACE inhibitors were the first drugs subject to comparison with a placebo to demonstrate a favorable effect on mortality in people with CHF. Since that time, the efficacy of the ACE inhibitor enalapril has been shown in canine patients with CHF due to acquired valvular disease and dilated cardiomyopathy. That activation of the RAAS in heart failure has important implications was suggested by a therapeutic trial that compared a combination of hydralazine and isosorbide dinitrate to enalapril in people with CHF. Despite the fact that the hydralazine had the predicted beneficial effects on stroke volume, mortality was lower in the group receiving enalapril.

At least initially, the effects of the RAAS are likely to be positive; they help to maintain blood pressure and cardiac output. However, there is strong evidence to believe that chronic activation of the RAAS contributes to the progressive nature of CHF. In people with CHF, markers of RAAS activation are associated with a poor prognosis but ACE inhibitors, which blunt the effect of the RAAS, reduce mortality. It is therefore likely that RAAS activation itself has a detrimental effect in chronic CHF.

9. If activation of the RAAS is "maladaptive," why is it tolerated by natural selection?

The RAAS and adrenergic nervous system have been preserved by evolution because they are well suited to the short-term maintenance of circulatory function. The neuroendocrine responses observed in heart failure are similar to those that result from acute hemorrhage. The effects of the RAAS and adrenergic nervous system are favorable when the cause of decreased cardiac performance is of short duration because vasoconstriction and sodium retention allow survival of acute circulatory embarrassment. Provided the cause of decreased cardiac performance resolves, homeostasis is restored and the compensatory mechanisms are again "turned off."

10. ACE inhibitors have demonstrated efficacy in the management of acquired valvular disease and dilated cardiomyopathy in dogs. Why are they thought to be superior to other vasodilators such as hydralazine?

Hydralazine is a more potent vasodilator than are the ACE inhibitors, and hydralazine is superior to the ACE inhibitors in terms of acute effects on cardiac performance. However, hydralazine results in reflex-mediated increases in adrenergic tone and activation of the RAAS, and this is probably the reason that clinical trials in people with CHF have demonstrated greater mortality reduction with the use of ACE inhibitors. The fact that survival studies demonstrate the superiority of ACE inhibitors over a more potent and seemingly effective vasodilator underscores the importance of the RAAS in the pathogenesis of CHF. It should be recognized that the clinical trial that compared hydralazine to ACE inhibitors was performed in people who suffered from systolic myocardial dysfunction. Whether or not ACE inhibitors are in fact superior to hydralazine in patients with mitral valve disease is not known.

11. Do beta-adrenergic antagonists have a role in the management of systolic failure?

Beta-adrenergic antagonists are negative inotropes, negative chronotropes, and negative dromotropes. That these drugs might be beneficial to patients with decreased contractility is counter-intuitive. However, recent clinical trials demonstrate that long-term use of beta blockers has favorable effects in people with systolic myocardial dysfunction. Specifically, the beta-blocker carvedilol reduces morbidity and mortality relative to placebo in patients with chronic heart failure. The reason for the improvement in clinical status and reduction in mortality is not known; it is likely that beta blockers protect the heart from the toxic effect of persistently elevated adrenergic tone. Caution must be exercised in extrapolating this new and encouraging information to the treatment of animals with heart failure. Animals are generally presented for veterinary evaluation with advanced myocardial dysfunction; some of these animals may be critically dependent on elevated adrenergic tone in order to maintain cardiac output and blood pressure. When this is the case, the negatively inotropic effects of beta blockers can have catastrophic results.

12. Diuretics are a mainstay in the management of acute CHF; do they have a role in chronic CHF?

Diuretics most definitely have a role in the management of chronic CHF. Although cats with hypertrophic cardiomyopathy seem to suffer from episodes of heart failure, the common acquired heart diseases in dogs result in progressive cardiac dysfunction and a persistent sodium-retaining state. While overly aggressive diuretic use can decrease cardiac performance and contribute to activation of the RAAS, most dogs with chronic CHF require lifelong diuretic therapy.

13. Why is digoxin different from other positive inotropes?

Digoxin is a positive inotrope that has clinically important effects on the autonomic nervous system. The positive inotropic effect is mediated through increases in intracellular calcium concentration that result from paralysis of the cellular sodium-potassium pump. The autonomic effects of digoxin are diverse but include increases in arterial baroreceptor sensitivity. In general, digoxin increases vagal tone and decreases sympathetic outflow; in so doing, digoxin slows the heart rate. Thus, digoxin is unique among inotropes in that it slows the heart rate; this feature of digoxin may limit myocardial oxygen demand and partly explain the beneficial effects of this drug. Based on clinical studies performed in people, the long-term effects of digoxin are favorable; digoxin improves clinical status and decreases hospitalization due to worsening congestion. While the effect of digoxin on mortality is, in fact, neutral, this is in contrast to the negative effect on long-term survival that is associated with the use of other positive inotropes. For this reason, it has been suggested that the beneficial effect of digoxin results not from inotropy but rather from the autonomic "sparing" effect of the drug.

The table below includes doses of drugs that may be of use in the medical management of chronic systolic failure. The most common causes of systolic failure in small animals are dilated cardiomyopathy and mitral valve regurgitation due to endocardiosis; thus, unless indicated, the doses listed apply to the dog only. Anitarrhythmic therapy is covered in greater detail in Chapter 15.

Drugs Used in the Management of Chronic Systolic Failure Due to Canine Dilated Cardiomyopathy/Mitral Valve Regurgitation

DRUG	PRIMARY MECHANISM OF ACTION	DOSE	ADDITIONAL NOTES
Furosemide	Decreases preload through potent loop diuretic effect	1–5 mg/kg PO q8–12h	Wide dose range; dosage and interval determined by clinical status and response

Table continued on following page

*Drugs Used in the Management of Chronic Systolic Failure Due to
Canine Dilated Cardiomyopathy/Mitral Valve Regurgitation (Continued)*

DRUG	PRIMARY MECHANISM OF ACTION	DOSE	ADDITIONAL NOTES
Spironolactone	Aldosterone antagonist that decreases preload through a potassium-sparing diuretic effect	1–2 mg/kg PO q12h	Relatively weak diuretic but antagonism of aldosterone may help to preserve myocardial function and prevent fibrosis; usually used in combination with other diuretics
Hydrochloro-thiazide	Decreases preload through diuretic effect	2–4 mg/kg PO q12h	Relatively weak diuretic; usually used in combination with other diuretics
Enalapril	Balanced vasodilator with important neuro-endocrine effects	0.5 mg/kg PO q12–24h	ACEIs have become standard therapy for systolic failure in dogs
Benazepril	Balanced vasodilator with important neuro-endocrine effects	0.25–0.5 mg/kg PO q24h	ACEIs have become standard therapy for systolic failure in dogs Excreted by renal and hepatic route, benazepril may be the preferred ACEI in the face of renal dysfunction
Hydralazine	Decreases systemic resistance through arteriolar dilation	0.5–3 mg/kg PO q12h	Potent vasodilator that is used when ACEIs are not tolerated or, occasionally, in addition to an ACEI in severe chronic systolic failure due to mitral valve endocardiosis A low dose is used initially and then titrated based on blood pressure and/or clinical response
Nitroglycerin	Decreases preload through venodilation	Small dogs: 0.1 mg/hr patch Large dogs: 0.2 mg/hr patch	Used most often in the management of fulminant congestive failure, occasionally in combination with diuretics for chronic failure For this purpose, the patches are probably preferable to the ointment; the smaller patch can be cut for very small dogs Because of possible nitrate tolerance, 12 hours on/12 hours off is used by some
Digoxin	Positive inotrope with important autonomic effects	Dogs < 15 kg: 0.005–0.011 mg/kg PO q12h Dogs > 15 kg: 0.22 mg/m² PO q12h Cats < 3 kg: 0.03125 mg PO q48h Cats 3–6 kg: 0.03125 mg PO q24h Cats > 6 kg: 0.3125 mg PO q 12 h	Vagomimetic effect often used to slow the ventricular rates of patients in whom supraventricular tachy-arrhythmias, particularly atrial fibrillation, complicate systolic heart failure Monitoring of therapy through determination of serum digoxin levels is advisable Renal function and serum potassium should be monitored

Table continued on following page

Drugs Used in the Management of Chronic Systolic Failure Due to Canine
Dilated Cardiomyopathy/Mitral Valve Regurgitation (Continued)

DRUG	PRIMARY MECHANISM OF ACTION	DOSE	ADDITIONAL NOTES
Diltiazem	Supraventricular anti-arrhythmic agent that slows the ventricular response to atrial fibrillation through effects on AV nodal conduction	0.5–1.5 mg/kg PO q8h	Sometimes used in addition to digoxin to slow ventricular rates in atrial fibrillation
Atenolol	Supraventricular anti-arrhythmic agent that slows the ventricular response to atrial fibrillation through effects on AV nodal conduction	0.25–1 mg/kg PO q12–24 h	Sometimes used in addition to digoxin (± diltiazem) to slow ventricular rates in atrial fibrillation Recent evidence suggests that beta-blockers may slow the progression of myocardial dysfunction

PO, orally; ACEI, angiotensin-converting enzyme inhibitor, AV = atrioventricular.

14. What agents are used in the management of chronic diastolic failure?

Hypertrophic cardiomyopathy (HCM) is the most common cause of diastolic failure in small animals. Decreased ventricular compliance and impaired myocardial relaxation increase diastolic ventricular pressures and potentially result in CHF. Therapeutic strategies include the use of drugs that speed myocardial relaxation and/or decrease heart rate. Diltiazem is used commonly in feline HCM. This drug has a modest effect on heart rate but is believed to improve myocardial relaxation. This latter property is known as a positive lusitropic effect. Beta-blocking drugs such as propranolol and atenolol are also used in the management of chronic diastolic failure resulting from HCM. These drugs effectively slow heart rate and are likely to be useful when rapid rates impair ventricular filling. Beta blockers do not appear to have a direct effect on myocardial relaxation, although they may increase ventricular compliance.

The table below includes doses of drugs that may be of use in the medical management of chronic diastolic failure. The most common causes of diastolic failure in small animals are restrictive and hypertorphic cardiomyopathies in the cat; thus, the doses listed apply to the cat only. Echocardiographic characterization of feline myocardial disease is recommended as a means to guide therapy; see Chapter 23 for further details.

Drugs Used in the Management of Chronic Diastolic Failure
Due to Feline Myocardial Disease

DRUG	PRIMARY MECHANISM OF ACTION	DOSE	NOTES
Furosemide	Decreases preload through diuretic effect	0.5–4 mg/kg PO q12–24h	Patients with diastolic failure tend to tolerate aggressive diuresis poorly; the lowest dose that limits clinical signs is optimal
Diltiazem	Positive lusitrope	Standard formulation: 7.5 mg/cat PO q8h Long-acting forms (Cardizem CD or Dilacor XR): 10 mg/kg PO q24h; must be reformulated to provide appropriate capsule sizes	Commonly used in the chronic management of feline patients with hypertrophic cardiomyopathy

Table continued on following page

*Drugs Used in the Management of Chronic Diastolic Failure
Due to Feline Myocardial Disease (Continued)*

DRUG	PRIMARY MECHANISM OF ACTION	DOSE	NOTES
Propranolol	Negative chronotrope and negative inotrope that may reduce intraventricular pressure gradients in patients with the obstructive form of feline hypertrophic cardiomyopathy	2.5–5 mg/cat PO q8h	Used in the chronic management of feline patients with hypertrophic cardiomyopathy Beta-blockers may have an advantage over calcium antagonists when intraventricular pressure gradients are present or when tachycardia persists following the resolution of congestive signs
Atenolol	Negative chronotrope and negative inotrope that may reduce intraventricular pressure gradients in patients with the obstructive form of feline hypertrophic cardiomyopathy	6.25–12.5 mg/cat PO q12h	Used in the chronic management of feline patients with hypertrophic cardiomyopathy Beta-blockers may have an advantage over calcium antagonists when intraventricular pressure gradients are present or when tachycardia persists following the resolution of congestive signs The pharmacokinetics of atenolol may represent an advantage over propranolol
Enalapril	Balanced vasodilator with important neuroendocrine effects	0.25–0.5 mg/kg PO q24h	ACEIs have become standard therapy for systolic failure in dogs; their role in patients with diastolic failure is not certain. The reduction in aldosterone levels might be helpful in cases that develop recurrent congestive signs despite standard therapy (furosemide + diltiazem and/or a beta-blocker)
Benazepril	Balanced vasodilator with important neuroendocrine effects	0.25–0.5 mg/kg PO q24h	ACEIs have become standard therapy for systolic failure in dogs; their role in patients with diastolic failure is not certain. The reduction in aldosterone levels might be helpful in cases that develop recurrent congestive signs despite standard therapy (furosemide + diltiazem and/or a beta-blocker)

PO, orally; ACEI, angiotensin-converting enzyme inhibitor.

15. What about diet in chronic heart failure?

CHF is a clinical syndrome that is associated with renal retention of salt and water, and so dietary salt restriction has long been an aspect of its medical management. The availability of potent diuretics and ACE inhibitors has perhaps decreased the importance of dietary sodium manipulation. However, decreased salt intake has a preload-reducing effect and moderate salt restriction is reasonable for patients with chronic CHF.

16. Furosemide is the diuretic that is used most commonly in CHF; are any others important?

The effect of diuresis is mechanical; reductions in intravascular volume decrease preload and limit the accumulation of edema. Furosemide is a potent loop diuretic that is widely used in the management of chronic CHF. Recent evidence indicates that spironolactone, an aldosterone antagonist, decreases morbidity and mortality in human patients with CHF who are receiving a combination of an ACE inhibitor and loop diuretic. Interestingly, this favorable effect was evident at a dose of spironolactone that did not cause diuresis. This is probably explained by the extrarenal effects of aldosterone. While this hormone stimulates the renal retention of sodium and water, it also promotes the development of myocardial fibrosis.

17. What is the prognosis?
Ultimately, the prognosis of patients with CHF is poor; unless the cause of heart failure can be identified and remedied, CHF is terminal and survival of 4–8 months is typical even with palliative medical therapy.

18. Is there anything new on the horizon for the treatment of heart failure?
In recent years, much attention has been directed toward the pharmacologic manipulation of the neuroendocrine responses that characterize CHF. The use of ACE inhibitors is well established and, at least in people, beta-adrenergic blockade now plays an important role in the management of chronic heart failure. Blunting of other hormonal responses to impaired cardiac performance might also have promise.

Plasma levels of endothelin and arginine vasopressin are both elevated in the setting of heart failure. Endotheline is a potent endogenous vasoconstrictor. Arginine vasopressin, also known as antidiuretic hormone (ADH), is a vasoconstrictor that contributes to the renal retention of solute-free water. The clinical importance of these hormones in the pathogenesis of heart failure is not certain; however, it may be that agents that antagonize their effects would benefit patients with CHF. Endothelin and arginine vasopressin antagonists are in the investigational stage.

Atrial natriuretic peptide (ANP) and related hormones, such as brain natriuretic peptide (BNP), are released in response to atrial and ventricular stretch; they contribute to vasodilation and renal sodium excretion. In a sense, they have effects that oppose those of RAAS and adrenergic nervous system. In CHF, the effect of the natriuretic peptides is overwhelmed by neuroendocrine responses that result in vasoconstriction and sodium retention. However, there might be a therapeutic role for agents that can increase the activity of these apparently "favorable" hormones. Antagonists of neutral endopeptidase, an enzyme that inactivates ANP and BNP, have been used experimentally in canine heart failure and shown a promising effect.

CONTROVERSY

19. Are positive inotropes useful in the management of CHF?
In patients with chronic CHF due to dilated cardiomyopathy, it seems reasonable that an effective positive inotrope would improve cardiac performance and therefore reduce mortality. However, clinical trials conducted in people do not uphold this supposition. For example, the administration of milrinone, a potent positive inotrope, increased mortality in a population of people with CHF due to systolic myocardial dysfunction. Other positive inotropes including xamoterol and vesvarinone have had detrimental effects when administered over long periods to people with CHF. In fact, the only positive inotrope that has been shown to have positive long-term effects in people is digoxin, and it is possible that the favorable effects of this drug is related as much to its autonomic effects as its inotropic property. The reason that positive inotropes are potentially harmful is not known, but it might relate to metabolic cost of increased contractility. Inotropes generally increase myocardial oxygen demand, which may hasten the deterioration of cardiac function. However, the lesson from numerous clinical trials conducted in people is apparently clear: in the long term, inotropes other than digoxin are harmful and effective therapies for heart failure are ones that "spare the heart" by blunting the effects of neuroendocrine activation.

The extrapolation of conclusions drawn in people to veterinary patients must always be undertaken with caution, however. While the effect of milrinone on mortality in animals with CHF is not known, this drug has been shown to improve clinical signs in dogs with dilated cardiomyopathy. More recently, preliminary evidence suggests that pimbobendan decreases mortality in some dogs with CHF due to dilated cardiomyopathy. Why positive inotropes may have different effects in people and animals is unclear, although it might relate to severity of myocardial dysfunction that is observed in animals; canine patients with dilated cardiomyopathy typically have advanced myocardial dysfunction. Perhaps in these cases it is more important to preserve cardiac performance than it is to "spare the heart." Additionally, many dogs with CHF are euthanized before they die of progressive pump failure. Treatments that reliably improve clinical signs might cause owners to delay euthanasia, which could partly explain mortality reduction associated with the administration of positive inotropes such as pimbobendan.

BIBLIOGRAPHY

1. Braunwald E, Colucci WS: Pathophysiology of heart failure. In Braunwald E (ed): Heart Disease: A Textbook of Cardiovascular Medicine, 4th ed. Philadelphia, W.B. Saunders, 1997, pp 394–420.
2. Cleland JGF, Bristow MR, Erdmann E, et al: Beta-blocking agents in heart failure: Should they be used and how? Eur Heart J 17:1629–1639, 1996.
3. Cody RJ: Hormonal alterations in heart failure. In Hosenpud JD, Greenberg BH (eds): Congestive Heart Failure: Pathophysiology, Diagnosis, and Approach to Management, 2nd ed. Philadelphia, Lippincott Williams & Wilkins, 2000.
4. The COVE Study Group: Controlled clinical evaluation of enalapril in dogs with heart failure: Results of the Cooperative Veterinary Enalapril Study Group. J Vet Intern Med 9:243–252, 1995.
5. The Digitalis Investigation Group: The effect of digoxin on mortality and morbidity in patients with heart failure. N Engl J Med 336:525–533, 1997.
6. Gheorghiade M, Pitt B: Digitalis Investigation Group (DIG) trial: A stimulus for further research. Am Heart J 134:3–12, 1997.
7. Hamlin RL: Pathophysiology of the failing heart. In Fox PR, Sisson D, Moise NS (eds): Textbook of Canine and Feline Cardiology: Principles and Clinical Practice, 2nd ed. Philadelphia, W.B. Saunders, 1999, pp 205–215.
8. Keene BW, Rush JE: Therapy of heart failure. In Ettinger SJ and Feldman EC (eds): Textbook of Veterinary Internal Medicine, 4th ed. Philadelphia, W.B. Saunders, 1993, pp 867–892.
9. Kittleson MD: Management of heart failure. In Kittleson MD, Kienle RD (eds): Small Animal Cardiovascular Medicine. St. Louis, Mosby, 1998, pp 149–194.
10. Kittleson MD: Pathophysiology of heart failure. In Kittleson MD, Kienle RD (eds): Small Animal Cardiovascular Medicine. St. Louis, Mosby, 1998, pp 136–148.
11. Knight DH: Efficacy of inotropic support of the failing heart. Vet Clin North Am Small Anim Pract 21:879–904, 1991.
12. Luis Fuentes V, Kleeman R, Justus C, et al: The effect of the novel inodilator pimobendan on heart failure status in cocker spaniels and dobermans with idiopathic dilated cardiomyopathy (abstract). Proceedings of the British Small Animal Veterinary Association Congress, Birmingham, UK, 1998.
13. Packer M, Cohn JN (eds): Consensus recommendations for the management of chronic heart failure. Am J Cardiol 83(2A):1A–38A, 1999.
14. Packer M, Bristow MR, Cohn JN, et al: The effect of carvedilol on mobidity and mortality in patients with chronic heart failure. N Engl J Med 334:1349–1355, 1996.
15. Pitt B, Zannad F, Remme WJ, et al: The effect of spironolactone on morbidity and mortality in patients with severe heart failure. N Engl J Med 341:709–717, 1999.
16. Sabbah HN, Shimoyama H, Kono T, et al: Effects of long-term monotherapy with enalapril, metoprolol, and digoxin on the progression of left ventricular dysfunction and dilation in dogs with reduced ejection fraction. Circulation 89:2852–2859, 1994.
17. Sisson D, Kittleson MD: Management of heart failure: Principles of treatment, therapeutic strategies and pharmacology. In Fox PR, Sisson D, Moise NS (eds): Textbook of Canine and Feline Cardiology: Principles and Clinical Practice, 2nd ed. Philadelphia, W. B. Saunders, 1999, pp 216–250.
18. Ware WA, Keene BW: Outpatient management of chronic heart failure. In Bonagura JD (ed): Kirk's Current Veterinary Therapy XIII: Small Animal Practice. Philadelphia, W.B. Saunders, 2000, pp 748–752.

29. VENTRICULAR TACHYARRHYTHMIA

Carl D. Sammarco, B.V.Sc., MRCVS

1. What are ventricular tachyarrhythmias?

A ventricular tachyarrhythmia is any electrical beat originating from the ventricle that occurs early or prematurely. This excludes escape beats due to AV node block and sinus pause/arrest.

2. What are ventricular premature complexes?

Ventricular premature complexes (VPCs) are depolarizations that originate from the ventricles and interrupt the cardiac rhythm because they occur prior to the expected normal complex. When ventricular depolarization begins within the ventricles, it is necessary for the ventricles to depolarize as a "functional syncytium"; this takes longer than a normal depolarization that follows the specialized conduction system and the resultant electrocardiographic complex is wider than normal. The electrocardiographic polarity of the ectopic depolarization depends on the anatomic site of origin. For example, a VPC that originates from the cardiac apex may result in a wave of depolarization that is directed cranially; the resultant electrocardiographic complex is predominantly negative in lead II. Therefore, VPCs are recognized electrocardiographically as premature complexes with wide and bizarre configuration; P waves, if seen, are not causally related to the QRS.

3. What is ventricular tachycardia?

Ventricular tachycardia is a series of three or more ventricular complexes. The "run" of ventricular tachycardia is initiated by a VPC. Ventricular tachycardias generally have a rate greater than 160 bpm and can be nonsustained or sustained. Nonsustained ventricular tachycardia lasts for less than 30 seconds, while sustained ventricular tachycardias last longer than 30 seconds.

4. What else can cause tachycardia with wide QRS complexes?

Supraventricular tachycardias with aberrant ventricular conduction or bundle branch block can be confused with ventricular arrhythmias; both result in wide-complex, monomorphic tachycardias with no obvious P waves. Slowing the heart rate may allow differentiation of these rhythms, revealing the patient's "normal" QRS configuration. Attempts to slow the heart rate can be made with vagal maneuvers, precordial thumps, or administration of intravenous antiarrhythmic therapy.

5. What is the diagnostic approach to a suspected ventricular tachyarrhythmia?

If the arrhythmia is frequent, running an ECG on a standard machine or chest-held device may be sufficient to document the arrhythmia and make the diagnosis. Chest-held devices such as the Vet Biolog (Micromedical, Australia) and the SDI VET/ECG Monitoring (Sensor Devices Inc., Waukesha, WI) can produce an ECG by applying the device to an alcohol-soaked haircoat/skin on the thorax. Monitoring of the ECG for a longer period of time or in a more directed way may be needed for less frequent arrhythmias. Holter and event monitors are useful in cases of such intermittent arrhythmias.

One of the pitfalls to avoid when investigating the cause of syncope is to conclude that ventricular tachycardia is the cause of syncope based solely on the presence of VPCs on a standard 2-minute ECG. In any syncopal dog, including Dobermans and boxers, the presence of VPCs on a 2-minute ECG does not always indicate the patient is fainting due to ventricular tachycardia. In the author's experience and in reported studies, syncope secondary to bradycardia can be occurring in patients who exhibit VPCs on a 2-minute ECG. Holter and event monitors are important diagnostic tools in evaluating these cases.

6. What causes ventricular arrhythmias?

Ventricular arrhythmias can occur due to primary heart disease, secondary to systemic disease, or can be idiopathic (a diagnosis of exclusion when no underlying systemic or cardiac disease is detectable by extensive evaluation). Full evaluation includes a thorough history, physical examination, complete blood count, serum chemistry profile, urinalysis, thoracic and abdominal radiographs, and ultrasound (chest and abdomen). When ventricular arrhythmias are present with no detectable underlying disease to cause the VPCs, the arrhythmia is assumed to be idiopathic.

In cats, cardiomyopathy and hyperthyroidism are common causes of ventricular arrhythmias. Ventricular arrhythmias secondary to other systemic diseases and idiopathic arrhythmias can occur, but are rare.

7. When are ventricular arrhythmias treated?

As with any treatment, the whole patient must be evaluated prior to starting therapy. Provided the clinical status of the patient allows it, any underlying disorder should first be treated directly. In many cases, if the patient is stabilized, the frequency of the ventricular arrhythmia may reduce or the arrhythmia may completely resolve.

When ventricular tachyarrhythmia results in hemodynamic compromise, pharmacologic antiarrhythmic therapy is generally indicated. Hemodynamic compromise can be seen with ventricular tachycardia but is not generally associated with frequent VPCs. The rate of the tachycardia and the length of its duration influence whether or not a ventricular tachycardia causes poor perfusion. Nonsustained ventricular tachycardia rarely causes signs of poor perfusion. Other factors that can affect perfusion, such as myocardial function, volume status, and the presence of drugs that cause vasodilatation, may predispose a patient to poor perfusion from a ventricular tachycardia.

Because antiarrhythmic drugs have not been clearly shown to reduce the risk of sudden death, the decision to treat an arrhythmia depends on the clinician's ability to determine whether or not the arrhythmia has a role in current clinical presentation. There is some evidence that beta blockers may help reduce sudden death in people, but no evidence for this has been established in veterinary patients.

In conclusion, treatment of ventricular arrhythmias is not based on any specific ECG criteria. In most cases, single VPCs seen on an ECG are not an indication to start antiarrhythmic therapy.

8. What is an accelerated idioventricular rhythm? Is it different from ventricular tachycardia?

Distinguishing between ventricular tachycardia and accelerated idioventricular rhythm (AIVR) is important. Although somewhat arbitrary in its definition, an AIVR has certain clinical and electrocardiographic differences from ventricular tachycardia. An AIVR typically is a more benign rhythm and frequently does not require direct antiarrhythmic therapy. An AIVR differs from a ventricular tachycardia mainly in rate of depolarization of the ectopic focus. An AIVR will typically be less than 180–200 bpm, and generally has a similar rate to the underlying sinus rate. It is common to see the underlying rhythm shift from the sinus rhythm to the ventricular focus as the sinus rate speeds up and slows down. A waxing and waning of the sinus rate allows the ventricular focus to capture the ventricles for a period of time until the sinus rate speeds up again. Fusion beats, hybrid beats of the sinus node, and ventricular focus are frequently seen as the rhythm changes from sinus to ventricular (see figure).

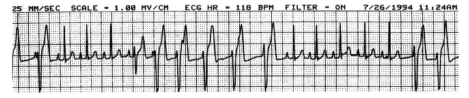

Accelerated idioventricular rhythm from a dog postoperative splenectomy. There are five ventricular beats in a row in the center of the strip. The beat prior to these is a fusion beat. There are three sinus beats prior to the-fusion beat. Note the sinus rate slows just prior to the ventricular focus capturing the heart. The ventricular rhythm terminates when the sinus rate elevates.

AIVRs are typically seen in patients with systemic disease. An AIVR is commonly seen in dogs that have had severe trauma (e.g., hit by a car), gastric dilatation and volvulus, following splenectomy, and in neurologic disease. In these cases supportive care for the underlying disease is the most important therapy. Since these rhythms usually do not compromise perfusion, antiarrhythmic therapy is rarely needed. Interestingly, if an AIVR is suppressed with an IV antiarrhythmic, such as a constant-rate infusion of lidocaine, the rhythm frequently becomes refractory to the antiarrhythmic and persists despite higher doses. If the rate of an AIVR is greater than 180–220 bpm, compromises perfusion, or is persistent, antiarrhythmic therapy may be necessary. The AIVR usually resolves in 3–5 days, with or without treatment.

9. What antiarrhythmic drugs are available?

Listed below are the commonly used antiarrhythmic drugs and their mechanisms of action. The various ion changes occurring in the conduction cells and the stages of the action potential are shown in the figure. Antiarrhythmics are classified based on their effect on the action potential (AP).

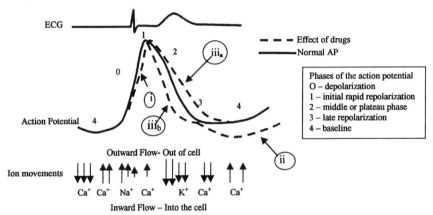

The mechanisms of antiarrhythmic agents can be classified relative to: fast sodium channel blockade (i); blockade of the electrophysiological effects of sympathetic excitation of the heart (ii); the effect on repolarization (iii$_a$ and iii$_b$); and the inhibition of slow calcium channels.

CLASS I: Fast Sodium Channel Blockers

Class I drugs are membrane stabilizers. They usually decrease automaticity, slow conduction, increase the refractory period, and have variable effects on the AP.

Class IA: Lengthen the effective refractory period and prolong the QT interval
- Depress phase 0 of the AP by inhibiting the fast sodium channels (i)
- Decrease conduction velocity (promote re-entry)
- Delay AP duration and repolarization by inhibiting K^+ current (iii$_a$)
- Examples: quinidine sulfate, procainamide, disopyramide

Class IB: Shorten the AP
- Inhibit the sodium channels but shorten the AP (i)
- No phase 0 effect or delay in conduction velocity in normal tissue, but may effect ischemic or abnormal tissue
- Shortens the AP (iii$_b$)
- Increase the threshold for ventricular fibrillation
- Examples: lidocaine, mexiletine, tocainide

Class IC: Block sodium channels but do not change AP duration
- Inhibit fast sodium channels and thus depress upstroke of the AP phase 0 (i)
- Inhibit the His-Purkinje conduction system to give QRS widening, which decreases conduction velocity
- Shorten the AP of Purkinje fibers only

• Do not effect the refractory period or repolarization
• Examples: flecainide, encainide

CLASS II: Sympathetic Blockers

Class II drugs produce antisympathetic or sympatholytic effects. These drugs may have specific beta-1 blocking or have combined beta-1 and beta-2 antagonistic activity. They lower the resting baseline (becomes more negative) of the AP and raise the ventricular fibrillation threshold (ii). Examples are propranolol, atenolol, and esmolol.

CLASS III: Inhibitors of Repolarization

Class III drugs increase the AP duration and the refractoriness without affecting phase 0. They are reported to be able to terminate and prevent ventricular fibrillation. Examples are amiodarone, bretylium, and sotalol.

CLASS IV: Calcium Antagonists

Class IV drugs inhibit the calcium influx through slow inward channels. These drugs are important in effecting the automaticity and conduction of the SA and AV nodes. Examples are diltiazem, verapamil, and adenosine.

The dosages for the most commonly used antiarrhythmic drugs are given in the table below.

Classification and Dosing of Antiarrhythmic Drugs

	DRUG	DOG DOSE	CAT DOSE
Class I			
IA	Disopyramide	6–15 mg/kg PO q 8 hr	
	Quinidine sulfate	5–10 mg/kg	
	Quinidine gluconate	6–20 mg/kg PO q 6–8 hr	
	Procainamide	8–20 mg/kg IM, PO QID (slow release—TID)	
IB	Lidocaine	2–8 mg/kg IV, CRI* 25–100 µg/kg/min, 6 mg/kg IM	0.25–0.75 mg/kg IV slowly
	Mexiletine	5–8 mg/kg PO q 8 hr	
	Tocainide	15–20 mg/kg pO q 8 hr	
IC	Flecainide	1–5 mg/kg PO BID–TID	
	Encainide	0.5–1 mg/kg PO TID	
Class II	Atenolol	0.25–1 mg/kg PO SID–BID	6.25–12.5 mg/cat PO SID
	Esmolol (short-acting)	0.25–0.5 mg/kg IV slowly	
	Propranolol	0.2–1 mg/kg PO TID, 0.02–0.06 mg/kg IV slowly	2.5–5 mg/cat PO BID–TID
Class III	Sotalol	1–4 mg/kg BID	2 mg/kg
	Amiodarone	10 mg/kg PO BID for 1 week, then 8 mg/kg SID Can be reduced to 5 mg/kg	
	Bretylium	5–10 mg/kg IV	
Class IV	Diltiazem	0.5–1.5 mg/kg PO q 8 hr, 0.1–0.2 mg/kg, CRI 5–10 mg/kg/hr	7.5 mg/cat TID, Dilacor (slow-release) 60 mg/cat PO SID
	Verapamil	0.05 mg/kg IV	1–3 mg/kg PO q 8 hr
	Adenosine	0.08–1.0 mg/kg IV	

IV, intravenously; IM, intramuscularly; PO, orally; BID, twice daily; TID, three times a day; QID, four times a day; CRI, continuous-rate infusion.
* A simple formula for making a CRI for lidocaine is to make a 2 mg/ml solution of lidocaine with a drip rate 1 ml/lb/hr to give a CRI of 67 µg/kg/min. For example, a 30-lb dog would receive the 2 mg/ml solution at 30 ml/hr. A 2 mg/ml solution of lidocaine is easily made by adding 1 ml of 2% lidocaine for every 10 ml of saline in bag.

10. Which drug do I pick first?

As mentioned, the underlying disease should be addressed initially. If the arrhythmia causes hemodynamic compromise, antiarrhythmic therapy should be initiated. The route of administration will be determined by the urgency of the need to suppress the arrhythmia. Rapid blood levels can be reached with intravenous dosing, but side effects of the drug can be more severe.

Drugs in classes I, II, and III are typically used for ventricular arrhythmias. Lidocaine and procainamide are good first-line therapy in the acute or early stage. If lidocaine is needed, it is initially given as a bolus at 2–4 mg/kg IV to see if it is effective at achieving conversion. If conversion to sinus arrhythmia is not achieved, repeat boluses can be given up to a total dose of 8 mg/kg over a 15-minute period; patients must be carefully monitored for signs of neurotoxicity, such as seizures, when high doses of lidocaine are administered. If conversion is achieved, but the ventricular tachycardia returns quickly, a constant-rate infusion (CRI) of lidocaine may be used. An antiarrhythmic drug delivered by CRI is best given with an infusion pump for safest and most accurate delivery. The CRI dosage for lidocaine is given in the table above. If a CRI of lidocaine is to be used, a repeat bolus of lidocaine needs to be given immediately prior to starting the CRI. The lidocaine bolus should be sufficient to cause conversion back to sinus rhythm. If lidocaine does not convert or control the arrhythmia, IV procainamide is a second choice. Procainamide can be initially loaded intravenously, then followed with oral dosing or intramuscular injections if the patient is vomiting or not allowed oral medications.

An intravenous beta blocker, esmolol or propranolol could be used as a third-line drug for resistant ventricular arrhythmias. These should be used with care in patients with myocardial failure and active congestive heart failure. In these cases, the heart failure may be more important to control first.

If maintenance therapy is needed, procainamide can be used. If procainamide does not control the arrhythmia, but lidocaine does, mexiletine or tocainide also can be used. They are more expensive than procainamide and all three can be proarrhythmic (see below). If the underlying disease is stabilized or controlled, the arrhythmia may cease or decrease to a level where antiarrhythmic therapy is not needed. For this reason, it is often worthwhile to try discontinuing the antiarrhythmic.

If beta blockers control the arrhythmia and long-term therapy is necessary, the trend is to continue to use a beta blocker. Beta blockers have been shown to reduce mortality in people and the risk for proarrhythmia is reduced compared to the class I antiarrhythmics. Class III antiarrhythmics are another option, but are far more expensive and their efficacy in veterinary medicine is still being evaluated. Sotalol may prove a useful drug in boxer dogs with ventricular tachycardia. Sotalol is useful in controlling ventricular arrhythmias, but its ability to prevent sudden death still unknown. Its effectiveness compared to class I drugs and beta blockers needs to be evaluated. Beta blockers and sotalol should be used with caution in dogs with underlying myocardial failure or dogs in active congestive failure. Removing sympathetic tone in these patients could cause symptomatic hypotension or worsen heart failure.

11. What is proarrhythmia?

Proarrhythmia refers to a drug's ability to promote an arrhythmia. Several types of proarrhythmia have been noted: (1) a change or worsening of the current arrhythmia, (2) the development of a new arrhythmia, and (3) the occurrence of a bradyarrhythmia resulting from depression of the sinus node or AV node conduction. In an individual case, it may be difficult to discern proarrhythmia from a worsening of the underlying disease and arrhythmia. It may be necessary to discontinue the drug to evaluate its role in the increased arrhythmia.

The class I antiarrhythmics have been shown to be proarrhythmic in people. A landmark study, Cardiac Arrhythmia Suppression Trial (CAST), demonstrated that people with asymptomatic premature ventricular complexes receiving the class IC antiarrhythmics encainide or flecainide actually had a higher mortality compared to placebo. Although this has not been demonstrated in veterinary patients, judicious use of these antiarrhythmics is recommended.

The proarrhythmia of class I drugs is the reason why beta blockers may be preferred in long-term management of arrhythmias. The CAST study did demonstrate that beta blockers might improve survival. Other clinical studies performed in people, mainly looking at beta blockers after myocardial infarction, have demonstrated a decrease in the number of sudden deaths in these patients.

CONTROVERSIES

12. How do we prevent sudden death?

This is truly a controversial issue. The bottom line is that definitive guidelines in people are poorly established, and even less is known in veterinary medicine. The problem lies in lack of specific ECG predictors for sudden death. There appear to be no definitive clues, outside of the extremes, to what arrhythmia will cause sudden death. Obviously a dog with no underlying cardiac disease and three VPCs in 24 hours is at much less risk for sudden death than a Doberman with dilated cardiomyopathy and ventricular tachycardia at 350 bpm. The cases that we see between these extremes present the problem. If we can determine which patient is at risk, we can evaluate a drug that will improve survival. Large patient population studies are needed to evaluate efficacy of any drug. An important fact to remember is that the ability of an antiarrhythmic to suppress the number of ventricular arrhythmias is not a predictor of its ability to prevent sudden death, as demonstrated by the CAST study. Hopefully in the future, other drugs that are not proarrhythmic may suppress the number of arrhythmias and also prevent sudden death. Possible candidates are beta blockers and class III agents, such as amiodarone and sotalol.

13. Can implantable defibrillators be used in dogs?

The use of implantable defibrillators in people has grown over the last 10 years. Technology has streamlined these devices and improved their capabilities. It is physically possible to implant these devices into dogs. Although newer devices are expensive, they are available from hospitals and defibrillator companies at minimal or no cost. The current difficulties with implanting defibrillators in dogs are that dogs can have large T waves and extremely variable heart rates compared to people and this can lead to misinterpretation by the defibrillator, resulting in inappropriate shocks. Improved software and algorithms in newer devices may overcome this in the future. Another consideration is the humane aspect. Cardioversion shock is painful. Intermittent and unexpected shocks may be disturbing to the dog and could cause poor behavioral responses. Other than research dogs, currently there are no reports of these devices being implanted in clinical veterinary patients.

BIBLIOGRAPHY

1. CAST Investigators: Preliminary report: Effect of encainide and flecainide on mortality in a randomized trial of arrhythmia suppression after myocardial infarction. N Engl J Med 321:227–233, 1989.
2. El-Sherif N: Polymorphic ventricular tachycardia. In Podrid PJ, Kowey PR (eds): Cardiac Arrhythmia: Mechanisms, Diagnosis, and Management. Baltimore, Williams & Wilkins, 1995.
3. Kittleson MD: Diagnosis and treatment of arrhythmias (dysrhythmias). In Kittleson MD, Kienle RD (eds): Small Animal Cardiovascular Medicine. St. Louis, Mosby, 1998, pp 474–486.
4. Mandel WJ: Sustained monomorphic ventricular tachycardia. In Podrid PJ, Kowey PR (eds): Cardiac Arrhythmia: Mechanisms, Diagnosis, and Management. Baltimore, Williams & Wilkins, 1995.
5. Rubin AM, Morganroth J, and Kowey PR: Ventricular premature depolarizations. In Podrid PJ, Kowey PR (eds): Cardiac Arrhythmia: Mechanisms, Diagnosis, and Management. Baltimore, Williams & Wilkins, 1995, pp 891–906
6. Sodowick BC, Buxton AE: Clinical significance of nonsustained ventricular tachycardia. In Podrid PJ, Kowey PR (eds): Cardiac Arrhythmia: Mechanisms, Diagnosis, and Management. Baltimore, Williams & Wilkins, 1995, pp 907–918.
7. Zipes DP: Specific arrhythmias: Diagnosis and treatment. In Braunwald E (ed): Heart Disease: A Textbook of Cardiovascular Medicine. Philadelphia, W.B. Saunders, 1997, pp 640–704.

30. SUPRAVENTRICULAR TACHYARRHYTHMIA

Kathy N. Wright, D.V.M.

1. How would you define the term "supraventricular tachyarrhythmia"?

In electrocardiographic terminology, the bifurcation of the AV bundle marks the division between supraventricular and ventricular. This is because the origin of a rhythm relative to this landmark determines QRS morphology. Under most circumstances, QRS complexes that arise proximal to the bifurcation are narrow or have a "normal" appearance. In contrast, QRS complexes that originate distal to the AV bifurcation are wide and have a bizarre configuration. Since electrocardiographic appearances cannot always distinguish atrial rhythms from those that arise from near the AV node—the junctional rhythms—the general term supraventricular has descriptive utility.

Therefore, supraventricular tachyarrhythmias (SVT) are rapid rhythms either originating in the atria or atrioventricular (AV) junction or using the atria or AV junction as a crucial component of the tachycardia circuit. The terms supraventricular tachycardia and supraventricular tachyarrhythmia are usually reserved for pathologic rhythms and exclude physiologic, sinus tachycardias. In this discussion, the term supraventricular tachyarrhythmia will refer to atrial and juctional premature complexes, atrial tachycardia, atrial fibrillation, atrial flutter, and to the junctional tachycardias.

2. Describe a vagal maneuver and its ideal result in the setting of atrial tachycardia and in the setting of junctional tachycardias.

Vagal maneuvers in small animals consist of ocular pressure (retropulsing the globes), carotid sinus massage, or stimulation of a gag reflex. Such a maneuver is done to abruptly increase vagal tone to the heart. The sinoatrial (SA) and AV nodes are particularly sensitive to changes in autonomic tone; therefore, vagal maneuvers primarily result in slowing SA nodal discharge and prolonging AV nodal conduction time and increasing refractoriness. Ideally (but rarely), a vagal maneuver produces a brief period of AV block. Atrial tachyarrhythmias do not require the AV node for their continuation; i.e., the atria can continue to rapidly depolarize even if AV block is present. A brief period of AV block would thereby allow you to recognize rapid atrial depolarizations that are not conducted through the AV node to the ventricles. During a tachyarrhythmia that does require the AV node as part of its circuit (the junctional tachyarrhythmias), a brief period of AV block would result in termination of the tachycardia.

SVT in which the QRS complexes are wide or bizarre are occasionally observed and this appearance results from rate-dependent aberrancy of ventricular activation or the presence of preexisting bundle branch block. In these cases, it can be difficult to determine whether or not the tachycardia orginates from the ventricles or from a supraventricular focus. Recognizing that in any given case a vagal maneuver may have no observable effect, a sudden termination or interruption by AV block strongly suggests that a wide QRS tachycardia originated from a supraventricular focus. In ventricular tachycardia, the origin and path of the rhythm are confined to the ventricles and vagal maneuvers do not typically alter the cardiac rhythm.

3. What is aberrancy of ventricular activation?

Aberrancy of ventricular activation describes a supraventricular impulse with an abnormal, bizarre QRS complex reflecting abnormal intraventricular conduction. Abnormal ventricular activation can result from intraventricular conduction abnormalities related to changes in heart rate, metabolic and electrolyte abnormalities, or conduction over accessory pathways.

4. How do you differentiate sinus tachycardia from a supraventricular tachyarrhythmia?

Sinus tachycardia is characterized by a gradual initiation and termination of a rapid rhythm with regular R-R intervals. Each QRS complex is preceded by a P wave with the same configuration and mean electrical axis as the P wave during normal sinus rhythm. Sinus tachycardia occurs in the setting of increased sympathetic tone, such as fear, pain, hypovolemia, hypotension, fever/hyperthermia, anemia, hyperthyroidism, pheochromocytoma, and congestive heart failure.

The P wave during an SVT, if it is visible at all, typically has a different configuration and axis than that during sinus rhythm. The only exception to this is an SVT that originates near the SA node and therefore has a configuration similar to a sinus P wave. Supraventricular tachyarrhythmias typically have an abrupt onset and termination (paroxysms) or are incessant. A successful vagal maneuver gradually slows the rate of sinus tachycardia; reentrant SVT either abruptly terminates (AV junctional-dependent SVT) or continues in the presence of AV block (atrial-based SVT). As mentioned above, however, vagal maneuvers are often ineffective.

5. What is the rhythm diagnosis for the ECG in the figure below from a 10-year-old domestic shorthaired cat being treated for restrictive cardiomyopathy?

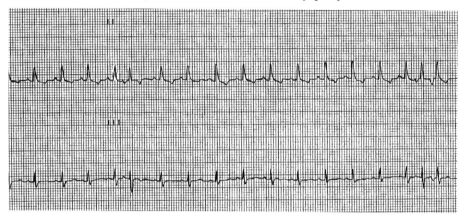

ECG from a 10-year-old domestic shorthaired cat being treated for restrictive cardiomyopathy. Paper speed 25 mm/sec; sensitivity 20 mm/mV.

To answer this, go through the following thought process:
- Is the ventricular rate too fast, too slow, or normal for a 10-year-old cat?
   The overall ventricular rate is low normal for a cat at 140 bpm. Note that this same rate is slow for a cat that is in the hospital with primary heart disease but not yet taking medications. Despite the overall rate, there are three complexes that come earlier than normal. The interval between the early QRS and the preceding QRS is 260 msec. This is known as the coupling interval.
- Is the rhythm regular or irregular? Is there a pattern to the irregularity?
   The rhythm is irregular due to the premature complexes mentioned above. There is a pattern to the irregularity. The majority of the QRS complexes occur at regular intervals, but are periodically interrupted by single or paired premature complexes that have consistent coupling intervals
- Is there a P wave for each QRS complex and a QRS complex for each P wave?
   Yes. A small positive deflection (look at lead II) can be seen within the T wave preceding the premature QRS complexes. These are atrial premature complexes or APCs.
- Are the P waves of normal configuration?
   No. Look at the sinus P waves on the ECG, and then examine the premature P waves. The atrial premature complexes (APCs) are narrower and slightly decreased in amplitude compared to the sinus P waves.

• Are any of the standard ECG intervals abnormal?

Yes. The sinus P-wave duration is prolonged for a cat at 70 msec. This is known as p-mi-trale and generally signifies left atrial enlargement. The PR interval is also of increased duration at 120 msec during sinus rhythm, constituting first-degree AV block. The QRS duration is increased at 80 msec, indicating an intraventricular conduction disturbance. Finally, the QT interval is increased at 220 msec, likely secondary to the relatively slow sinus rate and intraventricular conduction delay.

6. Suggest common causes of atrial premature complexes (APCs) in dogs and cats.

APCs are commonly associated with atrial dilation. This may be secondary to congenital heart disease, valvular disease, cardiomyopathies, or other myocardial diseases. Atrial masses, hyperthyroidism, hypoxia, electrolyte imbalances (particularly hypokalemia), acidosis, anesthetic agents, sympathomimetics (including beta agonists for asthma treatment, caffeine, and chocolate), and digitalis intoxication are other known causes.

7. If APCs are identified in a dog or cat, what other diagnostic tests should be performed?

First, you would want to ask careful historical questions, including a detailed medication history. It is important to identify associated disorders because APCs can regress once you eliminate precipitating causes. A complete blood count, serum biochemical profile (with electrolytes), blood gas analysis, and appropriate endocrine testing should be ordered if clinically indicated. To check for underlying structural heart disease, thoracic radiographs and an echocardiogram should be performed. If APCs are infrequent on a routine ECG, but you question their overall frequency throughout the day, Holter monitoring can answer that question.

8. Examine the ECG in the figure on page 188 from an 8-year-old male golden retriever presented to you for evaluation of weakness and one episode of collapse, and consider these questions.

• What is the heart rate?

The ventricular rate is 360 bpm.

• What is the term for alternation in QRS amplitude?

Electrical alternans is the term for alternation in QRS amplitude. For reasons that are not well understood, electrical alternans is occasionally observed in association with SVT. Electrical alternans is also observed in cases of cardiac tamponade which is, perhaps, a more familiar association.

• What is the cardiac rhythm diagnosis?

The ventricular rate is fast: this is a *tachyarrhythmia*. The QRS complexes are narrow and normal in configuration: this is a *supraventricular* tachyarrhythmia. The ST segment is deformed, making it likely that there are P waves within the ST segment. The QRS complexes occur at regular intervals, so this is a *regular* SVT.

9. The golden retriever in question 8 was given intravenous diltiazem, with the results as shown in the figure on page 189. What diagnostic information does this provide?

Second-degree AV block has resulted from the intravenous diltiazem infusion. This has helped you to identify abnormal P waves occurring at a rate of 360 per minute with variable conduction through the AV node to the ventricles. The SVT is able to continue despite the presence of second-degree AV block. Eliminated from your differential diagnostic list are those SVTs requiring conduction through the AV node as a critical part of their reentrant circuit. Atrial tachyarrhythmias, however, do not require AV nodal participation to continue. Thus, we can diagnose an atrial tachyarrhythmia (atrial flutter) in this case.

10. What is an accessory pathway?

An accessory pathway (AP) is a congenital connection between the atrial and ventricular myocardium. These act as "bypass tracts" because they can conduct an impulse from atria to ventricles or ventricles to atria without the normal delay that occurs within the AV node.

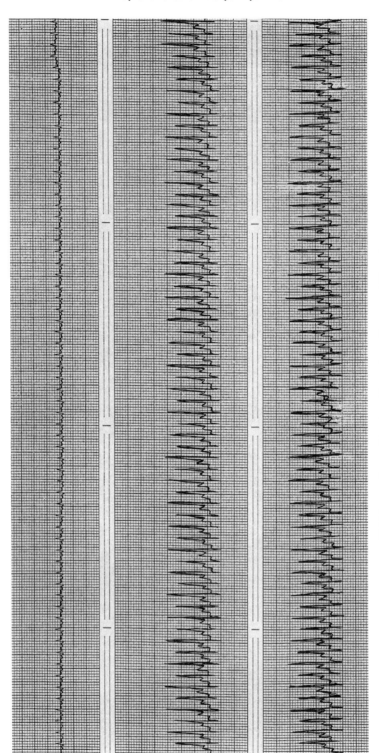

ECG from an 8-year-old male golden retriever. Paper speed 25 mm/sec.

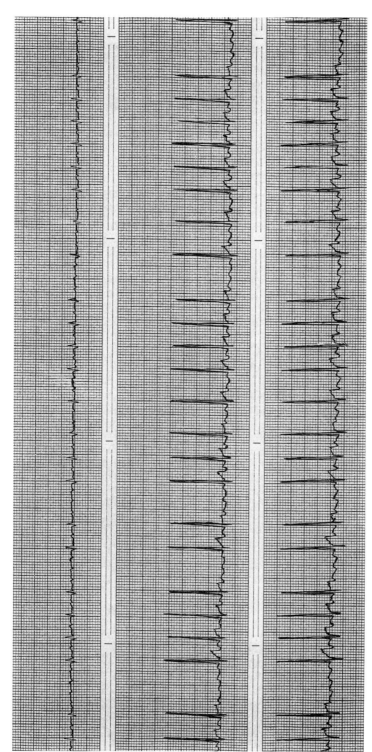

ECG from an 8-year-old male golden retriever, following intravenous diltiazem. Paper speed 25 mm/sec.

11. What is ventricular preexcitation?

Ventricular preexcitation is the early activation of part or all of the ventricular myocardium by a supraventricular impulse that conducts down an AP, bypassing the normal specialized conduction tissue.

12. Do all accessory pathways produce ventricular preexcitation?

No, not all accessory pathways produce ventricular preexcitation. Some pathways are only capable of retrograde conduction, i. e. from the ventricles to the atria. These are known as concealed accessory pathways. In order to produce ventricular preexcitation, an accessory pathway must be capable of anterograde conduction, i.e. from the atria to the ventricles.

13. Why is ventricular preexcitation clinically important?

Ventricular preexcitation is important because it is electrocardiographic evidence of an accessory pathway that can provide the substrate for the development of potentially dangerous SVT. Atrioventricular reciprocating tachycardia is the arrhythmia classically associated with an accessory pathway. Most commonly, the tachycardia impulse repeatedly conducts from the atria down the AV nodal-His-Purkinje system to the ventricles and then up the accesssory pathway from the ventricles to the atria; this circus movement is referred to as reentry. The association of SVT and ventricular preexcitation is sometimes known as the Wolf-Parkinson-White Syndrome.

14. Examine the ECG in the figure below from an 8-year-old male Doberman pinscher being treated for Doberman cardiomyopathy. What is your rhythm diagnosis?

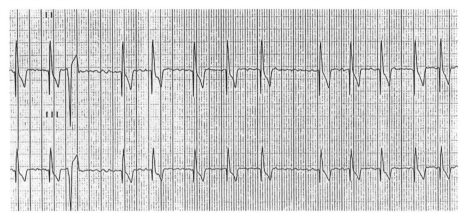

ECG from an 8-year-old male Doberman pinscher being treated for cardiomyopathy. Paper speed 25 mm/sec; sensitivity 5 mm/mV.

Ask the following questions to help determine the rhythm diagnosis:
- Are the R-R intervals regular in this case?
  No
- Are the QRS complexes normally conducted?
  To best answer this, you would like to examine an ECG containing conducted sinus complexes. This is not always available when an incessant tachyarrhythmia is present. All QRS complexes from this dog appear to be conducted (i.e., look exactly the same as those seen on a prior ECG of sinus tachycardia) except the fifth QRS complex, which is wider and bizarre (characteristics typical of a ventricular premature complex).
- Is there a pattern to the R-R interval irregularity, i.e., is it a regularly irregular rhythm?
  No

• Can you identify P waves in the leads provided?

No, merely irregular undulations in the baseline. Remember to run as many leads as possible (the more the better!), as P waves may be isoelectric in certain leads but more easily identified in others.

The above answers fit a diagnosis of atrial fibrillation.

15. Would atrial fibrillation more commonly occur in an Irish wolfhound or a Siamese cat? Why?

Atrial fibrillation would more commonly occur in a Irish wolfhound than in a Siamese cat. Atrial fibrillation typically results from multiple coexisting reentrant wavelets circulating within the atria and requires large atria to sustain itself. The atria of a normal Irish wolfhound are sizeable to begin with, but the normal atria in a Siamese cat are much smaller. The Siamese would have to develop severe atrial dilatation secondary to another heart disease (such as one of the cardiomyopathies) before atrial fibrillation could develop. The Irish wolfhound is predisposed to this arrhythmia already by virtue of its normally larger atria.

16. What conditions or diseases are most commonly associated with atrial fibrillation in the dog and cat?

Atrial fibrillation in small animals is most commonly associated with diseases causing atrial dilatation. Whenever a small animal practitioner encounters a patient with atrial fibrillation, serious underlying heart disease should be suspected until proven otherwise. Cardiomyopathies (dogs and cats), congenital heart diseases (dogs and cats), and degenerative valvular disease (dogs) are the most common causes of atrial dilatation in small animals. Rarely, atrial fibrillation can develop in an otherwise normal heart during or shortly following anesthesia or thoracic trauma. Remember that giant-breed dogs appear to sometimes develop "lone atrial fibrillation," not associated with structural heart disease or a known triggering event. Always first rule out structural heart disease in the giant-breed dog as well, as many will have this as an underlying cause of their atrial fibrillation (particularly if the ventricular response is rapid).

17. Name three classes of antiarrhythmic drugs commonly used to slow AV nodal conduction in small animals and give an example of each.

• *Digitalis glycosides:* digoxin
• *Calcium-channel blockers:* diltiazem or verapamil
• *Beta blockers:* propranolol, atenolol, esmolol, metoprolol, and many others

18. A Great Dane is brought to your thriving veterinary practice. The owner complains about her dog's lethargy and weight gain. She has read about hypothyroidism and believes that is her dog's problem. You, on the other hand, astutely diagnose dilated cardiomyopathy with atrial fibrillation and biventricular congestive heart failure, based on physical examination and diagnostic testing. What is your approach to managing atrial fibrillation in this dog?

Attempts to effect conversion to sinus rhythm in patients that develop atrial fibrillation due to structural cardiac disease are generally felt to be unrewarding. Therefore, your goal in this case is to slow the ventricular response to allow the failing ventricles more time to fill with blood. Thus, you want to increase the degree of second-degree AV block (block fibrillatory impulses from the atria in the AV node). One way to accomplish this is to decrease the level of sympathetic tone, i.e. treat the congestive heart failure!

Digoxin is used both to slow AV nodal conduction and give weak positive inotropic support in a dog with dilated cardiomyopathy (DCM). Digoxin alone in these cases is rarely adequate to slow the ventricular rate to less than 150 bpm. Diltiazem or a beta blocker are typically added to digoxin if the ventricular rate is still too high after the dog has been on digoxin for approximately 24–48 hours. Both calcium channel blockers and beta blockers have a negative inotropic effect and the patient's clinical status and ventricular rate must be carefully monitored. The chosen drug (or combination) should be titrated to the lowest dose that maintains an acceptable ventricular rate. After that dose is determined, the patient is discharged on long-term therapy.

19. What is the diagnostic and therapeutic approach to "lone," or idiopathic, atrial fibrillation?

Dogs with "lone" atrial fibrillation are typically of the large and giant breeds, with no identifiable cause for their arrhythmia. Your diagnostic aim is to search extensively for and uncover any contributing factor(s) for the rhythm disturbance, before labeling it "idiopathic." This includes thoracic radiographs and an echocardiogram to rule out structural heart disease such as DCM, atrial masses, or previously overlooked congenital heart disease. A complete biochemical profile is also advisable to determine if any electrolyte or metabolic disturbances are potentiating the arrhythmia. The owner should be carefully questioned regarding medications, both prescription and nonprescription, their dog is receiving and whether their pet has undergone anesthesia recently. All of these could contribute to an episode of atrial fibrillation in an otherwise normal giant-breed dog.

Treatment of idiopathic atrial fibrillation is controversial. The ventricular response rate is typically much slower than that of a dog in atrial fibrillation secondary to structural heart disease. During exercise, the ventricular response may climb higher than is considered ideal, but this is not the case in all dogs with idiopathic atrial fibrillation. Since atrial fibrillation is an abnormal rhythm, which can lead to electrical remodeling and an atrial myopathy, attempts at cardioversion for an animal with idiopathic atrial fibrillation are worthwhile. Cardioversion may be either electrical through a synchronized DC shock or chemical with agents like procainamide or quinidine. If cardioversion is unsuccessful, then repeated monitoring for the development of structural heart disease and the administration of a beta blocker to prevent rapid ventricular conduction when sympathetic tone is high (such as during exercise) are diagnostic and therapeutic choices of the author.

20. Name the Vaughan-Williams class and cardiac channels or receptors inhibited by each of these common antiarrhythmic drugs.

DRUG	VAUGHAN-WILLIAMS CLASS	CARDIAC CHANNELS OR RECEPTORS INHIBITED
Amiodarone	Class III	Potassium, calcium, and sodium channels; alpha- and beta-adrenergic receptors
Atenolol	Class II	Beta-adrenergic receptors
Diltiazem	Class IV	Calcium channels
Procainamide	Class IA	Sodium and potassium channels
Quinidine	Class IA	Sodium and potassium channels; alpha-adrenergic and muscarinic receptors
D,L-Sotalol	Class III	Potassium channels; beta-adrenergic receptors

21. Which of the above drugs prolong refractoriness in the atrial myocardium?

Antiarrhythmic drugs that block potassium channels prolong refractoriness with myocardial tissue. From the list of drugs in question 20, D,L-sotalol, procainamide, quinidine, and amiodarone all block potassium channels.

22. Rapid SVT can have dire clinical consequences. Reduced cardiac output can result in weakness or syncope; with chronicity, rapid tachycardias can result in impaired myocardial function. Suggest an approach to the medical management of rapid, regular SVT.

The acute management of a rapid, hemodynamically unstable SVT centers around slowing AV nodal conduction. If the SVT is AV nodal dependent, then second-degree AV block will terminate the arrhythmia. If the SVT is AV nodal independent, then second-degree AV block will slow the ventricular response rate and thus lessen the animal's hemodynamic compromise. Vagal maneuvers are used initially and after each intravenous drug administration. Intravenous diltiazem is the negative dromotrope of choice, as it has more potent AV nodal slowing effects than intravenous beta blockers and less negative inotropic effects than verapamil or beta blockers. A dose of 0.1–0.3 mg/kg is infused over 2 minutes. As mentioned earlier, the animal should be carefully monitored electrocardiographically and hemodynamically (hypotension can result from blockade of vascular calcium channels). Oral antiarrhythmic therapy can be initiated once the animal is stable. Long-term oral therapy most commonly includes a combination of a negative dromotrope (AV nodal slowing drug) and a class IA or class III agent to prolong refractoriness in atrial or accessory pathway tissue.

23. Your final appointment of a long, hard day is a 4-month-old Labrador retriever scheduled for her first rabies vaccination. Sensing your fatigue, the owner timidly mentions that her dog is not as rambunctious as she used to be. She also occasionally sees her heart "trying to jump out of her chest" when she is lying on the floor. Your physical examination of "Belle" is within normal limits—apart from her heart rate of 250 bpm. You obtain an ECG and thoracic radiographs. The thoracic radiographs are normal; the ECG (see figure) is not. Consider the following questions.

See broadside figure on next page.

- Describe your ECG findings.

The ventricular rate is rapid at 236 bpm; the rhythm is regular; and QRS complexes are narrow and sinus P waves are not identified. These three findings translate into a supraventricular tachyarrhythmia. *For advanced electrocardiographers:* If you look at leads II, aVR, aVF, and V1, you can see small deflections within the ST segment. These represent P waves (P′ waves). The RP′ interval is shorter than the P′R interval, making this a short RP′ SVT.

- What are the differential diagnoses?

Differential diagnoses include AV reciprocating tachycardia using an accessory pathway as described in question 9; an atypical form of AV nodal reentrant tachycardia (usually P′ waves cannot be identified in classic AV nodal reentry because they are buried within the QRS complex); and atrial tachycardia. In a puppy or young adult dog with this ECG pattern, AV reciprocating tachycardia ranks highest on your list. Labrador retrievers may have a breed predisposition for the development of AV reciprocating tachycardia, which might further strengthen the presumptive diagnosis.

- What additional tests should be performed?

Iatrogenic induction of second-degree AV block would help differentiate junctional-dependent versus atrial tachyarrhythmias, as described in question 8. You would also like to assess electrolytes, thoracic radiographs (looking for congenital heart disease), and an echocardiogram (looking more specifically for congenital heart disease and cardiac function that can be secondarily affected by a frequent tachyarrhythmia).

- What are the possible treatments?

Medical treatments are aimed at slowing AV nodal conduction and increasing refractoriness of the accessory pathway. Drugs that slow AV conduction include digitalis glycosides, calcium channel blockers, and beta blockers. Some cardiologists do not recommend digitalis glycosides in these patients because of fear of speeding anterograde conduction down the accessory pathway. Others believe this is a theoretical but not a practical concern. Drugs that slow conduction within an accessory pathway are also those that prolong refractoriness within atrial myocardium. These include class IA agents (procainamide, quinidine), class 1C agents (not used in veterinary medicine), and class III agents (sotalol, amiodarone). Because D,L-sotalol has beta-blocking actions and amiodarone has beta-blocking and calcium-channel blocking activity, these agents slow both limbs of the reentrant circuit in AV reciprocating tachycardia.

Medical therapy often is not effective in the long term in these dogs with frequent episodes of AV reciprocating tachycardia. The other alternative is to determine the exact location of the accessory pathway using multielectrode catheters positioned along the AV groove. Once the accessory pathway is precisely located, radiofrequency energy is delivered to destroy the pathway. This is a complex technique that is offered at a few referral centers.

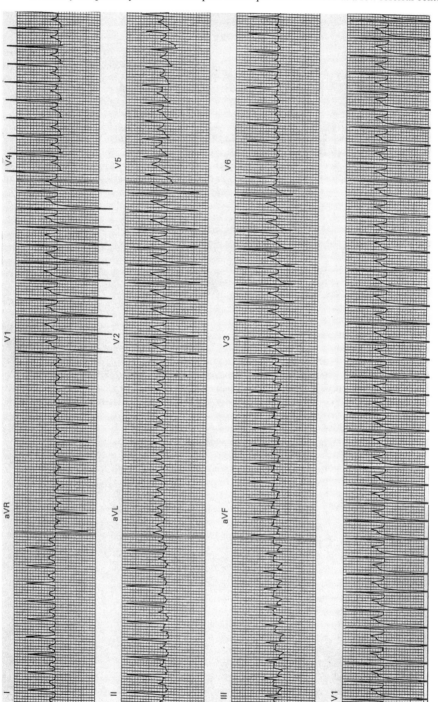

ECG from a 4-month-old Labrador retriever. Paper speed 25 mm/sec; sensitivity 10 mm/mV.

24. Define tachycardia-induced cardiomyopathy. What is *distinctive* about this cardiomyopathy?

Tachycardia-induced cardiomyopathy is a form of reversible myocardial dysfunction caused by chronic tachyarrhythmias. The distinctive feature of tachycardia-induced cardiomyopathy is its reversibility. Otherwise, it is indistinguishable from idiopathic dilated cardiomyopathy using available diagnostic techniques. We have documented cases of dogs in severe congestive heart failure with a diagnosis of "dilated cardiomyopathy" whose heart size and function returns to normal within weeks after successful radiofrequency catheter ablation of their arrhythmia.

25. Freckles, a 6-year-old domestic shorthaired cat, has been feeling dumpy lately. He does not want to play with his "Feline Flyer" and seems to have some difficulty breathing. His owner seeks your advice. After physical examination, thoracic radiographs, and a brief echocardiogram by a veterinary cardiologist, you diagnose hypertrophic cardiomyopathy, moderate left-sided congestive heart failure, and frequent paroxysms of atrial tachycardia. What is your management approach for the atrial arrhythmia?

The conceptual approach to treating atrial tachyarrhythmias in cats with hypertrophic cardiomyopathy involves controlling congestive heart failure and slowing AV nodal conduction of the tachyarrhythmia to the ventricles. In cats with this particular disease, however, digitalis glycosides are avoided for two reasons. First, inotropic support is not necessary and can be detrimental if dynamic aortic outflow obstruction is present. Second, digoxin has an especially narrow therapeutic index in cats, so is not used unless chronic inotropic support is required (as in dilated cardiomyopathy and some restrictive cardiomyopathies). First-line therapy for hypertrophic cardiomyopathy comes down to a calcium-channel blocker (a diltiazem preparation) or beta blocker (atenolol). Thankfully, these drugs also slow conduction through the AV node. Veterinary cardiologists are also beginning to investigate the use of D,L-sotalol in feline hypertrophic cardiomyopathy cases with frequent supraventricular or ventricular tachyarrhythmias. This drug has to be compounded down to a cat-sized dose. It has the advantage of prolonging atrial refractoriness through its class III effect, as well as slowing AV nodal conduction through its beta-blocking actions. Consult a veterinary cardiologist before using.

BIBLIOGRAPHY

1. Dhala A, Deshpande S, Blanck Z, et al: Supraventricular tachycardia: Electrophysiologic basis of the surface ECG pattern. In Podrid PJ, Kowrey PR (eds): Cardiac Arrhythmias: Mechanisms, Diagnosis, and Management. Baltimore, Williams & Wilkins, 1995, pp 1004–1021.
2. Harpster NK: Feline arrhythmias: diagnosis and management. In Kirk RW, Bonagura JD (eds): Current Veterinary Therapy XI: Small Animal Practice. Philadelphia, W.B. Saunders, 1992, pp 732–744.
3. Manolis AS, Estes NAM: Supraventricular tachycardia: Mechanisms and therapy. Arch Intern Med 147:1706–1716, 1987.
4. Pion PD: Current uses and hazards of calcium-channel blockers. In Kirk RW, Bonagura JD (ed): Current Veterinary Therapy XI: Small Animal Practice. Philadelphia, W.B. Saunders, 1992, pp 684–688.
5. Snyder PS, Atkins CE: Current uses and hazards of digitalis glycosides. In Kirk RW, Bonagura JD (ed): Current Veterinary Therapy XI: Small Animal Practice. Philadelphia, W.B. Saunders, 1992, pp 689–693.
6. Ware WA: Current uses and hazards of beta-blockers. In Kirk RW, Bonagura JD (eds): Current Veterinary Therapy XI: Small Animal Practice. Philadelphia, W.B. Saunders, 1992, pp 676–684.
7. Wathen MA, Klein GJ, Yee R, et al: Classification and terminology of supraventricular tachycardia. Cardiol Clin 11:109–120, 1993.
8. Wellens HJ: The value of the ECG in the diagnosis of supraventricular tachycardias. Eur Heart J 17(suppl C):10–20, 1996.
9. Wright KN: Assessment and treatment of supraventricular tachyarrhythmias. In Bonagura JD (ed): Current Veterinary Therapy XIII: Small Animal Practice. Philadelphia, W.B. Saunders, 2000, pp 726–730.
10. Wright KN, Atkins CE, Kanter R: Supraventricular tachycardia in four young dogs. J Am Vet Med Assoc 208:75–80, 1996.
11. Wright KN, Mehdirad AA, Giacobbe P, et al: Radiofrequency catheter ablation of accessory pathways in three dogs with subsequent resolution of tachycardia-induced cardiomyopathy. J Vet Intern Med 13:361–371, 1999.

31. BRADYARRHYTHMIA

Francis W.K. Smith, Jr., D.V.M.

1. What heart rates define bradycardia in dogs and cats?

Normal heart rates vary with the animal's state of arousal (adrenergic tone), level of fitness, body size, and age. Excited animals can have a rapid heart rate, while sleeping animals can have very slow heart rates (e.g., < 40 bpm in dogs). Athletic animals have slower resting heart rates and, at least in the hospital setting, large-breed dogs tend to have slower heart rates than small-breed dogs. Cats have higher heart rates than dogs and juvenile animals have higher heart rates than mature animals. The definitions of bradycardia listed below are based on heart rates of mature animals in a relaxed state.

Cats	Heart rate < 120 bpm
Large-breed dogs	Heart rate < 60 bpm
Small-breed dogs	Heart rate < 80 bpm

2. List various rhythms that would result in bradycardia.

- Sinus bradycardia
- Sinus arrest or sinus block
- Sick sinus syndrome
- Atrial standstill (persistent or hyperkalemic)
- Second-degree AV block
- Complete (i.e., third-degree) AV block

3. A slow heart rate is detected on physical examination. What physical findings may be helpful in differentiating AV block from sinus bradycardia?

Animals with sinus bradycardia maintain synchrony between the sinus impulse, atrial activation, and ventricular activation. Patients with AV block lose that synchrony on the nonconducted beats such that the atrial activation and ventricular activation are not coordinated. If the atrial contraction occurs simultaneously with the ventricular contraction, the AV valve will be closed and blood within the atria will not be able to enter the ventricle. As a result, the blood within the right atrium will be forced up the jugular vein, causing a large jugular pulse that is termed a cannon A wave. The presence of intermittent large jugular pulses supports AV block.

In some animals with advanced second-degree or complete AV block, you can hear fourth heart sounds associated with atrial contraction and fewer first and second heart sounds associated with ventricular contraction.

4. What clinical signs can be seen secondary to bradycardia?

Clinical signs, if any, generally relate to low cardiac output and consist of exercise intolerance, lethargy, and syncope. Chronic low cardiac output can eventually result in signs of congestive heart failure. Signs of right-sided failure (e.g., ascites) often precede those of left-sided heart failure (e.g., dyspnea secondary to pulmonary edema).

5. Define sinus bradycardia.

A heart rate that is slower than normal in which the slow rate is due to a depressed firing rate of the sinus node. In the absence of concurrent AV block, conduction through the AV node is normal so that there is a QRS complex for every P wave.

6. What is the differential diagnosis for conditions that result in sinus bradycardia?

- Sinus node disease (e.g., sick sinus syndrome)
- High vagal tone secondary to respiratory, gastrointestinal, or neurologic disease

- Hypothyroidism
- Hyperkalemia
- Hypothermia
- Athletic conditioning
- Drugs such as digitalis, beta-adrenergic blockers (e.g., propranolol), calcium channel antagonists (e.g., diltiazem), acepromazine, and xylazine

7. What is the appropriate therapy for sinus bradycardia?

In the absence of clinical signs therapy is generally not required. If bradycardia occurs secondary to a treatable underlying pathologic condition (e.g., hypothyroidism, hyperkalemia, hypothermia), therapy should be directed at correcting the underlying cause. Any drugs that slow the sinus rate should be discontinued. If there is no correctable underlying cause for the bradycardia and the animal is symptomatic, oral anticholinergic drugs (propantheline bromide), sympathomimetic agents (terbutaline or albuterol), or methylxanthine bronchodilators (aminophylline or theophylline) can be prescribed.

8. What is the difference between sinus arrest and sinoatrial block?

Sinus arrest and (second-degree) sinoatrial block result in pauses that are equal to or greater than twice the normal R-R interval on the ECG. Sinus arrest is the result of failure of sinus node impulse formation due to depressed automaticity in the sinus node. Sinoatrial block is the result of the sinus node impulse being blocked before it leaves the sinus node.

The pause may be followed by a normal P-QRS or, if the pause of sufficiently long, it may be followed by a junctional ventricular escape complex. It can be difficult to distinguish these two rhythms on the surface ECG but, fortunately, this distinction is seldom of clinical importance. If the pauses are always exactly twice the normal R-R interval, suspect sinoatrial block.

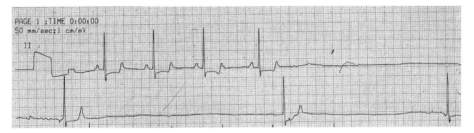

ECG of a dog with sick sinus syndrome.

9. The ECG shown above was obtained from a 10-year-old miniature schnauzer with a history of syncope. What is the rhythm diagnosis and what treatment options would you consider for this patient?

The ECG shows a sinus rhythm with prolonged episodes of sinus arrest or sinus block followed by junctional escape beats. Given the signalment and absence of historical findings to suggest high levels of vagal tone, the dog probably has sick sinus syndrome (SSS).

An atropine response test is suggested to evaluate sinus node function. To perform this test, atropine is administered at a dose of 0.04 mg/kg intramuscularly and the heart rate is determined 20–30 minutes later. If there is a good response to atropine, the patient can be treated with propantheline bromide. If there is no response to atropine, an oral bronchodilator such as aminophylline, theophylline, or albuterol can be prescribed. If the patient does not respond to medical therapy, pacemaker implantation is required.

10. Which breeds are at the highest risk for sick sinus syndrome?

Sick sinus syndrome is most prevalent in female miniature schnauzers. Other predisposed breeds include Pomeranians, boxers, cocker spaniels, and dachshunds.

11. In addition to sinus bradycardia and sinus arrest or sinoatrial block, what other ECG findings are commonly seen in patients with sick sinus syndrome?

While the classic findings of sick sinus syndrome reflect sinus node dysfunction, it is not uncommon to have concurrent disease in the AV node and bundle branches. As a result, patients with sick sinus syndrome can have very long periods of asystole because the junctional pacemaker does not initiate an impulse after a period of sinus arrest or block. Some animals with sick sinus syndrome will also have periods of supraventricular tachycardia resulting in what is termed bradycardia-tachycardia syndrome.

12. What are the differential diagnoses for the rhythm shown below?
- Atrial standstill (persistent or hyperkalemic)
- Atrial fibrillation with complete AV block
- Sinus bradycardia with small P waves lost in the baseline

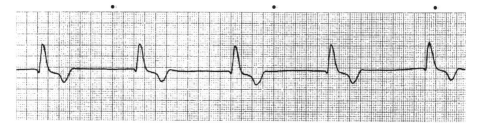

ECG of atrial standstill. (From Tilley LP, Miller MS, Smith FWK Jr: Canine and Feline Cardiac Arrhythmias. Philadelphia, Lea & Febiger, 1993, with permission.)

13. The ECG shown above was taken from a 3-year-old poodle with a history of intermittent anorexia, vomiting, and lethargy. The presenting complaints at the time the ECG was obtained were vomiting and collapse. What is the most likely diagnosis?

Atrial standstill secondary to hyperkalemia. The QRS complexes are wide, probably due to slowed intraventricular conduction caused by hyperkalemia. The dog is probably hyperkalemic and clinically ill due to hypoadrenocorticism (Addison's disease).

14. What tests should be conducted and what treatment should be initiated?

Blood should be obtained for a CBC and biochemical profile. Immediate determination of serum electrolytes is recommended. An ACTH response test should be performed. Initiate therapy with shock dosages of 0.9% saline. Depending on the patient's condition, other options to acutely lower potassium levels include sodium bicarbonate or insulin and dextrose. In the setting of life-threatening hyperkalemia, IV calcium gluconate can be administered slowly to block the effects of potassium at the cellular level. Calcium gluconate has no effect on serum potassium levels. Shock dosages of soluble corticosteroids are also recommended in the setting of hypoadrenocorticism. Steroids, however, will not affect the rhythm.

15. What are the causes of atrial standstill?

Atrial standstill is generally the result of hyperkalemia. In dogs, hyperkalemia is usually associated with hypoadrenocorticism. In cats, hyperkalemia is usually associated with urethral obstruction. Atrial standstill that occurs secondary to hyperkalemia is referred to as temporary atrial standstill in that the rhythm returns to normal after treatment is initiated and hyperkalemia resolves. The rhythm in patients with hyperkalemia and atrial standstill is termed a sinoventricular rhythm because the impulse is conducted from the sinus node to the AV node, although there is no atrial activation and hence no P waves.

Persistent atrial standstill is a rare condition that occurs in dogs with an atrial myopathy and cats with cardiomyopathy and severe atrial enlargement. This is most commonly reported in English springer spaniels and old English sheepdogs, but can be seen in any type of dog.

Electrolyte values in these patients are normal. Presenting signs are generally those of weakness or syncope due to bradycardia. Some animals present with signs of right or biventricular heart failure. Pacemaker implantation may control signs associated with bradycardia, but most dogs have a progressive myopathy that results in refractory heart failure despite pacemaker implantation.

16. What are the ECG characteristics that define first-, second-, and third-degree AV block?

First-degree AV block is caused by slow conduction through the AV node. On the ECG this results in a long PR interval. As conduction is only slow and not blocked in the AV node, there is a P wave for every QRS. Bradycardia does not develop unless there is a slow sinus rate as well.

Second-degree AV block is caused by the intermittent interruption of conduction through the AV node. On the beats where the impulses are not conducted through the AV node, there is a P wave without an associated QRS. The term advanced or high-grade second-degree AV block is used when there are two or more consecutive blocked P waves.

Complete AV block is caused by the inability of all electrical impulses to cross the AV node. There is no association between any of the P waves and QRS complexes. The ventricular rhythm arises from subsidiary pacemakers within the ventricles and is known as an escape rhythm. The inherent rate of ventricular pacemaker fibers is slow and, in the dog, ventricular escape rhythms typically have a rate between 40–60 bpm. In cats the rate is between 60–100 bpm.

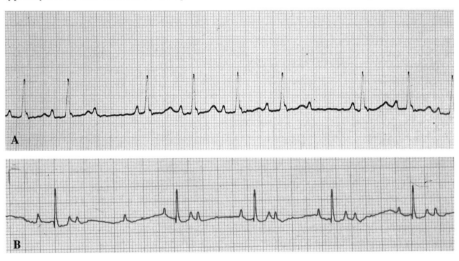

17. What is the rhythm diagnosis in the two ECGs shown above and how are the rhythms different?

Both ECGs demonstrate second-degree AV block. The A panel shows Mobitz type I AV block (Wenckebach block), which is classically associated with a progressive prolongation of the P-R interval, eventually leading to a nonconducted P wave (AV block). The B panel shows Mobitz type II AV block, which is associated with a constant P-R interval in the conducted beats with occasional nonconducted beats.

18. What are the clinically significant differences between Mobitz type I and Mobitz type II AV block?

Mobitz type I AV block is often associated with high levels of vagal tone or metabolic disturbances and rarely progresses to complete heart block. Mobitz type II AV block is commonly associated with structural heart disease and therefore more likely to progress to complete AV block than type I block.

19. What are the causes of AV block?

- High vagal tone
- Idiopathic fibrosis of the AV node
- Inflammation of the AV node
- Neoplastic infiltration of the AV node
- Drugs (digoxin, beta-blockers, diltiazem, verapamil, xylazine)
- Congenital disease
- Hypertrophic cardiomyopathy (cats)
- Infection (bacterial endocarditis, Lyme disease, Chagas' disease)
- Electrolyte disturbances (hyperkalemia, hypokalemia)

20. What treatment options exist for symptomatic AV block?

Atropine is administered to determine the role of vagal tone in the conduction disturbance. If the heart block resolves with atropine, oral anticholinergic agents such as propantheline bromide may be helpful. If there is no response to atropine, treatment with a pacemaker is recommended (see Chapter 59). If the patient is symptomatic and a pacemaker cannot be implanted right away, the patient can be stabilized with an isoproterenol drip or managed with bronchodilators such as theophylline, albuterol, or terbutaline. The oral bronchodilators will not accelerate the ventricular rate to the same extent as the isoproterenol drip.

When pacemaker implantation is indicated but not feasible, therapy with oral medications can be tried. If there is some improvement following an injection of atropine, prescribe propantheline bromide along with theophylline, albuterol, or terbutaline. If there is no response to atropine, use theophylline, albuterol, or terbutaline without the propantheline bromide. An anti-inflammatory dose of corticosteroids could also be prescribed for a week, in hopes that the AV block was associated with inflammation in the AV node that might respond to steroids.

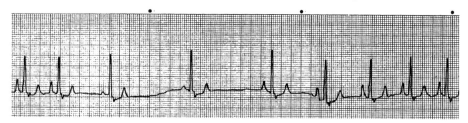

ECG of a dog with sinus arrhythmia. (From Tilley LP, Miller MS, Smith FWK Jr: Canine and Feline Cardiac Arrhythmias. Philadelphia, Lea & Febiger, 1993, with permission.)

21. A 10-year-old miniature poodle presented with a history of coughing. Physical examination findings included a III/VI holosystolic murmur that was loudest at the left heart apex, diffuse pulmonary crackles, heart rate of 80 bpm with an irregular rhythm that sped up on inspiration and slowed on expiration. The following ECG was obtained (see figure above). What is the likely cause of the cough and the heart rate and rhythm in this patient?

The ECG demonstrates a pronounced sinus arrhythmia with a heart rate of approximately 110. While a definitive diagnosis is not possible based on the available data, the findings described suggest that the clinical signs are likely due to pulmonary disease. While the murmur supports a diagnosis of chronic mitral valve disease in this old poodle, the heart rate and rhythm are not typical of heart failure. A pronounced sinus arrhythmia suggests high levels of vagal tone that are often seen with respiratory disease. Most patients presenting with congestive heart failure will have high levels of sympathetic tone, resulting in a sinus tachycardia. The crackles ausculted in this patient are probably associated with mucus in the airways rather than pulmonary edema. Thoracic radiographs are recommended to confirm the cause of the cough in this patient.

BIBLIOGRAPHY

1. Edwards NJ: Bolton's Handbook of Canine and Feline Electrocardiography, 2nd ed. Philadelphia, W.B. Saunders, 1987.

2. Kittleson MD: Electrocardiography. In Kittleson MD, Kienle RD (eds): Small Animal Cardiovascular Medicine. St Louis, Mosby, 1998, pp 72–94.
3. Miller MS, Tilley LP, Smith FWK, Fox PR: Electrocardiography. In Fox PR, Sisson D, Moise NS (eds): Textbook of Canine and Feline Cardiology. Philadelphia, W.B. Saunders, 1999, pp 67–106.
4. Smith FWK, Hadlock DJ: Electrocardiography. In Miller MS, Tilley LP (eds): Manual of Canine and Feline Cardiology, 2nd ed. Philadelphia, W.B. Saunders, 1995, pp 47–74.
5. Tilley LP: Essentials of Canine and Feline Electrocardiography, 3rd ed. Philadelphia, Lea & Febiger, 1992.

32. CARDIOPULMONARY RESUSCITATION

Steven L. Marks, B.V.Sc., M.S., MRCVS

1. Define cardiopulmonary arrest.
Cardiopulmonary arrest is the cessation of spontaneous cardiac and respiratory function.

2. Define cardiopulmonary resuscitation and list the phases of resuscitation.
CPR is a technique for providing ventilatory and circulatory support until advanced cardiac life support can be instituted. The three phases of CPR are: (1) basic cardiac life support; (2) advanced cardiac life support; and (3) post-resuscitative care.

3. What procedures are involved with each phase of CPR?
Basic cardiac life support

Airway	Assess the airway and if required clear and/or establish an airway
Breathing	Assess breathing and initially give 2 long breaths and wait for a response; if no response, start ventilating at a rate of 15–20 breaths per minute.
Circulation	Assess circulation and start thoracic compressions

Advanced cardiac life support

Drugs	The drugs administered are dependent on the ECG rhythm and the condition of the pet
ECG	The rhythm must be determined in order to know what procedures to perform
Fluid therapy	Conservative fluid therapy unless hypovolemia is the known cause of the cardiopulmonary arrest
Fibrillation control	Used for ventricular fibrillation only. Very time-dependent, the sooner applied the better chance of conversion.

Post-resuscitative care
Guiding cerebral recovery
Therapy guided toward cerebral resuscitation
How is the patient responding?
Patient monitoring is critical
Intensive care
Providing supportive care

4. What is CPCR?
This acronym stands for cardiopulmonary-cerebral resuscitation, emphasizing the importance of brain function for survival. It is now used synonymously with CPR.

5. List the clinical signs that may warn of impending cardiopulmonary arrest.

- Change in respiratory rate
- Change in character of pulse
- Bradycardia
- Hypotension
- Cyanosis
- Hypothermia
- Dilated pupils

6. What body position is best for CPR?
Ideally, right lateral recumbency for animals less than 7.0 kg and dorsal recumbency for larger animals. It is difficult to maintain dorsal recumbency unless a V-shaped trough is available.

7. How is CPR performed?

There are two basic techniques of CPR:

1. **Intermittent ventilation and compression:** This technique requires at least two people and involves performing five chest compressions followed by one artificial ventilation. This cycle is then continued.

2. **Synchronous high airway pressure ventilation:** This technique requires at least two people and involves performing chest compressions and ventilations simultaneously in a 1:1 ratio. This is now the most commonly performed technique in animals.

8. How is CPR performed by one person?

This technique has been shown to be very ineffective. The chest compressions and ventilations are performed in a 15:2 ratio.

9. List predisposing factors that may lead to cardiopulmonary arrest.

- Cellular hypoxia
- Excess vagal tone
- Acid base and electrolyte disturbances

10. What diseases most often lead to cardiopulmonary arrest?

- Respiratory disease
- Cardiac disease
- Trauma
- Sepsis
- Metabolic disorders, including pancreatitis, diabetic ketoacidosis, and oliguric renal failure

11. What does DNR stand for and when is it used?

DNR stands for "do not resuscitate." This is a no-code order. It implies that the pet should not have CPR performed. The clinician and the pet owner should carefully consider a DNR order. In most cases this order is used only when the pet has severe irreversible disease and quality of life issues arise.

12. What are advance directives?

Advance directives refer to discussions with the pet owner concerning what procedures can and should be performed in the event of catastrophic illness. These discussions may also involve the financial aspects of procedures to be performed. Although difficult, these issues should be discussed with the client prior to the life-threatening event.

13. How do we ventilate the patients during CPR?

- Several techniques can be used to artificially ventilate these patients.
- Mouth-to-mouth breathing
- Mouth-to-nose breathing
- Endotracheal intubation and anesthesia machine
- Endotracheal intubation and Ambu bag
- Mechanical ventilator

14. What two theories explain increased blood flow during thoracic compression?

1. **The cardiac pump:** Direct compression of the heart during thoracic compressions increases cardiac output and perfusion. Compression and subsequent elastic recoil simulates systole and diastole. The cardiac pump theory explains the increase in blood flow that results when direct cardiac compressions are used in animals weighing 7 kg or less. The compressions are performed directly over the heart (intercostal space 3–5) with the pet in right lateral recumbency.

2. **The thoracic pump:** Changes in intrathoracic pressures result in ventricular filling and ejection; this is the mechanism that explains the effect of thoracic compressions in larger dogs. The compressions are performed with the patient in dorsal or lateral recumbency. The

compression should lead to approximately a 30% change in the chest and be performed over the widest proportion of the thorax.

15. What are the priority areas for perfusion during CPR?
Coronary arteries and cerebral arteries.

16. How can we assess if adequate thoracic compressions are being performed?
Evaluating peripheral pulses can help monitor if the compressions are effective and leading to increased cardiac output. If a pulse is not generated by each thoracic compression, the position of the animal should be changed or the compression technique altered.

17. What are interposed abdominal compressions and why are they performed?
Interposed abdominal compressions are abdominal compressions performed between thoracic compressions. They can be used to augment venous return and potentially increase coronary perfusion pressure

18. What are the two drugs most commonly administered during CPR?
Atropine and epinephrine.

19. List the available routes for drug administration.
• Central vein
• Intratracheal
• Intraosseous
• Peripheral vein

20. What drugs can be administered via the intratracheal route?
The acronym LEAN can be used as a reminder: Lidocaine, Epinephrine, Atropine, Naloxone.

21. Describe the Jen Chung technique and why it is used.
Referred to as GV-26, this is an acupuncture site suggested for cardiopulmonary stimulation. A 25-gauge needle is placed cutaneously at the nasal philtrum. The needle is advanced until the periosteum is felt. Gentle twisting of the needle will stimulate this point and may be valuable in cases of respiratory arrest.

22. Give an approximate percentage of survival for patients undergoing CPR.
Overall survival for veterinary patients is approximately 10%. However, the prognosis depends to an important extent on the nature of the disease that resulted in cardiorespiratory arrest. CPR is reasonably effective when anesthetic accidents result in hypoxia and arrest in otherwise healthy animals. Similarly, if severe trauma causes arrest in a previously healthy animal, aggressive resuscitative efforts may be rewarded. In contrast, arrest resulting from severe metabolic derangements or overwhelming sepsis is generally associated with a poor prognosis. Attempts at resuscitation may be transiently effective; however, few of these patients are ultimately discharged from hospital.

23. What are the most common rhythm disturbances seen on the canine ECG during cardiopulmonary arrest?
• Ventricular fibrillation
• Ventricular asystole
• Electrical mechanical dissociation

24. Why is ventricular fibrillation such a concerning finding on the ECG?
Ventricular fibrillation is a nonperfusing rhythm and must be converted as soon as possible. The longer the patient is in this rhythm, the more difficult it is to convert. Electrical defibrillation is the treatment of choice; chemical defibrillation is generally ineffective.

25. What is electromechanical dissociation?

Electromechanical dissociation (EMD) is present when electrical cardiac activity fails to result in useful cardiac contractions. Electrocardiographically, a wide QRS bradycardia is typically present; arterial pulses and heart sounds are absent.

26. How is ventricular asystole or electromechanical dissociation addressed during CPR?

Epinephrine is administered in most attempts at CPR; this catecholamine is a potent positive inotrope and chronotrope. Additionally, epinephrine increases systemic vascular resistance so that perfusion pressure can be maintained when cardiac output is low. The use of atropine together with epinephrine and mechanical ventilation/cardiac compression is generally the initial approach when confronted with lethal bradycardia. In cases in which bradycardia is unresponsive to medical interventions, the emergent implantation of a temporary electronic cardiac pacemaker can be considered.

27. When should internal cardiac massage be used?

Internal cardiac massage should be used when thoracic compressions can not be used, i.e., with severe thoracic trauma or when thoracic compressions are not effective. The decision to use internal cardiac massage should be made as early as possible during CPR. It should not be used as a salvage procedure.

28. How is internal cardiac massage performed?

An emergency left intercostal thoracotomy must be performed. Shaving of hair and surgical scrub is not required. One gloved hand should cradle the heart and be able to compress the heart. Digital compression of the descending aorta against the thoracic vertebrae can be performed simultaneously.

29. What drugs should be included in the emergency or "crash cart"?

Epinephrine, atropine, naloxone, and lidocaine.

30. How do we monitor patients during the post-resuscitation period?

Patients should be closely monitored by daily physical and neurologic examinations. Other parameters to monitor daily may include:

- Body weight
- PCV/TP
- Blood glucose
- ECG
- Arterial blood pressure
- Arterial blood gas analysis
- Central venous pressure
- Urine output
- Acid base/electrolyte status

CONTROVERSIES

31. Should sodium bicarbonate be used during CPR?

For: During cardiopulmonary arrest patients become acidemic. Even when CPR is used appropriately, underperfusion of tissues leads to metabolic acidosis and hypoventilation leads to respiratory acidosis. Under these conditions myocardial contractility may be decreased, the myocardium may become irritable and prone to arrhythmia, and responses to emergency drugs may be dampened.

Against: The best treatment for acidemia during cardiopulmonary arrest is adequate ventilation. The metabolic acidosis that occurs is usually not significant during the first 15 minutes of the arrest and appropriate ventilation will prevent respiratory acidosis. The adverse side effects of sodium bicarbonate include volume overload, hypernatremia, and hyperosmolarity. In addition, bicarbonate acts as a carbon dioxide–producing substance, which may lead to myocardial hypercarbia and a failed resuscitation.

32. Can animals be resuscitated without establishing an airway?

For: In some circumstances an established airway may not be required for successful resuscitation. In a study evaluating by-stander CPR, ventricular fibrillation was initiated in two groups of pigs. In one group standard resuscitation was attempted and in the second group standard procedures were used without an established airway. The results indicated that pigs could be resuscitated without endotracheal intubation.

Against: Providing an airway is imperative to all successful resuscitations. It is part of the ABCs of CPR.

BIBLIOGRAPHY

1. Crowe DT: Cardiopulmonary resuscitation in the dog: A review and proposed new guidelines (Part I). Semin Vet Med Sug 3:32, 1988.
2. Crowe DT: Cardiopulmonary resuscitation in the dog: A review and proposed new guidelines (Part II). Semin Vet Med Sug 3:328, 1988.
3. Desforges JF: Current concepts: Cardiopulmonary resuscitation. N Engl J Med 127:1075–1080, 1992.
4. Hackett TB, Van Pelt DR: Cardiopulmonary resuscitation. In Bonagura JD (ed): Kirk's Current Veterinary Therapy XII: Small Animal Practice. Philadelphia, W.B. Saunders, 1995, pp 167–175.
5. Henik RA: Basic life support and external cardiac compression in dogs and cats. J Am Vet Med Assoc 200:1925–1939, 1992.
6. Janssens L, Altman S, Rogers PAM: Respiratory and cardiac arrest under general anesthesia: Treatment by acupuncture of the nasal philtrum. Vet Rec 105:273–276, 1979.
7. Kass PH, Haskins SC: Survival following cardiopulmonary resuscitation in dogs and cats. J Vet Emerg Crit Care 2:57, 1993.
8. Wingfield WE, Van Pelt DR: Respiratory and cardiopulmonary arrest in dogs and cats: 265 cases (1986–1991). J Am Vet Med Assoc 200:1993, 1993.

33. SYSTEMIC HYPERTENSION

Patti S. Snyder, D.V.M., M.S.

1. What is systemic hypertension?

Systemic hypertension is a sustained elevation in arterial blood pressure (systolic, diastolic, or both). Since blood pressure can increase significantly with restraint, and because factors such as excitement, exercise, the administration of certain medications, and ambient temperature can all affect blood pressure, a diagnosis of systemic hypertension should be made cautiously. Careful consideration should be given to the animal's history, physical examination findings, and factors such as those mentioned above. Because blood pressure can be affected by many diverse variables, a precise numerical definition of systemic hypertension is problematic. However, systemic hypertension is likely present in small animals when systolic pressures greater than 180 mmHg are repeatedly obtained by indirect measurement methods. If blood pressure is only minimally elevated, the blood pressure should be remeasured before a diagnosis of hypertension is made.

2. What is the best way to diagnose systemic hypertension?

Although the index of suspicion that a patient has systemic hypertension may be high based upon the history and physical findings, confirmation of the suspicion by measuring blood pressure is essential before making a final diagnosis or beginning antihypertensive medication. Direct arterial puncture is the most accurate measurement technique but the procedure is rarely tolerated in awake untrained animals; therefore, indirect measurement of blood pressure is the most common method used to document systemic hypertension.

3. What animals get systemic hypertension?

Hypertension that develops in the absence of underlying disease is known as primary, essential, or idiopathic hypertension. In veterinary medicine, systemic hypertension is most commonly associated with an underlying disease process. In cats, systemic hypertension is most often secondary to renal disease or hyperthyroidism. In dogs, hypertension has been reported most often in association with renal failure (especially glomerular disease), hyperadrenocorticism, diabetes mellitus and pheochromocytoma. Isolated cases of hypertension have been reported in animals with hypothyroidism, primary hyperaldosteronism, acromegaly, and obesity.

No significant breed predilections have been reported in animals with systemic hypertension. One study reported male cats to be at higher risk but this has not been uniformly accepted.

4. What is the prevalence of hypertension?

One study reported 61% of cats with chronic renal failure and 87% of cats with hyperthyroidism had mild elevations in their blood pressure; another study reported 65% of cats with chronic renal failure and 23% of cats with hyperthyroidism had elevated blood pressure. More than 50% of dogs with hyperadrenocorticism, 60% of dogs with renal disease, and 80% of dogs with glomerular disease were hypertensive in one review; in another, 46% of diabetic dogs were hypertensive.

5. What are the pathophysiologic mechanisms of systemic hypertension?

Systemic blood pressure is related to both cardiac output (CO) and systemic vascular resistance; if CO or vascular resistance increases and other conditions remain constant, blood pressure rises. The mechanisms responsible for the elevated blood pressure depend upon the cause of the hypertension. In some syndromes, the rise in blood pressure is related primarily to an increase in CO, as is the case in the hyperdynamic circulation that results from hyperthyroidism. In other cases, blood pressure rises due to increases in vascular resistance or a combination of increased output and vascular resistance. For primary hypertension the mechanisms are unknown, but in some dogs genetics play a role.

6. What are the mechanisms of hypertension in renal disease?

In renal disease, a failure to excrete adequate amounts of sodium and water subsequently leading to an increase in extracellular fluid volume is believed to be the primary reason for the elevation in blood pressure. However, in one group of hypertensive cats with chronic renal failure, the fractional excretion of sodium was decreased in some but increased or normal in others, suggesting that abnormal sodium excretion is unlikely to be the sole cause of hypertension in cats with chronic renal failure.

Increased activation of renin and therefore the renin-angiotensin-aldosterone-system (RAAS) and a reduction in vasodilatory substances are also suspected to be involved in the development of hypertension with renal failure. However, when plasma renin activity (PRA), angiotensin II, and aldosterone concentrations were evaluated in cats with chronic renal disease and hypertension, the results were variable. The concentrations of PRA were reduced in some but normal or increased in others. Aldosterone concentrations were increased but angiotensin II concentration did not differ significantly between normal and cats with renal failure and hypertension.

7. What are the mechanisms of hypertension in other conditions?

Hyperthyroidism results in an increase in metabolic rate, a decrease in vascular resistance, and a consequent increase in CO; an increase in the sensitivity of cardiac beta-adrenergic receptors leads to excessive beta-adrenergic stimulation and contributes to the increase in CO. There may also be increased sensitivity of renal beta-adrenergic receptors resulting in increased renin release and activation of the RAAS. These effects culminate in elevations in blood pressure.

In hyperadrenocorticism, hypertension likely results from the excess glucocorticoid enhancing catecholamine synthesis, thereby increasing the stimulation of beta and alpha-adrenergic receptors. Glucocorticoid excess may also increase the formation of angiotensinogen and thus activation of the RAAS.

The mechanism responsible for hypertension in diabetic patients is unclear and numerous possibilities have been postulated but unproven.

8. Do animals with heart disease have hypertension?

Secondary cardiac changes are common in hypertensive dogs and cats, but the reverse is not true because the cardiac abnormalities are the result rather than the cause of the hypertension. Inappropriately increased afterload, a feature of systolic heart failure, is not the equivalent of systemic hypertension. Thus animals with primary systolic cardiac disease have increased afterload but are not expected to have elevated systemic blood pressures.

9. Why are animals with hypertension presented to the veterinarian?

In cats, the most common presenting complaint is either blindness and/or pupillary dilation. In both situations, the cause is usually hypertensive retinopathy. Signs consistent with hypertensive encephalopathy such as seizures, disorientation, ataxia, circling, paresis, and nystagmus have been reported in some hypertensive cats and dogs.

Cats and dogs with systemic hypertension can develop cardiac murmurs, although this condition is not usually recognized by owners. Some hypertensive animals are presented for routine evaluation. Auscultation of the thorax may reveal a systolic murmur that subsequently leads to further cardiac evaluation and finally to a diagnosis of systemic hypertension with secondary hypertensive heart disease.

Animals may also be presented for clinical signs related to the primary disease process such as hyperthyroidism, renal failure, or hyperadrenocorticism.

10. What abnormalities are found on physical examination?

Hypertensive animals may have a completely normal physical examination. However, they could have abnormalities consistent with retinopathy, encephalopathy, or heart disease. In addition, abnormalities related to the primary disease process (e.g. renal failure, hyperthyroidism, or hyperadrenocorticism) may be recognized on physical examination.

11. What diagnostic evaluation should be performed in an animal suspected of having systemic hypertension?

Any animal that is suspected of being hypertensive should have an indirect blood pressure measurement performed. The finding of a normal blood pressure greatly reduces the likelihood that an animal is hypertensive. The exception to this is an animal with a pheochromocytoma, in which hypertension can be intermittent.

A serum biochemistry panel and urinalysis should be performed on all animals. In cats, it is probably prudent to evaluate the T_4 in all hypertensive cats older than 6 years of age. If the index of suspicion is still high that a cat is hyperthyroid despite a normal T_4, additional testing of thyroid function is indicated (i.e. repeat the T_4, consider a T_3 suppression test, perform nuclear scintigraphy). Adrenal function testing and possibly abdominal ultrasonography should be performed in dogs if the signalment, history, and physical examination are suggestive of hyperadrenocorticism. Urine catecholamine excretion is expected to be abnormal in dogs with pheochromocytomas but sample collection is difficult and the laboratory standards are not well established. Thoracic radiographs and an electrocardiogram are most useful in helping to exclude other diseases on the differential diagnosis list.

12. Is echocardiography indicated in animals with hypertension?

Echocardiography can be useful in determining if cardiac changes have occurred secondary to the hypertension. Since left ventricular hypertrophy has been documented in hypertensive cats that had normal cardiac auscultation, echocardiography is the best means to document these changes.

13. What abnormalities are found in clinicopathologic data?

If the animal has primary hypertension, the clinical pathologic data is often normal. When azotemia is present, it is impossible to know for certain which condition preceded the other. Azotemia, isothenuria, or proteinuria would likely indicate a renal cause for the hypertension. So far researchers have not shown a relationship between the degree of azotemia and the severity of hypertension in hypertensive veterinary patients.

Elevated hepatic enzymes, hypercholesterolemia, and minimally concentrated urine may increase the suspicion of hyperadrenocorticism in dogs. Hepatic enzyme elevation and minimally concentrated urine are commonly found in cats with hyperthyroidism.

14. What are the radiographic findings of systemic hypertension?

Thoracic radiographs in hypertensive cats may be normal or may show evidence of mild to moderate cardiomegaly. The pulmonary vasculature is usually normal and pulmonary edema and pleural effusion are rare. However, it should be emphasized that since hyperthyroidism is the underlying disease in many hypertensive cats, some degree of radiographic cardiac enlargement and pulmonary vessel enlargement are common in this patient population. Information regarding thoracic radiographs in dogs with systemic hypertension is lacking but congestive heart failure is rare.

15. What are the electrocardiographic findings of systemic hypertension?

Electrocardiograms in hypertensive cats may be normal or show a shift in the mean electrical axis consistent with a left anterior fascicular–type block. Cardiac arrhythmias and chamber enlargements are possible but uncommon. Information regarding electrocardiographic findings in dogs with systemic hypertension is scarce.

16. What are the echocardiographic findings of systemic hypertension?

Left ventricular hypertrophy has been identified in many cats with systemic hypertension. The hypertrophy may be symmetrical (but not usually severe) or may involve the interventricular septum predominantly. Left atrial enlargement may be present but is often not dramatic. The aortic diameter has also been reported to be enlarged in hypertensive cats compared with similar measurements in cats of comparable age. Left ventricular hypertrophy has been documented in experimental systemic hypertension in dogs. In a colony of hypertensive dogs, the left ventricular chamber size was increased but wall thickness was normal.

17. What are the goals in management of systemic hypertension?

Treatment should focus on managing the underlying cause of the hypertension, if possible. If "end organ" damage is apparent (e.g., retinopathy, cardiac disease, or neurologic disease), then both the primary disease and the hypertension should be treated. Dogs and cats with concurrent renal disease and systemic hypertension usually require medication indefinitely to control their hypertension. Hyperthyroid cats that are hypertensive with clinical signs attributed to the hypertension should be treated simultaneously for their hyperthyroidism and systemic hypertension. When the hyperthyroidism is controlled, the antihypertensive therapy may be discontinued in many cases. If the hypertension is not severe in dogs with hyperadrenocorticism, no antihypertensive medication is necessary. Since hypertension has been reported to occur with corticosteroid use in dogs and humans, discontinuation of corticosteroids is recommended if at all possible in animals with hypertension.

In instances where the cause for the hypertension cannot be found and corrected, specific antihypertensive therapy is usually necessary. Resolution of retinopathy, cardiac hypertrophy, and neurologic signs depends upon many factors including the severity and chronicity of the abnormality (e.g., retinal reattachment and return of vision is unlikely to occur if the detachment has been chronic) and the ability to control the hypertension.

18. What drugs are used in the management of the disease?

Amlodipine, a calcium channel blocker, has been shown to be an effective once daily, single agent antihypertensive medication in cats (cats: 0.18 mg/kg every 24 hr). Amlodipine has been used safely in cats with renal disease and in cats with hyperthyroidism. There are, however, scattered reports of worsening azotemia in a small population of hypertensive cats with concurrent renal disease when amlodipine was administered. For this reason, renal parameters should be monitored in cats receiving amlodipine or any other antihypertensive agent. The use of amlodipine in dogs is more limited; however, it has been effective in some dogs at a dose of 0.15–0.25 mg/kg every 24 hr. The angiotensin-converting enzyme (ACE) inhibitor, enalapril (dogs: 0.3–0.5 mg/kg every 12–24 hr; cats: 0.25–0.5 mg/kg every 12–24 hr) and the beta-adrenergic blocking agent, propranolol (dogs: 0.2–1 mg/kg every 8–12 hr; cats: 2.5–5 mg/cat every 8–12 hr) have been used with mixed results. Atenolol (dogs: 0.25–1 mg/kg every 12–24 hr; cats: 6.25–12.5 mg/cat every 12–24 hr) has also been substituted for propranolol. In some instances, phenoxybenzamine (2.5–7.5 mg/cat every 8–12 hr), an alpha-adrenergic blocking agent, has been used successfully alone or in combination with enalapril and propranolol in hypertensive cats. Another ACE inhibitor, benazepril, has been used successfully in some hypertensive cats (dogs and cats: 0.25–0.5 mg/kg every 24 hr). Other drugs such as prazosin, diltiazem, hydralazine and various diuretics have also been used.

19. Once antihypertensive medication is begun, how long does it take before blood pressure drops?

Statistically significant declines in blood pressure have been noted in hypertensive cats given oral amlodipine after one dose and blood pressure decreased into the normal range after one week of therapy. Blood pressure may drop more rapidly if parenteral medication is given. However, in response to chronic hypertension, adaptive changes in vascular structure are thought to cause an increase in cerebrovascular resistance. A precipitous decline in systemic blood pressure may result in relative cerebrovascular hypotension, which can compromise cerebral perfusion and place the patient at risk for the development of neurologic signs. Parenteral administration of antihypertensive medications is generally reserved for cases in which the risks of therapy are outweighed by the risk posed by persistent severe hypertension.

20. How often should animals with systemic hypertension be monitored?

Blood pressure should be monitored weekly until the blood pressure has been reduced into an acceptable range. Blood pressure measurements should be obtained at various times in the dosing schedule to insure that that medication is controlling the hypertension for the full 24-hour period. In addition, several measurements should be taken at each visit and averaged in an attempt to minimize the effect of a single high or low reading. After hypertension is controlled then the interval between follow-up visits may lengthen to approximately every 3-4 months or as dictated by the primary disease process.

21. What is the prognosis?

The long-term prognosis depends upon the cause of the hypertension. If blood pressure can be controlled, and there is no underlying cause for the hypertension, the prognosis is good.

CONTROVERSIES

22. Does severe hypertension accelerate the development or progression of renal failure?

In certain animal models of hypertension and in humans with essential hypertension, there is convincing evidence that an association exists between severe hypertension and the subsequent development of chronic renal failure. In humans, there is a strong relationship between elevations in mean arterial pressure and reduction in glomerular filtration rate. At this time, no such relationship has been identified in dogs or cats with naturally occurring renal disease.

23. Does controlling hypertension slow the progression of renal disease?

Research in hypertensive animal models and in human clinical trials has suggested that normalization of blood pressure does slow progression of renal disease but that the effect is dependent upon which antihypertensive agent is used. Not only does systemic arterial hypertension need to be controlled but intrarenal blood pressure needs to be lowered as well. ACE inhibitors appear to be renoprotective and recently there is also evidence that some of the newer calcium channel blockers, such as amlodipine, may have a renoprotective effect. Most of this research is based upon experimental models so whether this remains true in naturally occurring renal disease in companion animals is not known.

BIBLIOGRAPHY

1. Belew AM, Barlett T, Brown SA: Evaluation of the white-coat effect in cats. J Vet Intern Med 13:134–142, 1999.
2. Bodey AR, Michell AR: Epidemiological study of blood pressure in domestic dogs. J Small Anim Pract 37:116–125, 1996.
3. Bodey AR, Sansom J: Epidemiological study of blood pressure in domestic cats. J Small Anim Pract 39:567–573, 1998.
4. Dukes J: Hypertension: A review of the mechanisms, manifestations and management. J Small Anim Pract 33:119–129, 1992.
5. Epstein M: Calcium antagonists and renal hemodynamics: Implications for renal protection. Clin Invest Med 14:590–595, 1991.
6. Epstein M: Hypertension as a risk factor for progression of chronic renal disease. Blood Press Suppl 1:23–28, 1994.
7. Henik RA: Diagnosis and treatment of feline systemic hypertension. Comp Contin Educ Pract Vet 19: 163–179, 1997.
8. Jensen JL, Henik RA, Brownfield M, Armstrong J: Plasma renin activity and angiotensin I and aldosterone concentrations in cats with hypertension associated with chronic renal disease. Am J Vet Res 58:535–540, 1997.
9. Kobayashi DL, Peterson ME, Graves TK, et al: Hypertension in cats with chronic renal failure or hyperthyroidism. J Vet Intern Med 4:58–62, 1990.
10. Littman MP: Spontaneous systemic hypertension in 24 cats. J Vet Intern Med 8:79–86, 1994.
11. Morgan RV: Systemic hypertension in four cats: ocular and medical findings. J Am Anim Hosp Assoc 22:615–621, 1986.
12. Ortega TM, Feldman EC, Nelson RW, et al: Systemic arterial blood pressure and urine protein/creatinine ratio in dogs with hyperadrenocorticism. J Am Vet Med Assoc 209:1724–1729, 1996.
13. Snyder PS: Amlodipine: A randomized, blinded clinical trial in 9 cats with systemic hypertension. J Vet Intern Med 12:157–162, 1998.
14. Stiles J, Polzin DJ, Bistner SI: The prevalence of retinopathy in cats with systemic hypertension and chronic renal failure or hyperthyroidism. J Am Anim Hosp Assoc 30:564–572, 1994.
15. Tolins JP, Raij L: Antihypertensive therapy and the progression of chronic renal disease. Are there renoprotective drugs? Semin Nephrol 11:538–548, 1991.

34. DEGENERATIVE VALVULAR DISEASE

Jonathan A. Abbott, D.V.M.

1. What is myxomatous valvular degeneration?

Myxomatous valvular degeneration is one of many terms that refer to a sterile, degenerative disease that affects the cardiac valves of middle-aged and older dogs. Synonyms include endocardiosis, chronic degenerative mitral valve disease, and simply, chronic valve disease.

2. Describe the structure and function of the normal mitral valve apparatus.

The mitral valve apparatus consists of the mitral valve leaflets and the supporting structures : the left ventricular papillary muscles, chordae tendineae, and the mitral valve annulus. The mitral valve annulus is the fibrous ring that forms the left atrioventricular junction and the site at which the basilar aspect of the mitral leaflets are attached. There are two mitral valve leaflets. The cranial, or anterior, leaflet has fibrous continuity with the aortic valve and forms the caudal boundary of the left ventricular outflow tract; the caudal leaflet is more often referred to as the posterior mitral valve leaflet.

In a healthy animal, the leaflets are thin sheets of connective tissue covered by cardiac endothelium. The free edges of the leaflets are tethered by the chordae tendineae to the two left ventricular papillary muscles. These chords serve to anchor the mitral leaflets; during systole, they prevent prolapse of the leaflets into the left atrium. The function of the mitral valve is straightforward; it prevents the regurgitation of blood into the left atrium during ventricular systole and thus ensures that the force of ventricular contraction results only in useful flow into the aorta.

3. What is the pathologic nature of degnerative valvular disease? What is the post mortem appearance?

Degenerative valvular disease is characterized by the accumulation of mucopolysaccharides within the spongiosa and fibrosa layers of the mitral leaflets. Grossly, the leaflets are abnormally thick and have a nodular appearance. Lengthening of the chordae tendineae is also observed. Both atrioventricular (AV) valves can be affected; however, degenerative disease affecting the mitral valve is of greater clinical importance than degenerative tricuspid disease. Endocardiosis is a sterile degenerative process; inflammation or infection is not a feature.

4. What causes degenerative mitral valve disease?

Degenerative mitral valve disease (MVD) commonly affects chondrodystrophoid canine breeds that also have a high prevalence of collapsing trachea and intervertebral disc disease; consequently, it has been suggested that MVD is but one manifestation of a more generalized connective tissue disorder. The cause of MVD is unknown, although a genetic basis is likely. MVD is common in certain breeds of dog; in the cavalier King Charles spaniel, the age at which MVD becomes clinically apparent has a heritable basis.

5. What are the pathophysiologic consequences of MVD?

Distortion of the mitral valve leaflets prevents normal coaptation of the mitral valve leaflets and the consequence is mitral valve regurgitation. Lengthening and rupture of the mitral chordae tendineae predisposes to mitral valve prolapse, which can also contribute to mitral valve incompetence. Inadequate mitral valve apposition allows a portion of the left ventricular stroke volume to be ejected backward into the left atrium. This regurgitant volume is augmented by the pulmonary venous return and then returns to the left ventricle during diastole. Thus, incompetence of the mitral valve imposes a volume overload on the left atrium and the left ventricle. Volume loading of the left heart is a stimulus for eccentric hypertrophy (hypertrophy accompanied by dilation).

Small volumes of mitral valve regurgitation (MR) are usually well tolerated but two factors can potentially contribute to worsening of MR. Although the speed at which it does so is highly individual, MVD is generally a progressive disorder. Thus, ongoing alterations in valvular structure will worsen mitral valve incompetence. Additionally, dilation of the mitral annulus inevitably results from atrial/ventricular dilation and this further limits leaflet coaptation and worsens MR. Systolic myocardial function of the left ventricle tends to be largely unaffected by MR unless the valvular lesion is severe and longstanding. When substantial MR is present, the isovolumic phase of ventricular contraction does not take place because the ventricle can "unload" into the low-pressure reservoir provided by the left atrium. Thus, afterload and therefore myocardial oxygen demand is relatively low in the setting of MR; as a result, MR tends to be a lesion that is well tolerated at least in the sense that contractility can be preserved until late in the natural history of the disease. Longstanding, severe MR can, however, result in myocardial cell death, replacement fibrosis and myocardial dysfunction that is known as "cardiomyopathy of overload."

6. What signalment is typical of patients that develop MVD?

MVD is common in dogs; cats are rarely affected. Endocardiosis is a degenerative disease that develops primarily in older dogs. Valvular lesions may develop in dogs of virtually any breed; however, the clinical consequences of MVD are observed almost exclusively in older dogs of the toy and small breeds.

The prevalence of MVD is not known with certainty, but it can be as high as 33% in dogs older than 10 years. It is the most common cardiac disease in the dog. Miniature and toy poodles, pomeranians, bichon frise, miniature schnauzers, dachshunds, cavalier King Charles spaniels, as well as mixed-breed dogs are commonly affected.

7. What is distinctive about MVD that affects the cavalier King Charles spaniel?

Mitral valve pathology in the cavalier King Charles spaniel is indistinguishable from MVD that affects other breeds. However, MVD in this breed is distinctive in that the disease becomes clinically evident at a relatively early age and in some individuals the disease is severe and rapidly progressive. In other breeds, clinical signs related to MVD are uncommon in dogs that are younger than about 8 years. In the cavalier King Charles spaniel, murmurs of mitral valve regurgitation are occasionally encountered in dogs as young as 2 and 3 years. Pedigree studies performed by Haggstrom and Kvart have demonstrated that the tendency to develop mitral valve lesions at an early age is heritable; the age of onset of MR in individual dogs can be approximately predicted by the age at which MR became evident in the parents.

8. What are the clinical consequences of MVD?

It should be emphasized that murmurs due to MVD are more common than clinical signs related to the disease. Some patients develop mild and only slowly progressive valvular lesions and ultimately succumb to extracardiac disease before the development of clinically consequential MR.

When MR is substantial, it imposes a volume overload on the left atrium and left ventricle. If left atrial pressures become sufficiently high, they are reflected back upon the pulmonary venous circulation with the potential consequence of pulmonary edema or left-sided congestive heart failure (CHF).

9. What abnormalities are revealed by the patient history?

Cough is the clinical sign that is most commonly associated with MVD. Respiratory distress is usually a feature of the history of those patients that develop pulmonary edema. Other clinical signs such as syncope, ascites, weight loss, lethargy, and lack of appetite can also be observed.

10. What causes cough in patients with MVD?

The cause of cough in dogs with MVD is multifactorial. Cough is an explosive, reflex-mediated exhalation; the receptors that initiate this reflex are located primarily in the larger airways. Pulmonary edema can stimulate cough receptors but generally does so when edema fluid floods the small airways; when pulmonary edema is the cause of cough, dyspnea is usually evident.

Compression of the left mainstem bronchus by an enlarged left atrium is another important cause of cough in dogs with MVD. Cough due to bronchial compression resulting from left atrial enlargement seems to be unique to the patient population that is subject to MVD. This might be partly explained by the high prevalence of concurrent primary airway diseases such as collapsing trachea in the dogs that commonly develop MVD. The stimulation of juxtapulmonary receptors might also play a role in the pathogenesis of cough in some dogs with MVD. Stimulation of juxtapulmonary or J receptors by pulmonary venous distention results in reflex-mediated bronchoconstriction and increases in mucus production. Stimulation of J receptors might therefore contribute to cough in patients that have MVD but do not have overt CHF.

Regardless, it is important to recognize that patients with MVD can develop a cough in the absence of CHF; this cough can be explained by cardiac disease, although in some cases concurrent primary respiratory tract disease plays a role.

11. How is MVD detected on physical examination?
The development of subtle valvular lesions precedes the development of audible mitral valve regurgitation. MVD becomes clinically apparent when it results in a cardiac murmur. Mitral valve regurgitation results in a systolic murmur that is usually heard best over the left cardiac apex. The correlation between murmur intensity and MR severity is imperfect; however, mild MR resulting from MVD generally results in a soft murmur while severe MR most often results in a loud murmur. Thus a soft murmur is typically evident early in the course of MVD; the murmur becomes louder as the patient ages and develops progressively more severe MR. Early in the course of MVD, when MR may result primarily from leaflet prolapse, the murmur can be of short duration and begin in mid- or late systole. As MR increases in severity, the murmur is heard throughout systole. Mitral regurgitation continues as long as left ventricular pressure exceeds left atrial pressure; as a result, MR can persist beyond aortic valve closure and therefore the murmur can obscure the second heart sound. The murmur of moderate or severe MR has an intensity that typically changes little during the course of systole and the murmur is said to have a plateau-shaped configuration.

12. What is a midsystolic click?
In some patients, a high-frequency midsystolic sound known as a click may precede the development of audible MR. Clicks are associated with mitral valve prolapse.

13. What is the clinical importance of a gallop rhythm in association with MVD?
A gallop rhythm results from audibility of the third or fourth heart sounds. The third heart sound is associated with the termination of rapid ventricular filling during early diastole. In general, this sound is audible when atrial pressures are high and the ventricle is near its limit of compliance; the sudden increase in ventricular pressure during early diastole results in rapid deceleration of transmitral flow and an audible, low-frequency sound known as the third heart sound, or S_3. A gallop rhythm heard in association with MVD generally reflects severe mitral valve incompetence.

The gallop sound is relatively subtle and is usually heard in patients that have loud systolic murmurs; this creates a situation in which timing of auscultatory events can be challenging. However, careful auscultation performed with the bell of the stethoscope placed over the cardiac apex often reveals a gallop rhythm in patients with severe MR. Because the finding of a gallop rhythm usually indicates not only severe MR but also that left atrial pressures are elevated, it is an important clinical finding.

14. Small-breed dogs with MR are often presented for the evaluation of cough; however, it can be difficult to determine whether heart disease or respiratory disease is more contributory to the clinical presentation. What history and physical findings are helpful in making this determination?
In small-breed dogs with MVD, heart disease or heart failure can explain cough; in some cases, however, the murmur of MR is incidental to the clinical presentation and the cough results

from primary respiratory tract disease, such as collapsing trachea or chronic bronchitis. Although primary respiratory tract disease can certainly coexist, one of the two often dominates the clinical presentation.

A history of months or years of cough that occurs in the absence of dyspnea tends to support a diagnosis of airway disease. When MVD is sufficiently severe that it causes clinical signs, it is generally progressive. Therefore, untreated patients in whom cardiac disease contributes importantly to cough tend to have a relatively short history; the clinical course often progresses to include dyspnea.

The body condition of the patient can provide useful clues. Patients that cough due to heart disease or heart failure are often thin. While exceptions certainly occur, obesity is more commonly associated with primary respiratory disease. The vital signs may also be useful. Healthy dogs often have a respiratory-associated arrhythmia that is evident on auscultation. In accordance with phasic variations in autonomic traffic, heart rate increases during inspiration and decreases during expiration. This respiratory sinus arrhythmia results primarily from fluctuations in vagal tone. When cardiac performance is impaired by severe MR, vagal discharge is inhibited and sympathetic tone becomes dominant. Thus, in many patients with clinical signs related to cardiac disease, tachycardia develops and there is loss of physiologic, respiratory arrhythmia—the clinical finding of respiratory sinus arrhythmia is virtually incompatible with a diagnosis of heart failure. In contrast, many patients that cough primarily due to primary respiratory disease have preserved and sometimes accentuated sinus arrhythmia.

In geriatric small-breed dogs, the absence of a cardiac murmur is generally an assurance that coughing results from primary respiratory tract disease. Soft murmurs due to MVD are seldom of clinical consequence. In contrast, patients that develop clinical signs related to MVD almost always have loud cardiac murmurs.

It should be emphasized that these are guidelines only and exceptions do occur. Diagnostic studies, most particularly radiography, provide objective information that can help to solve the diagnostic dilemma. As a general rule, however, respiratory disease is likely to be responsible for a chronic cough in an overweight dog with a soft murmur and preserved sinus arrhythmia. In contrast, heart disease, or even heart failure, is more likely responsible for cough in a thin patient with a loud murmur and tachycardia.

15. What radiographic findings are typical of MVD?

The appearance of the thoracic radiograph in patients with MVD is highly variable. Patients with mild MR may have a normal cardiac silhouette. Moderate or severe MR results in radiographic cardiomegaly that has a left-sided emphasis. Left ventricular enlargement typically accompanies left atrial enlargement, although the latter is more noticeable radiographically. Left atrial enlargement is evidenced by separation of the mainstem bronchi and, in the lateral projection, loss of the "caudal waist" of the cardiac silhouette (Fig. 1). Engorgement of the pulmonary veins is sometimes observed in patients with elevated left atrial pressures although this sign is inconsistent. The presence of pulmonary opacities in the company of radiographic left atrial enlargement is evidence of CHF.

16. What methods are available to aid in the radiographic interpretation of heart size?

Assessment of radiographic heart size is largely subjective and accuracy of the determination is dependent upon observer experience. The dogs that suffer from MVD most commonly are small dogs that have a roughly cylindrical chest. This chest conformation results in a misleadingly large cardiothoracic ratio in the lateral projection. These factors complicate the subjective assessment of thoracic radiographs and can cause the practitioner to conclude that cardiac enlargement is present when it is, in fact, not.

The vertebral heart sum (VHS) is a useful method of cardiac mensuration and is a means by which to avoid some of the limitations of subjective radiographic assessment. Using the lateral radiographic projection, the ventrodorsal and craniocaudal dimensions of the cardiac silhouette are measured and then summed using the "scale" provided by the thoracic vertebrae; the measurement

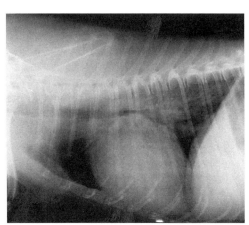
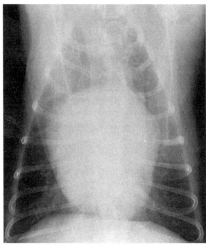

FIGURE 1. Lateral *(left)* and ventrodorsal *(right)* thoracic radiographs obtained from a 13-year-old male castrated Maltese dog. The cardiac silhouette is enlarged and there is evidence of left atrial enlargement. In the lateral projection, the trachea is elevated at the level of the carina, there is loss of the caudal waist, and the left atrium can be seen to compress the mainstem bronchi. In the ventrodorsal projection, a bulge at 3:00 represents the enlarged left atrial appendage.

is made from the fourth thoracic vertebra caudally (Fig. 2). Most normal dogs have a VHS that is less than 10.5 vertebral units.

17. What echocardiographic abnormalities result from mitral valve regurgitation?

MR causes a volume overload of the left atrium and left ventricle. Volume loading results in eccentric hypertrophy or dilation that is accompanied by an increase in myocardial mass; usually, the increase in wall thickness is proportional to the degree of dilation. When there is substantial MR, two-dimensional/M-mode echocardiography demonstrates left atrial and left ventricular dilation (Fig. 3). Often, the left ventricle and atrium enlarge to a similar degree. In some cases, the atrium is large when the ventricle is only mildly dilated; presumably this results when the compliance of the left atrium is relatively greater than that of the ventricle.

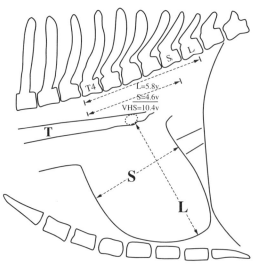

FIGURE 2. This schematic diagram illustrates the vertebral scale system for the radiographic measurement of canine heart size. L, Long axis; S, short axis; T, trachea; VSH, vertebral heart sum. (Adapted from Buchanan JW, Bucheler JB: Vertebral scale system to measure canine heart size in radiographs. J Am Vet Med Assoc 206:194–199, 1995.)

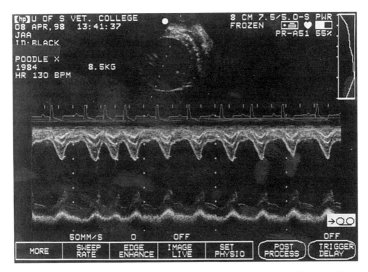

FIGURE 3. M-mode echocardiogram of the left ventricle obtained from a 14-year-old male castrated poodle cross. M-mode echocardiography provides a one-dimensional view of the heart; the ordinate measures distance from the transducer to the abscissa, time. The two-dimensional image from which this M-mode was derived is shown in the inset. There is marked left ventricular dilation and hypertrophy. Left ventricular systolic performance is hyperdynamic. The third and fourth cardiac cycles represent atrial premature complexes.

When systolic myocardial function (contractility) is preserved, measurements of left ventricular performance such as fractional shortening usually reflect hyperkinetic wall motion. When substantial MR is present, the forces that oppose early systolic myocardial shortening are decreased; this is because it is relatively "easy" to eject blood into the low pressure reservoir that is provided by the left atrium. Therefore, the finding of hyperkinesis does not imply that contractility is greater than normal; it suggests only that cardiac loading conditions have been altered by the presence of MR.

Abnormalities of valve structure are commonly observed when MR results from MVD. The leaflets may be thicker than normal and have a verrucous appearance. Systolic prolapse of the leaflets beyond the plane of the of the mitral annulus can be observed (Fig. 4); this finding can result from rupture or lengthening of chordae tendineae.

Variable degrees of right atrial/ventricular enlargement that reflect concurrent tricuspid valve involvement or the presence of pulmonary hypertension may also be observed.

18. What abnormalities are shown on Doppler echocardiography?

Doppler studies demonstrate the presence of disturbed flow within the left atrium during systole. MR is evident as a color-flow mosaic that extends a variable distance from the apposed mitral leaflets into the left atrium. Pulsed-wave Doppler interrogation of the left atrium reveals a high velocity, pansystolic jet; pulsed Doppler instruments cannot accurately describe high velocity flow and directional ambiguity known as aliasing is usually observed (Fig. 5). Continuous-wave Doppler studies demonstrate a high velocity jet directed away from the cardiac apex. The peak velocity of the jet is related to the instantaneous atrioventricular gradient; velocities approaching or exceeding 5 m/s are typical.

19. How is the severity of MR assessed?

The severity of MR can be evaluated semiquantitatively or quantitatively by Doppler echocardiography. The area of the MR jet observed during color-flow Doppler mapping is one means of assessing MR severity that is attractive in its simplicity; however, factors that

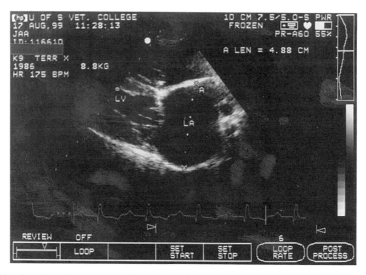

FIGURE 4. Systolic, right parasternal long axis echocardiographic image obtained from a 13-year-old male castrated terrier cross. The left atrium (LA) is markedly enlarged; prolapse of the mitral valve leaflets is evident.

relate to both Doppler technology and the physics of blood flow limit the accuracy of this method. The density of the continuous-wave Doppler trace is roughly proportional to the regurgitant volume and this index of MR severity is easy to obtain. Doppler echocardiography can also be used to quantify the regurgitant volume more precisely; the proximal flow convergence method and the use of velocity-time integrals can be used to calculate the regurgitant fraction. These methods are generally time consuming and seldom used in clinical practice.

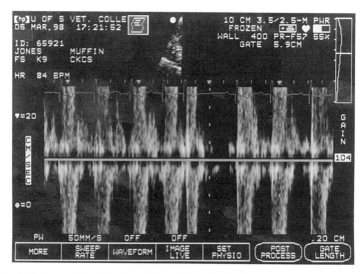

FIGURE 5. Pulsed-wave Doppler echocardiographic study obtained from an 8-year-old female spayed cavalier King Charles spaniel. The sample volume was placed in the left atrium. During systole, there is a high-velocity disturbed flow indicating mitral valve regurgitation; the fifth cardiac cycle is an atrial premature complex.

Surgical mitral valve repair is seldom performed in veterinary patients. Therefore, despite the availability of techniques that allow quantification of MR severity, it is probably of greater clinical importance to assess the *effects* of MR. The effect of MR can be assessed through the evaluation of heart size and by the determination of whether pulmonary edema is present. Thoracic radiographs alone are often adequate for this purpose although echocardiography is a useful adjunct.

20. What is the utility of echocardiography in the management of MVD?

Echocardiography can provide potentially useful information in all cases of MVD. However, in many cases the information is not essential. When an acquired, systolic apical murmur is heard in an elderly, small-breed dog, MVD is almost certainly the cause and echocardiographic confirmation of this suspicion is not necessary for case management.

Echocardiography is likely to be useful when it is uncertain from radiographic studies whether or not the heart is enlarged, when it is important to assess myocardial function, when pulmonary hypertension is suspected, and when there are historical or clinical findings that suggest that the cause of the patient's murmur is something other than MR.

21. What electrocardiographic abnormalities are associated with MVD?

In most affected patients, the electrocardiogram is normal. In some cases, electrocardiographic patterns suggesting left atrial enlargement or left ventricular hypertrophy are observed. Sinus tachycardia is typical for patients who are in overt congestive heart failure. Pathologic arrhythmias are observed in some severely affected patients; often, the origin of these arrhythmias is supraventricular. Atrial premature complexes are common; the onset of atrial fibrillation usually reflects marked left atrial enlargement.

22. What diagnostic tests are indicated and when?

As in any disorder, the diagnostic approach is dictated by the patient's clinical status and the utility of the available diagnostic tests. When subclinical MR is first detected, thoracic radiographs are potentially useful. Therapy of patients with subclinical disease can probably be justified in some cases, and thoracic radiographs may provide prognostic information. The information provided by echocardiography is probably of greatest use in cases in which clinical signs result from MVD. Thoracic radiographs are essential in patients in whom cough or dyspnea is part of the clinical presentation. Electrocardiography is indicated when pathologic arrhythmias are present or suspected.

23. Vasodilator drugs are often used in the management of MR; why is vasodilation beneficial?

When MR is present, the regurgitant volume depends on the size of the regurgitant orifice and the atrioventricular pressure difference, as well as the relationship between aortic impedance and the resistance imposed by the regurgitant orifice. Systemic vascular resistance (SVR) is one of the primary determinants of aortic impedance and pharmacologic dilation of the systemic arterioles results in a decrease in vascular resistance. When MR is present, a reduction in systemic vascular resistance favors an increase in forward stroke volume so that systemic blood pressure is maintained or is mildly diminished and the regurgitant fraction decreases. In effect, it becomes "easier" for the ventricle to eject blood into the aorta and less is regurgitated back into the left atrium.

24. What classes of vasodilators are used in the management of mitral valve disease?

The angiotensin-converting enzyme (ACE) inhibitors, which include enalapril, captopril, and benazepril, are drugs that inhibit the enzyme that converts angiotensin I to the active metabolite angiotensin II. Angiotensin II has numerous effects; it is a potent vasoconstrictor but the release of angiotensin II also stimulates the secretion of aldosterone and augments the activity of the adrenergic nervous system. Thus the decrease in angiotensin II levels that accompanies ACE inhibition results not only in vasodilation but also diverse neuroendocrine effects.

Hydralazine is an arteriolar dilator that acts directly on vascular smooth muscle; the precise mechanism of action is unknown. The administration of hydralazine can result in a reflex-mediated increase in adrenergic nervous system activity with the potential clinical consequence of tachycardia. The notion that chronic activation of the adrenergic nervous system and the renin-angiotensin-aldosterone system (RAAS) contributes to the progressive nature of the heart failure state is now widely accepted. ACE inhibitors blunt these compensatory mechanisms while hydralazine tends to augment them; it is primarily for this reason that ACE inhibitors have largely supplanted hydralazine as the vasodilator of first choice in patients with congestive heart failure due to MR. However, hydralazine still has a role in patients that do not tolerate ACE inhibiton and in patients with advanced CHF that is no longer responsive to diuretics and ACE inhibitors.

Similarly, the calcium channel antagonist amlodipine may have a role in the management of severe and chronic CHF due to MR. The nitrates, including nitroglycerin and nitroprusside, are used most often in the setting of acute or decompensated heart failure, although nitroglycerin is used by some in the chronic management of advanced CHF resulting from MR.

25. What is the role of medical therapy in subclinical (asymptomatic) MVD?

In the setting of MR, arterial vasodilators can potentially decrease mitral valve regurgitation and therefore slow the progression of associated cardiac enlargement. It is possible, although unproven, that ACE inhibitors might delay the onset of CHF in patients with subclinical MVD. However, it is likely that a therapeutic effect of these drugs requires activation of compensatory neuroendocrine mechanisms such as the adrenergic nervous system and the RAAS. Experimental studies demonstrate that RAAS activation is a feature of the heart failure state and that pharmacologic suppression of the RAAS is beneficial. However, there may be differences between experimental models and spontaneous CHF observed in dogs. Interestingly, in one study RAAS activation was not a feature of MVD in cavalier King Charles spaniels. Regardless, it seems unlikely that systemic RAAS is activated in patients that do not have substantial cardiac enlargement. Further, experimental and clinical studies would suggest that the benefits of ACE inhibition are most evident in patients with myocardial disease. MVD is primarily a mechanical disease; many patients develop overt CHF when systolic myocardial function is normal or only mildly diminished.

Hydralazine is a direct-acting vasodilator; while the favorable neuroendocrine effects that are associated with the ACE inhibitors have not been demonstrated for hydralazine, the latter is the more potent vasodilator. It may be that the mechanical vasodilatory property of hydralazine is of benefit to patients with MR due to MVD. The role of carvedilol, a relatively new beta-adrenergic antagonist with vasodilating properties, is yet to be assessed in patients with MVD.

Regardless, the role of medical therapy for subclinical MVD is at present uncertain. No agent has been proven to slow the progression of cardiac enlargement in spontaneous MVD. Further, the rate at which MR progresses is difficult to predict. Many patients that develop MVD never suffer morbidity related to heart disease and die of extracardiac disease long after the development of a murmur of MR. Vasodilators such as the ACE inhibitors, hydralazine, or possibly carvedilol may have a role in the management of subclinical MVD, although it seems likely that the benefits of therapy will only be evident in patients with relatively severe valvular disease and substantial MR.

26. What is the therapeutic approach to cough resulting from compression of the mainstem bronchi by an enlarged left atrium?

The cough that develops in patients that have a large left atrium but do not have pulmonary edema probably has a multifactorial etiology. Mechanical compression of the mainstem bronchi is at least partly responsible for cough in some patients. However, concurrent primary respiratory tract disease and perhaps the presence of high pulmonary venous pressures are other factors that can contribute to cough related to MVD. Vasodilators such as ACE inhibitors or possibly hydralazine can be used in patients such as this; it is hoped that systemic vasodilation will reduce regurgitant fraction and therefore decrease left atrial pressure and, possibly, size. When cough persists despite the use of a vasodilator, it is often important to consider the possibility that a concurrent,primary respiratory tract disease such as bronchitis is contributing to the pathogenesis of the cough. When this is the case, bronchodilators are sometimes helpful and, in the absence of pulmonary edema or infective respiratory disease, the use of antitussive agents can be considered. In general, the use of diuretics is avoided in patients that do not have radiographic evidence of pulmonary edema. However, a case might be made for diuretic use in patients with massive left atrial enlargement as these drugs tend to be quite effective in reducing cardiac size. Although preload reduction can have the undesirable consequence of RAAS activation, the decrease in the mitral annulus diameter might potentially decrease regurgitant fraction.

27. What therapy is indicated for patients that develop congestive heart failure due to MVD?

The results of a multicenter, double-blind placebo controlled trial attest to the efficacy of ACE inhibitors in CHF due to MVD; arguably, all patients with CHF due to MVD should receive an ACE inhibitor provided the drug is tolerated. The concurrent use of diuretic agents is indicated when pulmonary edema results from MR. Furosemide is the diuretic used most commonly and the dose and dosage interval are tailored to relieve congestive signs without excessive reduction in ventricular filling pressures. An initial dose of 1 mg/kg orally every 12 hours is often adequate for patients that are receiving ACE inhibitors. Thus, standard therapy for CHF due to MVD consists of an ACE inhibitor together with a diuretic, usually furosemide. Digoxin is used concurrently in some cases.

28. Is digoxin useful in the management of MVD?

Digoxin has a modest inotropic effect that is mediated through an increase in intracellular calcium availability. Additionally, digoxin has important effects on the autonomic nervous system; specifically, it increases vagal discharge and this serves to slow the rate of sinus node discharge and AV nodal conduction velocity. The latter effect is commonly used to control the ventricular response rate of patients that develop atrial fibrillation.

Increases in baroreceptor sensitivity are thought to be at least partly responsible for the therapeutic effect of digoxin in heart failure. The arterial baroreceptors are pressure-sensitive nerve endings located in the aorta and carotid arteries; stimulation of these receptors by increases in arterial pressure initiates a reflex arc that results in vagal discharge and inhibition of adrenergic tone. In heart failure, the sensitivity of the baroreceptors is diminished and this contributes to heightened and unopposed sympathetic tone that is characteristic of CHF. There is evidence that digoxin increases baroreceptor sensitivity and, in so doing, partially normalizes baroreceptor function, resulting in increased vagal discharge.

The use of digoxin in patients that develop myocardial dysfunction (cardiomyopathy of overload) or atrial fibrillation as a complication of long-standing MR is almost universally accepted. However, overt CHF often results from MR when systolic myocardial function is apparently preserved; in these patients, the role of digoxin is debatable. Controlled studies of efficacy of digoxin in these patients are lacking. However, despite extensive evaluation of alternative agents, only digoxin, which is unique by virtue of its autonomic effects, has favorable long-term effects in humans. This suggests that the neuroendocrine effects of digoxin, which include normalization of baroreceptor function and reduction of renin levels, might be more important than the relatively weak inotropic effects of this drug. For this reason, some advocate the use of digoxin in all patients with moderate or severe CHF resulting from MR.

29. What medical therapy is indicated in cases of refractory or severe CHF?

When congestive signs are no longer controlled by standard therapy, or when the diuretic doses required to free the patient of congestive signs result in unacceptably low cardiac output, CHF can be considered to be refractory. Because of their proven efficacy, ACE inhibitors have become standard therapy for CHF due to MVD. However, these drugs are not potent vasodilators. For this reason, the use of hydralazine or possibly amlodipine in addition to ACE inhibitors can be considered for patients with refractory CHF resulting from severe MVD. This step should be undertaken with caution; monitoring of blood pressure is advisable as excessive vasodilation can result in dangerous hypotension.

The use of triple diuretic therapy—the administration of a potassium-sparing diuretic such as spironolactone and a thiazide in addition to furosemide—can also be considered for patients with severe or refractory CHF. Triple diuretic therapy utilizes the principle of sequential nephron blockade; each of the drugs act at functionally distinct sites of the nephron and this may help to overcome the development of resistance to single agent diuresis. Additionally, the use of triple diuretic therapy can allow the use of lower doses of the component drugs, which may limit some of the adverse effects associated with aggressive diuresis. In addition to its diuretic effect, spironolactone may have favorable neurohumoral effects; this drug antagonizes the effect of aldosterone, a hormone that is implicated in the development of myocardial fibrosis.

30. Can MVD be treated surgically?

MVD is primarily a mechanical disorder and is well suited to surgical approaches that include mitral valve replacement and repair. Unfortunately, surgical exposure of the mitral valve apparatus requires cardiopulmonary bypass. While this technique is successfully practiced at a few referral institutions, surgical therapy of MVD is in its infancy. The necessary expertise is not widely available and the costs associated with open heart surgery further limit the application of surgical approaches to this disease.

31. What catastrophes can explain sudden clinical deterioration in patients with MVD?

It should be recognized that CHF in veterinary patients often has an apparently sudden onset. Many pet dogs are relatively sedentary; because of this, cardiac disease can progress unnoticed until a point when even minimal exertion results in severe dyspnea. Additionally, subtle changes in respiratory rate and character can be difficult for owners to recognize. These and possibly other factors delay recognition of CHF in animals until it is well advanced. However, patients with MVD are subject to catastrophes that can result in acute decompensation.

Rupture of a chorda tendineae is a relatively common acute complication of MVD; the severity of the resultant clinical signs is dependent on the functional importance of the ruptured chord and the compliance of the left atrium. Rupture of a first-order mitral chorda tendineae causes acute and severe mitral valve regurgitation and the resultant increase in left atrial pressure may result in fulminant pulmonary edema that is refractory to medical therapy. If a third-order chord ruptures in a patient with a compliant and capacious atrium, it may go undetected. In fact, ruptured chordae are sometimes found on postmortem examination of patients with MVD that succumb to extracardiac disease. Rupture of mitral chordae is most common in patients that have preexisting mitral valve regurgitation and associated cardiac enlargement. The result is clinical decompensation, the severity of which is determined by factors stated above. Occasionally, rupture of a first-order mitral valve chorda is observed in patients that have only mild mitral valve disease. In these cases, the acute elevation in left atrial pressure is catastrophic and severe pulmonary edema results. This is one of the few clinical scenarios in veterinary medicine that results in truly acute heart failure; radiographically, the cardiac silhouette is only minimally enlarged in the presence of florid edema. Sometimes the pulmonary hypertension that develops subsequent to acute increases in left atrial pressure can result in right-sided CHF manifest clinically as ascites.

Rupture of the left atrium is an uncommon complication of MVD. Although surgical treatment of atrial rupture has been described, most often the result is death due to tamponade. Rarely, rupture of the atrial septum results in an acquired atrial septal defect.

32. What is the cause of ascites in patients with degenerative valvular disease?

Although the effects of MR usually dominate the clinical presentation of patients with degenerative valvular disease, the tricuspid valve can also be affected. In some cases, tricuspid valve regurgitation results in right-sided CHF. In dogs, right-sided CHF is typically manifest as ascites. Pulmonary hypertension related to high left atrial pressures increases right ventricular afterload and this may contribute to the development of right-sided CHF in some patients.

BIBLIOGRAPHY

1. Buchanan JW: Chronic valvular disease (endocardiosis) in dogs. Adv Vet Sci Comp Med 21:75, 1979.
2. The COVE Study Group: Controlled clinical evaluation of enalapril in dogs with heart failure: Results of the Cooperative Veterinary Enalapril Study Group. J Vet Intern Med 9:243, 1995.
3. The Digitalis Investigation Group: The effect of digoxin on mortality and morbidity in patients with heart failure. N Engl J Med 336: 525–533, 1997.
4. Ettinger SJ, Benitz AM, Ericsson GF, et al: Effects of enalapril maleate on survival of dogs with naturally acquired heart failure: The Long-Term Investigation of Veterinary Enalapril (LIVE) Study Group. J Am Vet Med Assoc 213:1573–1577, 1998.
5. Gheorghiade M, Pitt B: Digitalis Investigation Group (DIG) trial: A stimulus for further research. Am Heart J 134; 3–12, 1997.
6. Haggstrom J, Hansson K, Kvart C, et al: Effects of naturally acquired decompensated mitral valve regurgitation on the renin-angiotensin-aldosterone system and atrial natriuretic peptide concentration in dogs. Am J Vet Res 58:77–82, 1997.
7. Haggstrom J, Hansson K, Kvart C, Swenson L: Chronic valvular disease in the cavalier King Charles spaniel in Sweden. Vet Rec 131:549–553, 1992.
8. Hamlin RL: Pathophysiology of the failing heart. In Fox PR, Sisson D, Moise NS (eds): Textbook of Canine and Feline Cardiology: Principles and Clinical Practice, 2nd ed. Philadelphia, W.B. Saunders, 1999, pp 205–215.
9. Keene BW, Rush JE: Therapy of heart failure. In Ettinger SJ, Feldman EC (eds): Textbook of Veterinary Internal Medicine, 4th ed. Philadelphia, W.B. Saunders, 1993.
10. Kittleson MD: Myxomatous atrioventricular valvular degeneration. In Kittleson MD, Kienle RD (eds): Small Animal Cardiovascular Medicine. St. Louis, Mosby, 1998, pp 297–318.
11. O'Grady MR: Acquired valvular disease. In Ettinger SJ, Feldman EC (eds): Textbook of Veterinary Internal Medicine, 4th ed. Philadelphia, W.B. Saunders, 1993.
12. Opie LH, Poole-Wilson PA, Sonnenblick EH, Chatterjee K: Angiotensin-converting enzyme inhibitors and conventional vasodilators. In Opie LH (ed): Drugs for the Heart, 4th ed. Philadelphia, W.B. Saunders, 1997, pp 105–144.
13. Sisson D, Kittleson MD: Management of heart failure: Principles of treatment, therapeutic strategies and pharmacology. In Fox PR, Sisson D, Moise NS (eds): Textbook of Canine and Feline Cardiology: Principles and Clinical Practice, 2nd ed. Philadelphia, W.B. Saunders, 1999, pp 216–250.

35. INFECTIVE ENDOCARDITIS

Clay A. Calvert, D.V.M.

1. What is infective endocarditis?

Infective endocarditis is the infection of the endocardium by bacteria or fungi. For all intents and purposes, infective endocarditis is a bacterial colonization of the heart valves and adjacent endocardium with associated tissue destruction.

2. Which valves are most often infected?

The valves of the high-pressure left ventricle, the aortic and mitral, are most often involved. The aortic is the single most affected valve, and in some cases both the aortic and mitral valves are infected. The pulmonic and tricuspid valves are seldom infected.

3. Why are the heart valves almost exclusively infected rather than other endocardial surfaces?

The natural trauma encountered by valves during each cardiac cycle probably results in microscopic damage to the endothelium.

4. What is the incidence of bacterial endocarditis (BE) in dogs and cats?

Cats are rarely diagnosed with BE. Bacterial endocarditis is relatively uncommon in dogs as well, and the exact incidence is unknown and sporadic. Bacteremia alone is far more common than BE.

5. Are certain types of dogs more likely to acquire BE than others?

In general, bacteremia seems to be more common in tropical and semitropical regions and in medium- to large-sized dogs. Some reports cite a 2:1 male preponderance. German shepherd dogs, boxer dogs, and golden retrievers seem to be predisposed.

6. Have any predisposing factors been identified?

Chronic infections, including pyodermas, abscesses, foreign body infections, bacterial gingivitis and stomatitis, perianal infections, prior surgery (especially extensive or protracted procedures), bone infections, and bacterial prostatitis have been commonly associated with BE. Addtionally, the presence of congenital aortic stenosis is a risk factor for the development of infective endocarditis.

7. Does immunosuppression predispose to BE?

The use of corticosteroids has been associated with BE. Debilitation from cancer and cancer chemotherapy may predispose to BE.

8. Other than corticosteroid use, can veterinary procedures or therapy cause BE?

Clearly, bacteremia can develop secondary to procedures such as indwelling intravenous and urinary catheters. Furthermore, manipulation of infected tissue, causing increased interstitial pressure, can force bacteria into veins and lymphatics. The body's defense mechanisms (macrophages in the liver and spleen, as well as spleen and capillary neutrophils) are generally adequate to eradicate this type of bacteremia. Debilitated and immunosuppressed patients may develop persistent bacteremia, and some of these will develop BE.

9. Should prophylactic antibiotic therapy be administered to dogs undergoing invasive procedures, such as dentistry or ovariohysterectomy?

There is little evidence supporting a need for such an approach in normal dogs. Dogs with congenital subaortic stenosis should receive antibiotics during dentistry. Ampicillin, penicillin, and amoxicillin are not good choices since coagulase-positive staphylococci, the most frequent culprits, are usually resistant to these agents.

10. What are the most common bacteria involved in BE?
Coagulase-positive staphylococci and beta-hemolytic streptococci are most often isolated from blood or heart valves. However, many different bacteria have been isolated, including *E. coli* and *Pseudomonas* spp.

11. Does preexisting heart disease predispose to BE?
Most dogs confirmed to have BE do not have known prior heart disease. Neither congenital heart defects nor myxomatous degeneration of the mitral valve are high-risk factors. However, congenital subaortic stenosis predisposes to BE.
Some bacteria, including some pathogenic staphylococci and streptococci, produce proteases that damage the endothelium and result in platelet-fibrin deposition that predisposes to bacterial colonization in the absence of prior endothelial damage.

12. What is involved in the differential diagnosis between bacteremia alone and BE?
Positive blood culture results, preferably more than one, are required for the diagnosis of bacteremia. Also, clinical signs and laboratory data consistent with bacteremia are important. Bacteremia is distinguished from BE by the presence of endocardial bacterial colonization; this can be demonstrated or inferred through the detection of a recent-onset cardiac murmur or by the discovery of cardiac vegetations on echocardiographic examination. Echocardiography greatly facilitates the diagnosis of BE, particularly of the aortic valve.

13. Isn't it true that blood cultures are often unrewarding?
The most common causes for negative blood culture results are the absence of bacteremia and inadequate sampling. Excluding the possibility of contamination, if one performs blood cultures on dogs without bacteremia, the results will be negative. However, when multiple (preferably three samples over a 24-hour period) blood samples of 7–10 ml each are obtained from dogs with a strong likelihood of bacteremia, positive results are obtained in the majority of instances.

14. What factors contribute to negative blood culture results in dogs that are truly bacteremic?
The primary factors are:
• Technique and diligence of the microbiology laboratory
• Prior antibiotic therapy
• Inadequate sample volume (< 7 ml) or too few samples obtained
• Failure to culture for or the laboratory's inability to harvest anaerobic organisms (unknown significance)
• Fastidious bacteria

15. How do we know that a bacterium isolated by blood culture is not a contaminant?
Strict attention to disinfection of the venipuncture site is critical. Isolating the same pathogen from multiple samples indicates that it is the culprit. Isolating that same organism from a suspected site of infection, although seldom accomplished, is very strong evidence of a causal relationship. Isolating a nonpathogenic strain of bacteria known to be a skin commensal from only one sample, or isolating different such organisms from different samples, suggests contamination. This is particularly likely if poor technique of sample acquisition or contamination of the blood sample during transfer to blood culture medium is suspected.

16. In dogs with possible acute bacteremia, should one allow 24 hours to pass so that three blood culture samples can be obtained prior to initiation of antibiotic therapy?
Clinical judgment is required. Usually three samples can be obtained over a 3-hour period without compromising the likelihood of successful treatment.

17. Since urine cultures are easier to obtain, can they be substituted for blood cultures?

While it is true that the offending bacteria in dogs with bacteremia and BE are often filtered into the urine where they may be somewhat concentrated in the bladder, urine cultures should not be substituted for blood cultures. However, since the urinary tract, including the prostate gland, can be the source of bacteremia, urine and ejaculate culturing are important in selected cases.

18. Doesn't the advent of echocardiography facilitate the diagnosis of BE?

The vegetative lesions of aortic valve BE are usually very easy to recognize during echocardiography. Those of the mitral valve are more difficult to differentiate from myxomatous degeneration; however, the age and breed type of the patient can help distinguish BE from the latter. Supportive clinical signs and laboratory data are important.

19. What clinical signs are associated with BE?

All signs and symptoms of bacteremia, such as fever, trembling, injected sclera, vomiting, diarrhea, and malaise, can be associated with BE. Vague clinical signs such as lethargy and lack of appetite are common. Lameness, which may result from infective arthritis (or immune-mediated arthropathy), is observed fairly commonly. Some patients are presented for veterinary evaluation after the development of dyspnea related to congestive heart failure.

20. Are there any characteristics of the heart murmurs of BE?

Infection of any valve can result in a systolic heart murmur of variable intensity. Aortic valve BE results in aortic valve insufficiency or regurgitation that also produces a decrescendo diastolic murmur. This type of murmur is often of low frequency and low intensity, may be heard best approximately midway on a line between the auscultation point for the tricuspid valve and the manubrium (but is often audible over the left heart base with the stethoscope head under the upper leg), and is strongly indicative of aortic valve BE.

21. Are there any changes in the peripheral pulse characteristics associated with BE?

The femoral pulses of dogs with severe aortic valve BE are very abnormal and strongly indicative of the diagnosis. The volume overload associated with aortic regurgitation results in a high systolic pulse pressure and the rapid diastolic runoff back into the left ventricle causes a low diastolic pulse pressure. Thus, the characteristic pulse can be described as quick (short) and bounding or quick and hyperdynamic. The femoral pulse associated with advanced mitral valve disease is not unusual, other than possibly being weak.

22. Does the absence of fever rule out BE?

No! Chronic and low-grade bacteremia may be associated with a normal body temperature and very few clinical signs.

23. How often is shifting leg lameness associated with BE?

Intermittent lameness, possibly involving multiple or shifting limbs, is common, but is by no means present in all cases, and can be subtle. This lameness can be the result of septic arthritis but is often thought to result from immune-mediated mechanisms. In fact, the signs and symptoms of immune arthritis and that of arthritis secondary to bacteremia and BE are similar.

24. What causes the immune-mediated complications of BE?

Presumably circulating immune complexes are deposited along the glomerular basement membrane, in joint capsules, and in the enthothelium of vessels. Inflammatory responses to these can be considerable. Occasionally, a positive antinuclear antibody (ANA) test or systemic lupus erythematosus preparation is encountered.

25. What laboratory data are typical of BE?

An inflammatory leukogram and mild to moderate thrombocytopenia are commonly associated with bacteremia of any cause. Likewise, low or low-normal serum albumin, increased serum alkaline phosphatase activity, and low or low-normal serum glucose concentration, singularly or in combination, are associated with but not exclusive to bacteremia/BE. Proteinuria, pyuria, and bacteriuria are often detected in BE patients.

Chronic bacteremia/BE may be associated with a normal leukogram or a mature neutrophilia of varying degree. Monocytosis is present in as many as 90% of dogs with BE.

26. Are there any easily recognizable physical findings that should greatly increase the index of suspicion of BE?

A loud systolic heart murmur in an adult large-breed dog is an uncommon finding with dilated cardiomyopathy (assuming a congenital heart defect can be ruled out). Since severe myxomatous degeneration of the mitral valve is uncommon in large dogs, the likelihood of a loud murmur being due to BE is increased. The hyperdynamic (hyperkinetic), bounding femoral pulses sometimes associated with aortic valve BE are a good clue. Although often difficult to hear, an acquired decrescendo diastolic component to the heart murmur strongly suggests aortic regurgitation and BE.

27. What are the sequelae to BE?

Bacterial endocarditis can result in congestive heart failure and usually does when the aortic valve is involved. Arthropathy, myositis, vasculitis, protein-losing glomerulopathy, renal failure, and embolic complications involving various organs and tissues including limbs, brain, and myocardium are common.

28. Is the electrocardiogram useful in the diagnosis of BE?

Premature ventricular contractions occur in most dogs with BE but are not always detected by short recordings. Even then, such findings are nonspecific. A careful study of ST-segment changes in dogs with BE has not been reported, but elevation or depression of the ST segment, while possible, is not commonly detected. Evidence of chamber enlargement may be evident with chronic BE.

29. Do the sequelae of BE make the diagnosis more difficult?

Although the sequelae of BE should alert one to that possibility, often the presence of complications, such as renal failure, may distract one's attention away from the underlying cause. Bacterial endocarditis is a polysystemic disease and may be difficult to differentiate from immune-mediated disease, especially in the absence of positive blood cultures, a detected heart murmur, and echocardiography.

30. How can we really be certain that a dog has BE?

Ultrasound identification of valve lesions consistent with BE is the best method. Supportive clinical and laboratory findings that are most important are:
- Positive blood cultures
- Diastolic heart murmur (recent onset)
- Loud systolic heart murmur (recent onset) in a dog not prone to myxomatous degeneration

Clinical findings of lesser specificity include fever, inflammatory leukogram, lameness, and proteinuria.

31. Why is BE more difficult to eradicate than most bacterial infections?

The vegetative lesions of BE are composed of a platelet-thrombus-fibrin mass that contains bacteria; consequently, the pathogens are somewhat protected not only from neutrophils and macrophages, but also from antibiotics, which may fail to reach optimal concentrations within the vegetation. In addition, septic embolization from the vegetations to many organs and tissues, most notably the spleen and kidneys, establishes satellite infections that may also be difficult to eradicate.

32. What antibiotics are the best choice for treating BE?

Since most infections are the result of staphylococci and streptococci, and knowing the general antibiotic sensitivity patterns of the commonly involved organisms, an antibiotic regimen likely to be effective can usually be predicted. Cephalosporins, ticarcillin, ticarcillin-clavulanic acid, fluoroquinolones, clindamycin, and aminoglycosides are usually effective against coagulase-positive staphylococci. With the exception of the aminoglycosides and fluoroquinolones, these same antibiotics are usually effective against streptococci. The fluoroquinolones, aminoglycosides, and ticarcillin possess a good gram-negative spectrum.

For immediately life-threatening bacteremia, a combination of ampicillin, cephalosporin, or ticarcillin plus an aminoglycoside provides excellent coverage. An alternative combination is clindamycin plus a fluoroquinolone, the former also providing excellent anaerobic activity.

33. Does the route of administration matter?

High serum concentrations must be established and maintained. Thus, the intravenous route is superior to the oral route.

34. What about dosage?

Higher than normal dosages should be administered. This is seldom a problem with ampicillin and ticarcillin. High-dose (20 mg/kg 3 times/day) cephalosporin administration is associated with an increased risk of vomiting, anaphylactoid reactions, blood dyscrasias, and nephrotoxicity, but is nonetheless often administered.

The parenteral dosage of enrofloxacin is 5–6 mg/kg 2 times/day. This must be diluted 1:4–1:9 with a non–saline-containing fluid, injected over a 10-minute period, and not injected into an intravenous line containing Ringer's or saline solution.

The systemic dosage of gentamicin and amikacin is 1–2 mg/kg 3 times/day, which must not be exceeded. Good hydration must be maintained, and even then administration beyond 5–10 days is associated with a high risk of nephrotoxicity.

The antibiotic regimen should be adjusted, if necessary, based on antibiogram results.

35. Doesn't the duration of therapy need to be protracted?

Yes! Because of sanctuary sites of infection on the heart valves, kidneys, bone/intervertebral disc, and potentially multiple septic emboli, treatment must be continued for 6 weeks or longer. Intravenous therapy is maintained as long as practical and at least until there is clinical and laboratory evidence of dramatic improvement. Then the subcutaneous route of administration of a drug such as ceftiofur can be substituted. Oral antibiotics should only be prescribed after laboratory and clinical signs have normalized and after at least 3 weeks of parenteral therapy. Bacteriostatic antibiotics should not be used.

36. What other therapeutic measures may be required?

Supportive therapy involves fluid and electrolyte balance and nutritional support (which may include nasogastric feeding). Possible sources of infection such as wounds, abscess, and stomatitis must be treated appropriately. Catheters that are indwelling at the time of diagnosis must be removed and cultured.

37. What if congestive heart failure develops?

Congestive heart failure is usual with aortic valve BE, and it may be present at the time of diagnosis. If not, it usually occurs within one to several months. Treatment of congestive heart failure is conventional with digoxin, an ACE inhibitor, diuretic, low-sodium diet, and severe restriction of activity. In addition, a potent afterload reducer, such as hydralazine or amlodipine, may be considered after appropriate regulation with conventional therapy is established (1–3 weeks).

38. Is there any hope of long-term survival?

The best chance is if the diagnosis is made quickly, aggressive therapy applied, and if the aortic valve is not involved. Virtually 100% mortality, due to congestive heart failure, is associated with all but the earliest diagnosed cases of aortic valve BE.

Although latent congestive heart failure can occur one or more years after the diagnosis of mitral valve BE, the incidence is less than that associated with aortic valve BE.

Corticosteroid use, late diagnosis, and inadequate therapy all worsen the prognosis. Latent renal failure is an occasional outcome.

39. Are infections that lead to BE always obvious or severe?
No. The initial infection that eventually leads to BE is often subtle and the outcome, BE, is not expected.

40. Can BE be prevented?
Yes, at least sometimes. Good principles of antibiotic therapy should be applied to all bacterial infections. Also, the cavalier, unwise, or unnecessary use of corticosteroids in dogs with fever, an inflammatory leukogram, or vague illness that could be due to infection will lead to BE in some cases.

BIBLIOGRAPHY

1. Bennett D, Taylor DJ: Bacterial endocarditis and inflammatory joint disease in the dog. J Small Anim Pract 29:347–352, 1987.
2. Calvert CA: Valvular bacterial endocarditis in the dog. J Am Vet Med Assoc 180:1080–1084, 1982.
3. Calvert CA, Greene CE, Hardie EM: Cardiovascular infections in dogs: Epizootiology, clinical manifestations, and prognosis. J Am Vet Med Assoc 187:612–616, 1985.
4. Dow SW, Curtis CR, Jones RL, et al: Bacterial culture of blood from critically ill dogs and cats: 100 cases (1985–1987). J Am Vet Med Assoc 195:113–117, 1989.
5. Elwood CM, Cobb MA, Stepien RL: Clinical and echocardiographic findings in 10 dogs with vegetative bacterial endocarditis. J Small Anim Pract 34:420–426, 1993.
6. Lombard CW, Buergelt CD: Vegetative bacterial endocarditis in dogs; echocardiographic diagnosis and clinical signs. J Small Anim Pract 24:325–331, 1983.
7. Sisson D, Thomas WP: Endocarditis of the aortic valve in the dog. J Am Vet Med Assoc 184:570–578, 1984.
8. Thomas WP: Update: Infective endocarditis. In Kirk RW, Bonagura JD (eds): Kirk's Current Veterinary Therapy XI: Small Animal Practice. Philadelphia, W.B. Saunders, 1992, pp 752–755.

36. CANINE DILATED CARDIOMYOPATHY

Jonathan A. Abbott, D.V.M.

1. What is a cardiomyopathy?

Cardiomyopathy is a disease of the heart muscle that is associated with cardiac dysfunction. In the past, this term was reserved for idiopathic or primary heart muscle diseases. More recently, a task force of the World Health Organization (WHO) adopted the more general definition stated above. This was prompted by the growth of knowledge that has blurred the distinction between idiopathic myocardial disease and what were previously known as specific heart muscle diseases. The current WHO scheme classifies the cardiomyopathies based on pathophysiology and, when it is known, etiology. The following morphopathologic designations are accepted: dilated cardiomyopathy, restrictive cardiomyopathy, hypertrophic cardiomyopathy, arrhythmogenic right ventricular cardiomyopathy, and unclassified cardiomyopathy. Each of these basic types of heart muscle disease can be described as idiopathic or as a specific cardiomyopathy when the cause is known.

2. What is dilated cardiomyopathy?

Dilated cardiomyopathy (DCM) is a morphopathologic and functional designation; DCM is characterized by ventricular and atrial dilation that is a consequence of systolic myocardial dysfunction. Most often, left ventricular or biventricular dilation is present. Dilated cardiomyopathy in which the right ventricle is primarily affected occurs occasionally.

3. What is the pathogenesis of DCM?

Loss of systolic myocardial function causes ventricular hypokinesis and initiates a series of events that lead to progressive ventricular dilation. Systolic myocardial dysfunction can result from loss of cardiomyocytes due to necrosis or from functional disorders that affect the contractile apparatus. However, the hemodynamic consequences of impaired systolic myocardial function are generally the same regardless of the cause of myocardial dysfunction.

When stroke volume declines as a result of systolic myocardial dysfunction (decreased contractility), the end-systolic ventricular volume increases. This residual volume augments the pulmonary venous return and results in ventricular dilation and elevated end-diastolic wall stress. In addition, activation of the renin-angiotensin-aldosterone system (RAAS) occurs as a consequence of diminished cardiac output. One effect of RAAS activation is the retention of salt and water, which serves to expand the intravascular volume. This increase in intravascular volume further increases preload and contributes to progressive ventricular dilation. Elevated ventricular filling pressures together with atrioventricular valve incompetence resulting from dilation of the valve annulus cause atrial dilation.

4. What are the causes of dilated cardiomyopathy?

DCM is a syndrome rather than a specific disease; in a sense, it is an "end-stage" heart disease and likely represents the common expression of virtually any pathologic insult to the myocardium. This insult could take the form of viral infection, a toxin, a metabolic derangement, or a nutritional deficiency. For example, taurine deficiency has been associated with the development of DCM in cocker spaniels. In some dogs, myocardial carnitine deficiency likely has a role in the pathogenesis of DCM. In addition, antineoplastic agents such as doxorubicin can result in irreversible myocardial dysfunction. Spontaneous DCM in dogs is generally idiopathic.

5. What is a typical signalment for a patient with dilated cardiomyopathy?

Large- and giant-breed dogs including Doberman pinschers, Labrador retrievers, Great Danes, and boxer dogs are most commonly affected. There is a predisposition for males, and dogs with DCM are often middle-aged or older. A 5-year-old male Doberman pinscher is a typical signalment for DCM.

6. Are there differences in presentation among the breeds commonly afflicted?

In general, the course of DCM is similar in affected dogs. However, the boxer dog and the Doberman pinscher develop myocardial diseases that are sufficiently distinctive in their clinical presentation to warrant mention.

7. What typifies boxer dog cardiomyopathy?

Cardiomyopathy in boxer dogs is characterized by a high incidence of ventricular tachyarrhythmias and sudden death. Harpster classified the manner of presentation of boxer dogs with cardiomyopathy. Boxer dogs in category 1 have ventricular arrhythmias but do not have associated clinical signs. In category 2 the syndrome is manifest as syncope that is presumably related to ventricular tachyarrhythmia. Category 3 is characterized by congestive heart failure (CHF) due to systolic myocardial dysfunction. Progression from one category to the next does not appear to be inevitable, and ventricular tachyarrhythmia in the absence of overt myocardial dysfunction is common in boxer dogs. The arrhythmogenic form of cardiomyopathy in boxer dogs likely has a genetic basis; recent data suggests that it is autosomal dominant trait, at least in some cases.

8. What typifies DCM in Doberman pinschers?

There are some similarities between the cardiomyopathy of boxer dogs and that of Doberman pinschers. The incidence of ventricular tachyarrhythmia in affected Dobermans is high as is the incidence of sudden cardiac death. CHF in Doberman pinschers with DCM is often associated with a short and rapidly progressive course.

9. What is occult DCM?

Studies performed in the Doberman pinscher demonstrate that DCM is a slowly progressive and insidious disorder. A long subclinical phase of the disease precedes the development of overt myocardial dysfunction; in some dogs, sudden death interrupts this progression. Working independently, O'Grady and Calvert have provided criteria that define subclinical or occult DCM in Doberman pinschers. Quantitative echocardiographic variables that predict the development of overt myocardial dysfunction or sudden death have been published. In some Doberman pinschers, electrocardiographic abnormalities precede the development of myocardial dysfunction. The finding of premature ventricular complexes (PVC) during a resting electrocardiogram or more than 100 PVCs recorded during 24-hour ambulatory electrocardiographic (Holter) monitoring also predict the development of overt DCM in Dobermans.

10. What is distinctive about DCM in cocker spaniels?

The cocker spaniel is the only small-breed dog that commonly develops DCM. The syndrome in cocker spaniels is further distinguished by the prevalence of low plasma taurine levels in affected dogs. Some cocker spaniels with DCM also have plasma or myocardial carnitine deficiency.

Taurine is an amino acid; the precise function of this nutrient relative to cardiovascular function is not known. However, an association between nutritional taurine deficiency and feline dilated cardiomyopathy was made in 1987. Subsequent supplementation of commercial cat foods resulted in a radical decrease in the prevalence of feline dilated cardiomyopathy. Taurine is not an essential amino acid in the dog and decreased intake alone does not explain low plasma taurine levels in this species; a metabolic defect, perhaps in the ability to synthesize taurine, might explain the low plasma levels in affected dogs.

The Multicenter Spaniel Trial (MUST) was a double-blind clinical trial that compared the effect of nutritional supplementation with taurine and carnitine to placebo in cocker spaniels with DCM. All cocker spaniels enrolled in the study had low plasma taurine levels. Improvement in echocardiographic parameters was observed in patients that were randomized to receive taurine and carnitine. The investigators were unblinded after four months; taurine and carnitine supplementation was then initiated in patients that had received placebo. Ultimately, it was possible to withdraw cardiovascular drugs from all patients that received taurine and carnitine. The improvement in myocardial function was apparently sustained and many of the dogs included in the study ultimately died of extracardiac disease. The importance of carnitine deficiency was not determined. However, it can be stated that taurine deficiency is prevalent in cocker spaniels with DCM and that nutritional supplementation with taurine and carnitine is likely to result in substantial clinical improvement. When DCM is observed in cocker spaniels, it is advisable to evaluate the plasma taurine level. In patients in whom this value is low, nutritional supplementation with taurine and possibly carnitine is recommended. If the plasma taurine level cannot be obtained, or a delay in obtaining the result is anticipated, empirical supplementation is suggested.

11. What prompts the owner of a dog with DCM to seek veterinary attention?

Patients with DCM are usually presented for evaluation of clinical signs related to CHF. The history may reveal dyspnea, cough, abdominal distention due to the presence of ascites, and syncope. In addition, the owner of a dog with DCM may observe exercise intolerance, weight loss, depression, and lack of appetite.

12. The physical findings in dilated cardiomyopathy often suggest the diagnosis. What might be expected on auscultation?

Patients with DCM are often presented when in CHF. Consequently, tachycardia is commonly present and arrhythmia may be evident on auscultation. Often, but not invariably, there is a murmur of functional AV valve incompetence that results from dilation of the AV valve annulus. The murmur is plateau shaped and occurs during systole. It is usually soft and heard best over the left cardiac apex.

In some affected dogs, audibility of the third heart sound results in a gallop rhythm. Rapid deceleration of early diastolic transmitral flow is the hemodynamic event associated with the occurrence of an S_3 gallop. Thus the gallop rhythm results from accentuation of a physiologic event. The rapid deceleration of early diastolic flow is probably related to the presence of a large end-systolic volume, high atrial pressures, and reduced ventricular compliance. In the presence of an audible third heart sound, pulmonary crackles suggest pulmonary edema.

13. What is the most specific abnormality detected on physical examination?

In small animals, audibility of the third heart sound is usually a specific indicator of myocardial dysfunction. The presence of a gallop rhythm in a dog is an indication for detailed cardiovascular evaluation even if it occurs in the absence of other clinical signs. Care must be taken to differentiate a gallop from arrhythmias and from transient sounds such as splitting of the first or second heart sound and clicks (which usually occur during midsystole).

14. Describe the expected radiographic findings.

The cardiac silhouette is usually enlarged and most often there is radiographic evidence of left atrial enlargement (see figure at top of following page). When the left atrium is enlarged, pulmonary opacities indicate the presence of pulmonary edema and CHF. Initially, pulmonary edema results in an interstitial pulmonary infiltrate. With the accumulation of greater amounts of liquid in the lung, the alveoli are flooded and an alveolar pulmonary infiltrate is observed. Often, cardiogenic pulmonary edema has a symmetrical and central distribution. However, pulmonary edema of acute onset may have a patchy or generalized distribution. It should be noted that the ability of plain chest x-rays to resolve specific cardiac chambers is limited and that the radiographic appearance of DCM is variable. Some affected Doberman pinschers, for example, have minimal radiographic evidence of cardiac enlargement. In some affected dogs of this breed there may be only loss of the caudal cardiac waist, indicating left atrial enlargement, and alveolar pulmonary infiltrates of edema.

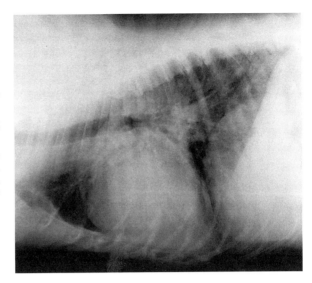

Lateral thoracic radiograph of a 12-year-old male castrated Labrador retriever cross with dilated cardiomyopathy. The cardiac silhouette is enlarged and there is evidence of left atrial enlargement. Cranially, there is the suggestion of pulmonary venous distention. Caudally, pulmonary vascular detail is poor, suggesting the presence of interstitial pulmonary edema.

15. What abnormalities are detected on electrocardiographic examination?

The electrocardiogram (ECG) provides information concerning heart rate, rhythm, and cardiac size. The elucidation of disturbances of cardiac rhythm is the primary utility of electrocardiography. In DCM, the ECG may reveal premature ventricular complexes, ventricular tachycardia, atrial premature complexes, atrial or junctional tachycardia, or atrial fibrillation. Sometimes there is evidence of ventricular hypertrophy, intraventricular conduction disturbances such as left bundle branch block, or evidence of left atrial enlargement. Broadening of the P wave beyond 40 msec suggests left atrial enlargement. The presence of concurrent P-wave notching may increase the specificity of P-wave broadening as a marker of left atrial enlargement.

16. When is echocardiography indicated?

Echocardiography provides a noninvasive assessment of cardiac chamber dimensions and myocardial function. It is the means by which to obtain a definitive noninvasive diagnosis of DCM and should be considered in all patients in which myocardial disease is suspected. In some instances, echocardiography can be performed with the patient standing or in sternal recumbency with minimal restraint and therefore little stress to the patient. When available, echocardiography can be considered prior to radiography in the dyspneic patient with physical findings that suggest DCM. Although echocardiography cannot provide a diagnosis of CHF it can be used to determine if the patient has structural cardiac abnormalities that might reasonably represent a substrate for the development of CHF.

17. What echocardiographic findings typify dilated cardiomyopathy?

In DCM, echocardiography demonstrates atrial and ventricular dilation with hypokinesis (see figures on next page). Usually, there is left ventricular or biventricular dilation; occasionally, the right ventricle is preferentially affected. Shortening fraction (SF), an index of systolic myocardial function, is low; often, it is very low and in the range of 5–15%. It should be emphasized that extracardiac disorders such as sepsis can impair myocardial function and result in a decrease in SF. Despite what can be a rapid clinical course, the development of DCM is usually a gradual process. Therefore, diminished SF in the absence of ventricular and atrial dilation may be related to extracardiac disease or measurement methodology; it is unlikely to explain signs of CHF. In DCM, the valves are structurally normal although Doppler studies often demonstrate mitral and tricuspid valve regurgitation.

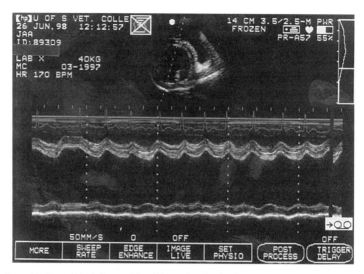

M-mode echocardiogfam of the left ventricle of the patient in the figure on page 233. M-mode echocardiography provides a one-dimensional view of the heart; the ordinate measures distance from the transducer and the abscissa, time. The two-dimensional image from which this M-mode was derived is shown in the inset. The echocardiogram demonstrates moderate left ventricular dilation and hypokinesis. The cardiac rhythm is atrial fibrillation.

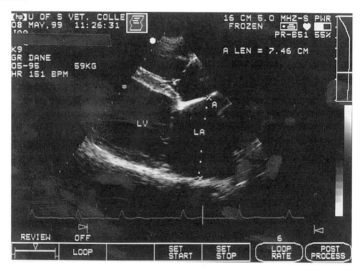

Systolic right parasternal long-axis echocardiographic image obtained from a 4-year-old male Great Dane with dilated cardiomyopathy and atrial fibrillation. The left atrium (LA) and left ventricle (LV) were dilated.

18. What medications are appropriate for the management of chronic CHF due to DCM?

A regimen that includes digoxin, an ACE inhibitor, and furosemide has become accepted for the management of CHF resulting from DCM. ACE inhibitors include captopril, enalapril, benazepril, and others. These drugs inhibit the enzyme that catalyzes the conversion of angiotensin I to angiotensin II. Angiotensin II is a vasoconstrictor that has numerous other effects that include modulation of the adrenergic nervous system, stimulation of antidiuretic hormone (ADH) and aldosterone release, and trophic effects on myocardium. The administration of enalapril to dogs with CHF due to DCM results in an improved quality of life and likely a favorable effect on mortality.

19. What is the role of digitalis in DCM?

Digitalis compounds have a positive inotropic effect and modulate the function of the adrenergic nervous system. They are unique in that they exert a positive inotropic effect yet lower heart rate and control the ventricular response rate in atrial fibrillation.

20. Furosemide is the diuretic that is used most commonly in CHF; are any others important?

The effect of diuresis is mechanical; reductions in intravascular volume decrease preload and limit the accumulation of edema. Furosemide is a potent loop diuretic that is widely used in the management of chronic CHF. Recent evidence indicates that spironolactone, an aldosterone antagonist, decreases morbidity and mortality in human patients with CHF who are receiving a combination of an ACE inhibitor and loop diuretic. Interestingly, this favorable effect was evident at a dose of spironolactone that did not cause diuresis. This is probably explained by the extrarenal effects of aldosterone. While this hormone stimulates the renal retention of sodium and water, it also promotes the development of myocardial fibrosis.

21. Should patients with subclinical or occult DCM be treated?

The efficacy of therapy for canine patients that have subclinical DCM has not been established. However, there is ample clinical evidence from studies of people in addition to experimental evidence to suggest that that the use of ACE inhibitors slows the progression of myocardial disease. Beta blockers may also have a role in the management of subclinical DCM. The use of these agents is consistent with the now accepted view that activation of the adrenergic nervous system and the RAAS contributes to the progressive nature of CHF due to systolic dysfunction. The use of an ACE inhibitor is reasonable when subclinical myocardial dysfunction has been demonstrated echocardiographically. Beta-blockers may also have a role but the use of these drugs in patients with systolic myocardial dysfunction must be undertaken only with caution.

22. Does L-carnitine supplementation have a role in the management of DCM?

L-carnitine is a quarternary amine that is synthesized from the amino acids lysine and methinonine; the D-isomer of this compound is toxic and further remarks refer to only to L-carnitine. Carnitine plays an integral role in cardiac energy metabolism; it is required for the transfer of long chain fatty acids across the mitochondrial membrane. Additionally, carnitine functions as a metabolic "scavenger," esterifying toxic metabolites.

In 1991, Keene et al. documented myocardial carnitine deficiency in a family of boxer dogs affected by DCM. In two of these dogs, nutritional supplementation with carnitine resulted in clinical and echocardiographic improvement that allowed the discontinuation of cardiovascular medications. Later, carnitine supplementation was stopped and myocardial dysfunction and signs of congestive heart failure returned. This work demonstrated that DCM in a family of boxer dogs was the result of myocardial carnitine deficiency. While myocardial free-carnitine deficiency is prevalent in dogs with DCM, resolution of myocardial dysfunction had not been documented subsequent to the initial report. It is likely that in many dogs with DCM myocardial carnitine deficiency is simply a marker of another, yet to be discovered metabolic defect.

The diagnosis of carnitine deficiency is made difficult by the complex disposition of this compound. Carnitine is concentrated in the myocardium so that plasma or serum carnitine levels do not necessarily reflect myocardial carnitine concentrations. Quantification of myocardial free- and esterified-carnitine levels can be performed on samples obtained by endomyocardial biopsy samples. However, the technique of endomyocardial biopsy is not widely practiced and the diagnosis of carnitine deficiency is generally a presumptive one that is made based upon clinical response.

In most dogs with DCM, carnitine supplementation is unlikely to effect a cure; however, some dogs with DCM seem to improve clinically following administration of this neutraceutical. High doses (1–2 g orally 3 times/day for large-breed dogs) are generally recommended. The cost of carnitine is relatively high although the use of a powdered form rather than tablets may reduce the cost. Because adverse effects other than possibly diarrhea have not been observed in association with the administration of carnitine, supplementation can be considered on an empiric basis when the financial burden can be borne by the pet owner.

23. How is atrial fibrillation (AF) managed in the setting of DCM?

Experimentally, it requires a critical mass of atrial myocardium to support the arrhythmia of atrial fibrillation. Only a few breeds of dog are sufficiently large to develop atrial fibrillation in the absence of cardiac disease. In dogs, atrial fibrillation usually signifies the presence of marked and possibly irreversible atrial enlargement. Because the predisposing cause of atrial fibrillation generally cannot be corrected in DCM, attempts to effect conversion to sinus rhythm are seldom successful in the long term. Further, the risk of thromboembolism, which sometimes complicates atrial fibrillation in people, seems to be low in dogs. Therefore, conversion to sinus rhythm is not generally attempted. Therapy of atrial fibrillation in the setting of DCM is directed towards optimizing stroke volume and myocardial oxygen demand through slowing of the ventricular response rate.

24. What are the roles of calcium channel antagonists, beta blockers, and digitalis in AF due to DCM?

Digoxin is used to control the ventricular response rate in AF associated with DCM. In some patients with DCM, slowing of the heart rate does not occur despite control of congestive signs. Here, the cautious use of diltiazem, a calcium channel blocker, or a beta-adrenergic antagonist such as atenolol or propranolol can be considered as adjunct therapy. Recent evidence obtained in clinical studies of humans indicates that the long-term use of beta-adrenergic antagonists in CHF due to systolic myocardial dysfunction has a beneficial effect on hemodynamics and survival. For this reason, these agents may be preferred when it is necessary to use drugs in addition to digoxin for slowing of heart rate in AF associated with DCM; however, caution must be exercised, as drugs other than digoxin that slow heart rate are negative inotropes and beta-blockers are potent in this regard.

25. What is the prognosis in DCM?

The prognosis when CHF results from DCM is generally poor. If the patient survives beyond the initial presentation, survival for 6–12 months and occasionally longer is possible with careful medical management. A few patients may respond favorably to supplementation with nutrients such as carnitine or taurine. A small number of patients with DCM seem to recover spontaneously. However, DCM in dogs is usually terminal.

CONTROVERSY

26. Do beta-adrenergic antagonists have a role in the management of DCM?

Beta-adrenergic anatgonists (beta blockers) reduce heart rate and decrease inotropic state. However, despite a pharmacodynamic profile that is apparently at odds with the pathophysiology of DCM, these agents have demonstrated efficacy in people with systolic myocardial dysfunction; in patients that tolerate them, the long-term use of beta-blockers decreases mortality and improves hemodynamics and clinical status. The reason for this unexpected favorable response is unknown; however, it is likely that beta blockers protect the heart from the cardiotoxic effect of prolonged elevations in sympathetic tone.

Extrapolation of this encouraging information to the therapy of dogs with DCM must be cautious. Patients with canine DCM are often presented for veterinary evaluation when myocardial dysfunction is advanced. It must be recognized that some patients with marked systolic dysfunction are critically dependent upon elevations in sympathetic tone to maintain perfusion pressure and cardiac output. In these individuals, beta blockers are apt to be very poorly tolerated. However, when suitable caution is exercised, there may be a role for beta blockers in some canine patients with DCM.

BIBLIOGRAPHY

1. Calvert CA, Chapman WL, Toal RL: Congestive cardiomyopathy in Doberman pinscher dogs. J Am Vet Med Assoc 191:598–602, 1982.
2. Calvert CA, Hall G, Jacobs G, et al: Clinical and pathologic findings in Doberman pinschers with occult cardiomyopathy that died suddenly or developed congestive heart failure: 54 cases (1984–1991). J Am Vet Med Assoc 210:510–511, 1997.
3. Calvert CA, Jacobs G, Smith DD, et al: Association between results of ambulatory electrocardiography and development of cardiomyopathy during long-term follow-up of Doberman pinschers. J Am Vet Med Assoc 216:34–39, 2000.
4. Calvert CA, Meurs KM: CVT update: Doberman pinscher occult cardiomyopathy. In Bonagura JD (ed): Kirk's Current Veterinary Therapy XIII: Small Animal Practice. Philadelphia, W.B. Saunders, 2000, pp 756–760.
5. Cleland JGF, Bristow MR, Erdmann E, et al: Beta-blocking agents in heart failure: Should they be used and how? Eur Heart J 17:1629–1639, 1996.
6. Cobb MA: Idiopathic dilated cardiomyopathy: Advances in aetiology, pathogenesis and management. J Small Anim Pract 33:113–118, 1992.
7. The COVE Study Group: Controlled clinical evaluation of enalapril in dogs with heart failure: Results of the Cooperative Veterinary Enalapril study group. J Vet Intern Med 9:243–252, 1995.
8. Ettinger SJ, Benitz AM, Ericsson GF, et al: Effects of enalapril maleate on survival of dogs with naturally acquired heart failure: The Long-Term Investigation of Veterinary Enalapril (LIVE) Study Group. J Am Vet Med Assoc 213:1573–1577, 1998.
9. Harpster NK: Boxer cardiomyopathy. In Kirk RW (ed): Current Veterinary Therapy VIII: Small Animal Practice. Philadelphia, W.B. Saunders, 1983, pp 329–337.
10. Keene BW, Panciera DP, Atkins CE, et al: Myocardial L-carnitine deficiency in a family of dogs with dilated cardiomyopathy. J Am Vet Med Assoc 198:647–650, 1991.
11. Kittleson MD: Primary myocardial disease leading to chronic myocardial failure (dilated cardiomyopathy and related diseases). In Kittleson MD, Kienle RD (eds): Small Animal Cardiovascular Medicine. St. Louis, Mosby, 1998, pp 319–347.
12. Kittleson MD: Taurine and carnitine responsive DCM in American cocker spaniels. In Bonagura JD (ed): Kirk's Current Veterinary Therapy XIII: Small Animal Practice. Philadelphia, W.B. Saunders, 2000, pp 761–762.
13. Kittleson MD, Keene B, Pion PD, Loyer CG: Results of the Multicenter Spaniel Trial (MUST): Taurine- and carnitine-responsive dilated cardiomyopathy in American cocker spaniels with decreased plasma taurine concentration. J Vet Intern Med 11:204–211, 1997.
14. Meurs KM, Spier KV, Miller MV, et al: Familial ventricular arrhythmias in boxers. J Vet Intern Med 13:437–439, 1999.
15. O'Grady MR, Horne R: Occult dilated cardiomyopathy: An echocardiographic and electrocardiographic study of 193 asymptomatic Doberman pinschers (abstract). J Vet Intern Med 6:112, 1992.
16. Packer M, Bristow MR, Cohn JN, et al: The effect of carvedilol on morbidity and mortality in patients with chronic heart failure. N Engl J Med 334:1349–1355, 1996.
17. Pitt B, Zannad F, Remme WJ, et al: The effect of spironolactone on morbidity and mortality in patients with severe heart failure. N Engl J Med 341:709–717, 1999.
18. Richardson P, McKenna W, Bristow M, et al: Report of the 1995 World Health Organization/International Society and Federation of Cardiology Task Force on the definition and classification of cardiomyopathies. Circulation 93:841–842, 1996.
19. Sabbah HN, Shimoyama H, Kono T, et al: Effects of long-term monotherapy with enalapril, metoprolol, and digoxin on the progression of left ventricular dysfunction in patients with heart failure. Circulation 89:2852–2859, 1994.
20. Sisson D, O'Grady MR, Calvert CA: Myocardial diseases of dogs. In Fox PR, Sisson D, Moise NS (eds): Textbook of Canine and Feline Cardiology: Principles and Clinical Practice. Philadelphia, W.B. Saunders, 1999, pp 581–620.

37. CANINE IDIOPATHIC HYPERTROPHIC CARDIOMYOPATHY

Donald P. Schrope, D.V.M.

1. What is idiopathic hypertrophic cardiomyopathy (HCM)?

Cardiomyopathy by definition is an abnormality of the myocardium. Cardiomyopathy can be broken down into *specific* cardiomyopathies and *idiopathic* cardiomyopathies. Specific cardiomyopathies are diseases of the myocardium due to definitive etiologies. Common specific cardiomyopathies would include taurine-deficient cardiomyopathy, hyperthyroid cardiomyopathy, and hypertensive cardiomyopathy. Idiopathic cardiomyopathies are diseases of the myocardium with unknown etiologies. Idiopathic cardiomyopathies are generally broken down into three groups: dilated cardiomyopathy, restrictive cardiomyopathy, and hypertrophic cardiomyopathy. Therefore, idiopathic hypertrophic cardiomyopathy is an abnormal thickening (hypertrophy) of the myocardium of unknown origin.

2. What are the possible etiologies of canine idiopathic HCM?

In many cases of human idiopathic HCM, a genetic defect can be identified. In most cases, the defect leads to abnormalities in various proteins associated with contraction, such as beta-myosin heavy chains, tropomyosin, and troponin-T. Genetic transmission of HCM has been documented in the cat, but not in the dog at this time. Theoretically, other abnormalities could stimulate myocardial hypertrophy; these include an increased sensitivity of the heart to catecholamines, an increased number of myocardial calcium channels, or abnormalities in coronary arteries causing compensatory hypertrophy.

A fixed obstruction to blood flow out of the left heart can also lead to secondary left ventricular hypertrophy (LVH) and it is important to try to differentiate subaortic stenosis (SAS) from HCM. Although it is not always obvious, the age and breed of the patient as well as the echocardiographic findings can help differentiate HCM from SAS.

3. Describe what is meant by outflow obstruction and systolic anterior motion (SAM) of the mitral valve as it pertains to HCM.

Left ventricular outflow tract (LVOT) obstruction can be broken down into two categories: *fixed* outflow tract obstruction and *dynamic* outflow tract obstruction. *Fixed* LVOT obstruction implies an *anatomic* obstruction to flow out of the left ventricle (LV) that is present throughout systole. A *dynamic* LVOT obstruction is an obstruction varies in intensity throughout systole. Usually, the obstruction is minimal during early systole, but worsens during mid- to late systole. Dynamic LVOT obstruction involves an abnormality in the motion of the mitral valve during systole. Normally, the mitral valve remains closed during systole. With a dynamic LVOT obstruction, however, the mitral valve falls across the LVOT beneath the aortic valve, obstructing blood leaving the LV (see figure on following page). Because the mitral valve leaflet is pulled out of its normal position, this also causes mitral regurgitation. In humans, this shifting of the mitral valve leaflet occurs in an anterior direction (i.e., toward the septum); therefore, this is called systolic anterior motion of the mitral valve.

There are various theories for the cause of SAM. It has been shown that malposition of the papillary muscles that support the mitral valve could predispose to SAM. Malposition of the papillary muscles could be secondary to hypertrophy of the LV, pushing the papillary muscles toward the septum, or due to a congenital malformation of the mitral valve apparatus. It has also been suggested that high-velocity flow out of the LVOT and abnormal flow patterns within the LV secondary to HCM may suck or push the mitral valve into the LVOT. In many cases where both SAM and LVH are present, it is unclear whether the dynamic obstruction caused the LVH or was itself induced by the LVH.

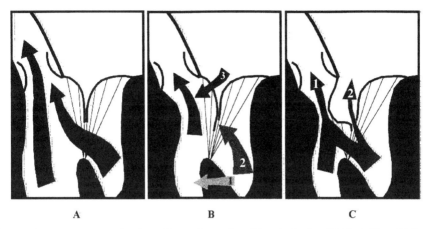

A   B   C

Diagram of the causes and results of systolic anterior motion of the mitral valve (SAM). *A*, Normal left ventricular (LV) systolic flow. No narrowing of the outflow tract is present. Note the normal position of the mitral valve (MV) with normal coaptation of the leaflets. The septal leaflet is a normal distance from the septum. *B*, Diagram of the theorized causes of SAM. Hypertrophy of the LV and the papillary muscles can cause a shift of the papillary muscles toward the septum (1). This pulls the MV toward the outflow tract. Additionally, this malposition may cause malalignment of the MV leaflets. This malalignment of the leaflets may cause blood flow within the LV to push the septal leaflet toward the outflow tract (2). Blood flowing at high velocities through the outflow tract due to LVH may pull the septal leaflet of the MV into the outflow tract (3). This is called the Venturi effect. Shifting of the septal MV leaflet toward the outflow tract resulting from (1) and (2) may also predispose to the Venturi effect. *C*, The resultant shift of the septal leaflet of the MV into the outflow tract causes outflow tract obstruction (1). The malposition of the MV leaflets also results in mitral regurgitation (2).

4. What is the signalment of a typical case of canine idiopathic HCM?

Canine idiopathic HCM appears to have a male predisposition, and is usually identified in dogs less than 3 years of age. There may be a breed predisposition in the German shepherd dog, Boston terrier, rottweiler, and dalmatian.

While SAM is commonly associated with HCM, it can also complicate the presentation of anatomic subaortic stenosis and this contributes to the difficulty in distinguishing these disorders. In addition, HCM has been observed most commonly in large-breed dogs such as the German shepherd dog and the rottweiler, breeds that have an established predisposition for the development of anatomic subaortic stenosis, and this further complicates the issue.

5. What are the typical results of chest radiographs, electrocardiogram, and echocardiogram in cases of canine idiopathic HCM?

Radiographs may show evidence of left atrial (LA) and left ventricular (LV) enlargement. Evidence of congestive heart failure (CHF), such as pulmonary venous congestion and pulmonary edema, may be seen but appears to be uncommon.

The ECG may show evidence of LA and LV enlargement. Ventricular arrhythmias have been identified in some patients.

An echocardiogram will show evidence of concentric LVH (i.e., thickening of the ventricular wall). The distribution of LVH can be broken down into two categories: *symmetric* and *asymmetric*. *Symmetric* LVH implies a homogeneous thickening of the septum and LV free wall. In cases of *asymmetric* LVH, there are areas of the LV myocardium that are significantly thicker than others. Asymmetric LVH usually appears as a significantly thickened septum, with a normal to mildly thickened LV free wall. The term asymmetric LVH implies that the septum is greater than 1.3 times the thickness of the LV free wall. Asymmetric LVH appears to be less common than symmetric LVH in cases of canine idiopathic HCM. Thickening of the papillary muscles may also be seen in conjunction with symmetric or asymmetric LVH. Hyperechogenicity of the subendocardial myocardium and papillary muscles has also been associated with LVH. This is most likely due to hypoxia of the affected muscle or the presence of myocardial fibrosis. (See figure below for diagrams of the different classifications.)

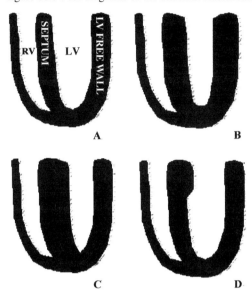

Diagram of different classifications of left ventricular hypertrophy (LVH). *A*, Normal left ventricle with normal symmetrical septal and free wall thickness. *B*, Symmetric LVH with uniform hypertrophy of septum and free wall. *C*, Asymmetric septal LVH. The septal wall thickness is greater than 1.3 × the free wall thickness. *D*, Proximal septal bulge, a specific type of asymmetric LVH with focal thickening of the septum inferior to the aortic valve in which the remainder of the septum is often normal or thickened to a lesser degree. LV, left ventricle; RV, right ventricle.

Other echocardiographic findings include narrowing of the LVOT and evidence of SAM. SAM may be identified on M-mode or 2D echocardiography. Doppler evaluation may show an increased peak flow velocity out the LVOT if obstruction is present. If an elevated LVOT velocity is due to SAM, the spectral Doppler envelope may take on a characteristic "ski-slope" appearance (see figure below). This is secondary to an acute increase in outflow velocity in midsystole due to the onset of the dynamic obstruction. If SAM is present, mitral valve regurgitation may also be identified.

Mitral valve inflows may also show abnormalities suggesting the presence of diastolic dysfunction. LA enlargement may be present.

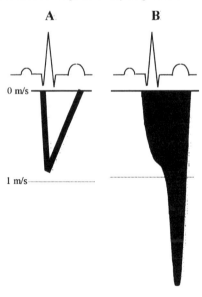

A, A normal aortic outflow spectral Doppler envelope. Notice the initial acute rise in velocity to nearly 1 m/s, with a gradual decline in velocity near the end of systole. The well-defined borders of the envelope with minimal density under the curve suggests a normal, uniform increase and decrease in velocity of all blood cells. *B*, An aortic outflow spectral Doppler envelope in a patient with dynamic outflow tract obstruction. Initially, the envelope appears fairly normal. As the velocity begins to level off in mid-systole, it acutely increases again due to the onset of the dynamic obstruction. Note that the borders of the envelope and the area under the curve are fairly uniform in density. This is called "spectral dispersion." Spectral dispersion occurs because of marked variation in the velocity and direction of red blood cells secondary to turbulence in the LV outflow tract and aorta due to the obstruction.

6. What is the pathophysiology of heart failure associated with canine HCM?

Thickening of the myocardium causes stiffening of the muscle of the affected ventricle. Contractility is essentially normal with this disease. The hypertrophy, however, makes it difficult for the myocardium to relax normally. This interferes with the filling phase of the ventricle (diastole) and potentially increases left atrial pressure. Unfortunately, the increased atrial pressure increases the pressure in the veins entering the atrium causing congestion. If there is increased pressure in the left atrium, then pulmonary edema can result. If there is increased pressure in the right atrium, systemic congestion can result. In some cases of HCM, significant mitral valve regurgitation may be present, which can also contribute to increased left atrial pressure.

7. How does canine idiopathic HCM compare to idiopathic HCM identified in cats and humans?

HCM has been identified in cats and humans and appears to be much more common in these species than in the dog. There appear to be certain pathologic differences among the three species. First, asymmetric LVH appears to be more common in humans and dogs. Second, the degree of myocardial interstitial fibrosis or replacement fibrosis appears to be more severe in humans than in cats or dogs. Finally, there is a significant difference in the prevalence of myocardial fiber disarray among these species. Myocardial fiber disarray is a malalignment of myofibrils relative to each other. Normally, myocardial fibers lie parallel to each other. With myocardial fiber disarray, bundles of myofibrils may lie perpendicular to each other or the myofibrils may have even less organization, giving the myocardium a "pinwheel" appearance on histopathologic examination. Myocardial fiber disarray is very common in humans, but it is fairly uncommon in cats and dogs. The prevalence of diseased coronary arteries associated with HCM appears to be similar among all three species.

8. Explain the appropriate acute therapy for CHF associated with idiopathic HCM.

If CHF is present, furosemide should be administered. Note that over-diuresis as a result of furosemide overdosage may greatly decrease LA pressure, which will worsen LV filling. Nitroglycerin paste may be administered initially, and might be beneficial. The paste should be applied to a bare area of the skin, and gloves should be worn, since the paste can be absorbed through the skin of the administrator. Tolerance to nitroglycerin may develop over 24 to 48 hours; therefore, it is rarely useful beyond this time period. Until the CHF is controlled, oxygen should be administered (if possible) in order to improve the comfort level of the patient. Fluids should not be administered in the face of pulmonary edema.

CONTROVERSY

9. What is the most appropriate therapy for the long-term management of HCM?

Canine HCM is uncommon and the efficacy of therapy for this disease is unknown. In general, treatment is based upon what is known of the pathophysiology of this disorder and what is known of the therapeutic responses of affected cats and people. Therapy for HCM generally involves the use of calcium channel blockers or beta blockers. Diltiazem is the most commonly used calcium channel blocker for the therapy of HCM in veterinary medicine. Atenolol and propranolol are the most commonly used beta blockers. Both classes of drugs act to decrease the heart rate, although the effect of beta blockers tends to be more profound in this regard. A decrease in heart rate gives the hypertrophied heart more time to fill by prolonging diastole. This can improve LV stroke volume and decrease LA pressure.

At least in cats, it has been suggested that calcium channel blockers (specifically diltiazem) may be more effective for HCM because they have been shown to directly improve myocardial relaxation (a positive lusitropic effect). Although beta blockers do not have a direct positive lusitropic effect, they have been shown to significantly improve oxygen delivery to the myocardium and also to improve myocardial oxygen usage by the myocardium. Because relaxation is oxygen dependent, these effects have an indirect positive lusitropic effect.

Both classes of drugs also cause a decrease in contractility (a negative inotropic effect). This negative inotropic effect may decrease the stress on the hypertrophied heart and may also decrease the severity of SAM, if present.

It has been suggested that diltiazem may cause regression of LVH in cats with HCM. It is the author's experience that similar effects can be seen with beta blockers in cats.

The aforementioned effects of both classes of drugs on lusitropy, inotropy, and LVH regression suggest that calcium channel blockers and beta blockers are fairly similar in their beneficial effects on HCM.

The last factor in the debate regarding calcium channel blockers and beta blockers is their effects on outflow tract obstruction. It has been shown that drugs with arterial vasodilatory effects (including diltiazem) can worsen existing LVOT obstruction in humans. Other human studies have shown that relieving LVOT obstruction through various means, such as surgery, can greatly improve cardiac function and resolve clinical signs. These findings would suggest that it is beneficial to improve or resolve LVOT obstruction, and likely detrimental to use drugs that would worsen the degree of LVOT obstruction. Calcium channel blockers such as diltiazem cause variable degrees of arterial vasodilation and therefore may worsen LVOT obstruction; beta blockers do not. It appears therefore that beta blockers may be a better choice for therapy of HCM if LVOT obstruction is present. If LVOT obstruction is not present, either calcium channel blockers or beta blockers could be considered.

BIBLIOGRAPHY

1. Betocchi S, Piscione F, Losi MA, et al: Effects of diltiazem on left ventricular systolic and diastolic function in hypertrophic cardiomyopathy. Am J Cardiol 78:451–457, 1996.
2. Levine RA, Vlahakes GJ, Lefebvre X, et al: Papillary muscle displacement causes systolic anterior motion of the mitral valve. Circulation 91:1189–1195, 1995.
3. Liu SK, Maron BJ, Tilley LP: Canine hypertrophic cardiomyopathy. J Am Vet Med Assoc 174:708–713, 1979.
4. Liu SK, Roberts WC, Maron BJ: Comparison of morphologic findings in spontaneously occurring hypertrophic cardiomyopathy in humans, cats, and dogs. Am J Cardiol 72:944–951, 1993.
5. Marks CA: Hypertrophic cardiomyopathy in a dog. J Am Vet Med Assoc 203:1020–1022, 1993.
6. Maron BJ, Bonow RO, Cannon RO, et al: Hypertrophic cardiomyopathy: Interrelations of clinical manifestations, pathophysiology, and therapy. (First of two parts.) N Engl J Med 316:780–789, 1987.
7. Maron BJ, Bonow RO, Cannon RO, et al: Hypertrophic cardiomyopathy: Interrelations of clinical manifestations, pathophysiology, and therapy. (Second of two parts.) N Engl J Med 316:844–852, 1987.
8. Richardson P, McKenna W, Bristow M, et al: Report of the 1995 World Health Organization/ International Society and Federation of Cardiology task force on the definition and classification of cardiomyopathies. Circulation 93:841–842, 1996.
9. Schwammenthal E, Nakatani S, Shengqiu H, et al: Mechanism of mitral regurgitation in hypertrophic cardiomyopathy. Circulation 98:856–865, 1998.
10. Sherrid MV, Perle G, Gundsburg DZ: Mechanism of benefit of negative inotropes in obstructive hypertrophic cardiomyopathy. Circulation 97:41–47, 1998.
11. Sisson DD, O'Grady MR, Calvert CA: Myocardial diseases of the dog. In Fox PR, Sisson DD, Moise NS (eds): Textbook of Canine and Feline Cardiology. Philadelphia, W.B. Saunders, 1999, pp 581–620.
12. Sisson DD, Thomas WP: Myocardial diseases. In Ettinger AJ, Feldman ED (eds): Textbook of Veterinary Internal Medicine. Philadelphia, W.B. Saunders, 1995, pp 1005–1009.
13. Spiritio P, Seidman CE, McKenna WJ, et al: The management of hypertrophic cardiomyopathy. N Engl J Med 336:775–785, 1997.
14. Wynne J, Braunwald E: The cardiomyopathies and myocarditidies. In Braunwald E (ed): Heart Disease: A Textbook of Cardiovascular Medicine. Philadelphia, W.B. Saunders, 1997, pp 1414–1426.

38. FELINE HYPERTROPHIC CARDIOMYOPATHY

Janice McIntosh Bright, B.S.N., M.S., D.V.M.

1. What is hypertrophic cardiomyopathy?

Hypertrophic cardiomyopathy (HCM) is a common cause of heart failure, arterial thromboembolism, and sudden death in cats. HCM is a primary disorder of the myocardium characterized by unexplained left ventricular hypertrophy (LVH) and impaired myocardial relaxation.

2. What causes feline HCM?

In most cats the etiology of HCM is unknown. In Maine coon cats the disease is a heritable, autosomal dominant disorder with complete penetrance. Recently this disease has also been shown to be inherited in Persian cats and in some American shorthair cats. Cats with heritable HCM may develop severe LVH at a young age, often as early as 4 months. In people, familial HCM is usually associated with inherited sarcomeric gene mutations, most commonly mutations of the β-myosin heavy chain. However, gene mutations cannot account for the regional hypertrophy often noted in people and in cats with this disease. Furthermore, specific sarcomeric gene mutations have not yet been identified in cats with inherited HCM. In most cats, the etiology of HCM remains an enigma. It is likely that various sarcomeric gene mutations as well as numerous other etiologic mechanisms result in primary pathologic cardiac hypertrophy with diastolic dysfunction.

3. Describe the pathophysiologic mechanisms of feline HCM.

The pathophysiology of feline HCM involves systolic abnormalities, diastolic abnormalites, and myocardial ischemia. However, diastolic dysfunction is thought to be primarily responsible for the clinical and hemodynamic manifestations of this disease. Diastolic dysfunction refers to impaired capacity of the left ventricle to accept blood or to fill without a compensatory increase in left atrial pressure. Impaired left ventricular (LV) filling may cause dyspnea as a result of pulmonary edema, or it may cause lethargy, syncope, or sudden death as a result of reduced stroke volume. In addition, LV diastolic dysfunction impedes normal left atrial flow predisposing to left atrial enlargement, circulatory stasis, and thromboembolism.

4. Is the diastolic dysfunction in cats with HCM due solely to LV hypertrophy?

Impaired diastolic function in cats with HCM occurs as a result of increased chamber stiffness (reduced compliance) as well as impaired myocyte relaxation. Increased LV chamber stiffness results from increased passive stiffness of the myocardium as a consequence of tissue fibrosis and myocyte disarray and also from increased ventricular mass (reduced volume-mass ratio). Reduced LV compliance shifts the end-diastolic pressure-volume relationship such that a greater diastolic pressure is required to achieve a given diastolic volume (see figure on following page).

Impaired myocardial relaxation in feline HCM patients also contributes to diastolic dysfunction. In cats with HCM the rate at which tension declines in the myofibers is reduced, resulting in a decreased rate of LV pressure decline and a diminution or absence of the early rapid-filling wave on LV pressure recordings.

5. Why do cats with HCM have myocardial ischemia and why is ischemia important?

Myocardial ischemia is present in patients with HCM as a result of reduced capillary density, narrowed intramural coronary arteries, and increased extravascular resistance. Myocardial ischemia is important because it may be responsible for malaise and lethargy caused by anginal pain. More definitively, myocardial ischemia is important because ischemia further impairs the energy-dependent process of myocardial relaxation, thereby further compromising diastolic function. Finally, myocardial ischemia undoubtedly predisposes to lethal arrhythmias.

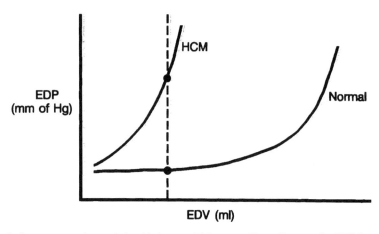

Left ventricular pressure–volume relationship in cats with hypertrophic cardiomyopathy (HCM) compared to normal. In a patient with HCM a given end-diastolic volume (EDV) is associated with a much greater end-diastolic pressure (EDP) than in a normal cat. (From August JR (ed): Consultations in Internal Medicine, 2nd ed. Philadelphia, W.B. Saunders, 1994, p 256, with permission.)

6. What systolic abnormalities are noted in cats with HCM?

Although diastolic abnormalities are primarily responsible for the clinical signs and hemodynamic features of feline HCM, some systolic abnormalities are also associated with this disorder. Echocardiographic, radionuclide, and angiocardiographic indexes of systolic function are usually normal or increased in cats with HCM. Occasionally, however, impaired systolic performance may be observed that is most likely the result of extensive myocardial fibrosis that occurs with chronic disease. Other systolic abnormalities noted in some cats with HCM include mitral regurgitation and the development of intraventricular systolic pressure gradients. Mitral regurgitation is most likely secondary to altered LV geometry or to abnormal systolic movement of the mitral valve leaflets caused by high-velocity flow in the LV outflow tract (Venturi effect).

7. How is the diagnosis of feline HCM made?

The diagnosis of feline HCM is made by echocardiographic or angiographic demonstration of a hypertrophied, nondilated left ventricle in the absence of an identifiable cause of LVH. All other features of the disease, including histopathology, are variable. In clinical practice, echocardiography has replaced angiography as the primary means by which to diagnose myocardial disease in the cat. In fact, echocardiography is the only noninvasive way to characterize feline myocardial disease.

8. List the differential diagnoses for feline HCM.

The differential diagnosis for primary HCM in cats includes other disorders known to produce secondary left ventricular hypertrophy, such as valvular or discrete subvalvular aortic stenosis, thyrotoxicosis, systemic hypertension, and hypersomatotropism. Infiltrative myocardial diseases such as lymphosarcoma may produce thickening of the LV wall or septum that mimics hypertrophy. With the exception of discrete subaortic stenosis, it is not possible to reliably distinguish primary from secondary forms of concentric LVH based on radiographic, echocardiographic, and Doppler features.

9. What usually brings owners of cats with HCM to seek veterinary care?

Cats with HCM are commonly brought to the veterinarian because of respiratory distress (tachypnea and/or dyspnea) that results from pulmonary edema, pleural effusion, or both.

Coughing is quite unusual. Cats with secondary thromboembolic disease are usually presented because of acute rear limb paralysis or paresis. Lameness of the right forelimb due to thromboembolism is somewhat less common. Less frequently, owners of cats with HCM seek veterinary care for their pet because of syncope or because of nonspecific signs of lethargy and lack of appetite. Many cats with HCM are asymptomatic and are brought to the veterinarian for unrelated reasons. Sudden death without preceding clinical signs may occur with HCM, and some owners may bring the body to the veterinarian for postmortem examination in such cases.

10. What cardiac ascultatory abnormalities are found with this disease?
   Cardiac auscultatory abnormalities are common but not universal in cats with HCM. Murmurs, gallop rhythms, and/or arrhythmias are often heard. Murmurs are systolic and usually reflect either secondary mitral regurgitation or turbulent flow in the LV outflow tract (see figure below). Not infrequently, systolic murmurs in affected cats are the result of a composite of multiple sources of intracardiac and intravascular turbulence.
   Because of the rapid heart rate in many cats with this disease, it is often difficult to distinguish whether a gallop is caused by an audible S_3, S_4, or by a summation of these two sounds. Fortunately, this distinction is not important diagnostically or therapeutically. Occasionally, the heart sounds are muffled because of the presence of pleural or pericardial effusions. The heart rate is often normal although tachycardia may develop as a compensatory response to reduced stroke volume, hypoxemia, or pain. A small number of cats (approximately 10%) with HCM have sinus bradycardia.

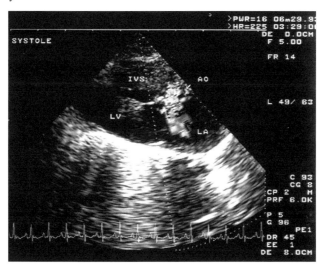

Still-frame color Doppler image obtained during systole from a cat with hypertrophic cardiomyopathy. The image reveals a jet of mitral regurgitation as well as high-velocity turbulent flow in the aortic root. AO, aorta; IVS, interventricular septum; LA, left atrium.

11. What electrocardiographic (ECG) findings are found in cats with HCM?
   A wide variety of ECG abnormalities including ventricular and supraventricular tachyarrhythmias, premature ventricular contractions, chamber enlargement patterns, and conduction disturbances may be present in cats with HCM. Some cats have multiple ECG abnormalities (see figure on following page). Intraventricular conduction abnormalities consistent with left anterior fascicular block occur frequently. Hemodynamically significant arrhythmias may occur intermittently, necessitating a Holter monitor or event monitor recording for diagnosis.

FE057611

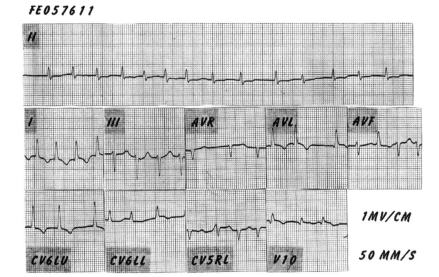

Electrocardiogram recorded from a cat with hypertrophic cardiomyopathy showing atrial fibrillation, left anterior fascicular block, and a probable premature ventricular contraction in lead AVF.

12. What are the survey radiographic features of feline HCM?

Like many aspects of feline HCM, the survey radiographic findings may vary depending upon the extent of hypertrophic change, the degree of myocardial dysfunction, the presence of secondary chamber enlargement, and the severity of circulatory congestion. Because cardiac hypertrophy occurs in a concentric manner, some cats may have no appreciable enlargement of the cardiac silhouette. Typically, however, survey thoracic radiographs reveal mild to moderate LV enlargement with more severe left atrial enlargement. Less frequently, generalized enlargement of the cardiac silhouette is noted due to development of substantial pericardial effusion or to secondary right-sided heart failure. When clinical signs are associated with HCM, pulmonary venous distention and pulmonary edema are common radiographic abnormalities, and pleural effusion may also be noted.

13. What clinically useful information can be gained from the echocardiographic study of cats with suspected HCM?

Echocardiography is the only noninvasive method for confirming a diagnosis of HCM and assessing the severity and distribution of the cardiac hypertrophy. Typical echocardiographic features of feline HCM include symmetric hypertrophy of the interventricular septum and LV caudal wall, normal to reduced LV chamber dimensions, and secondary left atrial enlargement. There may also be hypertrophy of the papillary muscles and right ventricular wall. The diagnosis is straightforward in cats with severe hypertrophic change, but in cats with more subtle hypertrophy and more normal sized chambers, the distinction between mild disease and normal may be less straightforward. Although some cardiologists use more conservative criteria, most consider M-mode measurements of the septum and LV wall abnormal if greater than 5.5 or 6 mm during diastole and 9.0 mm during systole.

Whereas many cats with HCM have global, symmetric LV hypertrophy, the hypertrophy may be asymmetric or regional, affecting only the septum or the caudal wall. It is not uncommon to find only the basilar portion of the septum affected (see figure at top of next page). Standard M-mode echocardiographic measurements may be misleading in cats with regional hypertrophy if used as the sole diagnostic criterion.

Although there does appear to be some correlation between the severity of hypertrophy and the severity of clinical signs, some cats with severe LV failure have ventricular wall and septal

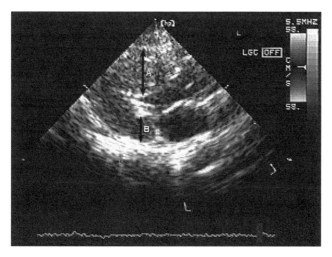

Still-frame two-dimensional echocardiographic image obtained from a Persian kitten with hypertrophic cardiomyopathy showing asymmetric hypertrophy of the interventricular septum. A, width of interventricular
septum; B, width of left ventricular caudal wall.

measurements that are only slightly increased. Conversely, severe hypertrophy and lumen attenuation have been observed in some asymptomatic cats.

Some cats with HCM, particularly those with asymmetric septal hypertrophy, have abnormal
ventral (anterior) movement of the mitral valve apparatus toward the septum during systole (see
figure below). This echocardiographic abnormality is called systolic anterior motion (SAM) of
the mitral valve. SAM is associated with the development of a late systolic pressure gradient
across the left ventricular outflow tract and mitral valve regurgitation. The pressure gradient may
reflect dynamic obstruction of the left ventricular outflow tract.

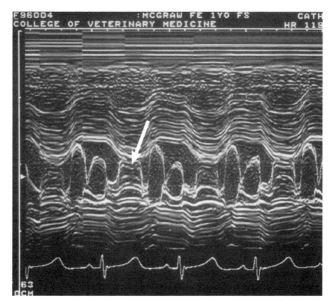

M-mode echocardiogram recorded from a 1-year-old cat with hypertrophic cardiomyopathy showing systolic
anterior motion (SAM) of the mitral valve *(arrow)* in addition to hypertrophy.

14. What information can Doppler echocardiography provide in cats with HCM?

Because Doppler echocardiography provides a noninvasive examination of the direction and velocity of blood flow, it may provide a nearly complete hemodynamic assessment of cats with HCM. However, the small cardiac size and rapid heart rate of feline patients makes acquisition of quantitative Doppler data technically difficult. Also, it is yet to be determined whether the Doppler measurements obtained from cats with HCM will affect prognosis or therapeutic management. Color Doppler imaging may demonstrate high-velocity turbulent blood flow in the right ventricular and/or left ventricular outflow tracts, and pressure gradients may be estimated from continuous Doppler velocity measurements. Yet these velocities and derived gradients are significantly affected by inotropic state and loading conditions and are of no clearly defined clinical significance. Color and spectral Doppler may also be used to confirm mitral regurgitation, which is a secondary event noted in some feline patients.

15. Can Doppler be used to evaluate diastolic function in cats with HCM?

Because Doppler echocardiography provides a noninvasive method of assessing blood flow, it provides a way of quantifying left ventricular filling and myocardial relaxation. Measurements of early and late LV inflow velocities may be obtained using pulsed Doppler if the heart rate is sufficiently slow. Because the rate of LV relaxation is delayed in affected cats, the pulsed Doppler LV inflow pattern usually shows a reduced early filling velocity and an increased atrial systolic filling velocity (see figure below). In addition, the isovolumic relaxation time can be measured from pulsed Doppler recordings showing LV inflow and outflow simultaneously. The isovolumic relaxation time is increased (> 50 msec) in most cats with HCM. It should be noted that while pulsed Doppler assessment of LV diastolic function may provide useful information regarding the severity of functional impairment, pulsed Doppler indexes of diastolic function are affected by a wide array of factors such as heart rate, loading conditions, and Doppler technique.

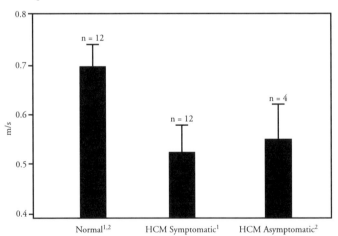

Normal[1,2]   HCM Symptomatic[1]   HCM Asymptomatic[2]

[1]Significantly Different (p = 0.026)
[2]Not Significantly Different

Bar graph illustrating the peak velocity of early left ventricular filling determined using pulsed Doppler in a group of normal cats and in a group of asymptomatic and symptomatic cats with HCM. The velocity is significantly lower in the symptomatic cats compared tothe normal group (data are mean ± standard error).

16. What are the goals of medical management for cats with HCM?

Medical management of feline HCM should be directed toward improving diastolic function, reducing myocardial ischemia, alleviating circulatory congestion/hypoxemia, and suppressing hemodynamically signficant arrhythmias (see table). Because some cats have intraventricular pressure gradients that exacerbate ischemia and therefore diastolic dysfunction, therapeutic interventions to reduce systolic gradients might be beneficial. Consideration should be given to treatment and prevention of arterial thromboembolism and to reversal of hypertrophy. At this time, however, there are no pharmacologic agents that consistently and universally reverse hypertrophy or prevent arterial thromboembolism.

Therapeutic Goals and Appropriate Interventions for Cats
with Hypertrophic Cardiomyopathy

THERAPEUTIC GOAL	INTERVENTION(S)
Improve myocardial relaxation	Diltiazem
Increase coronary flow	Diltiazem
Decrease myocardial O_2 demand	Diltiazem, beta blockers
Relieve edema/hypoxemia	Diuretics, nitroglycerin, thoracentesis, O_2, ACE inhibitors
Reduce systolic gradients	Diltiazem, beta blockers
Prevent thromobembolism	Coumadin (?), aspirin (?)
Reverse hypertrophy	ACE inhibitors (?), diltiazem (?)

17. What medications and interventions are used to achieve these management goals?
Both beta-adrenergic antagonists and calcium channel antagonists can be used to relieve myocardial ischemia and reduce systolic gradients in cats with HCM. However, only the calcium channel blockers have a direct beneficial effect on myocardial relaxation and coronary blood flow (see table above). Diltiazem is a calcium channel blocker that is safe and effective in most cats. This drug is given at a dose of 1.75–2.5 mg/kg orally 3 times/day when standard preparations are used, but a dose of 10 mg/kg is needed for sustained-release products. The sustained-release products are administered once daily. Specific sustained-release diltiazem preparations that have been safely used in cats for treatment of HCM include Cardizem CD (Hoechst Marion Roussel) and Dilacor XR (Rhone-Poulenc Rorer).

Diuretics are used to relieve circulatory congestion in cats with pulmonary edema. Furosemide is administered immediately to cats with severe respiratory distress at a dose of 2–3 mg/kg intramuscularly. Relief of edema may be enhanced by the simultaneous administration of 2% nitroglycerin ointment, 0.5–1.0 cm transdermally. Supplemental oxygen also should be administered. When the respiratory status of the patient has stabilized and the diagnosis of HCM has been confirmed, furosemide administration is continued orally, usually at a dose of 1 mg/kg once or twice daily until the pulmonary edema has resolved radiographically. Administration of diltiazem or a beta-blocking agent is begun as soon as oral medication can be given. When pulmonary edema has resolved, furosemide administration may be discontinued cautiously in many cats. Immediate thoracocentesis of acutely dyspneic cats should be done in addition to administering furosemide, nitroglycerin ointment, and oxygen if auscultation reveals muffled heart and lung sounds or if fluid lines are detected with percussion. Thoracocentesis is done with the animal in sternal position using a sterile 19- or 21- gauge butterfly needle introduced into the seventh or eighth intercostal space at the level of the costochondral junction.

At the recommended dose, diltiazem does not directly suppress sinoatrial (SA) automaticity. Therefore, this drug should not be dosed according to heart rate. With long-term diltiazem administration, the resting heart rate usually decreases indirectly as a result of improved cardiac performance. Cats with persistent resting tachycardia, atrial fibrillation, or paroxysmal tachyarrhythmias may need the cautious addition of a beta-adrenergic blocking agent, such as propranolol or atenolol, to the treatment regimen if diltiazem alone fails to control clinical signs.

18. Are beta-adrenegic antagonists more effective than calcium channel antagonists for treatment of cats having significant outflow tract gradients?

Some authors claim that beta-blockers should be used rather than calcium channel blockers in cats with large LV outflow tract gradients. The tendency to develop SAM and outflow tract gradients is related to cardiac loading conditions and contractility. Specifically, the afterload reduction that results from vasodilation, preload reduction, and enhanced contractility tends to provoke or augment SAM. Beta-adrenergic antagonists have a more potent negative inotropic effect than does diltiazem. Additionally, the commonly used beta-adrenergic antagonists have little effect on systemic vascular resistance. In contrast, diltiazem has a relatively weak vasodilatory effect. For these reasons many have suggested that beta-adrenergic antagonists are superior to calcium channel blockers when SAM is present. However, there is no evidence that beta-blockers are any more effective than calcium channel blockers for reducing intraventricular gradients, provided excessive vasodilation is avoided. Further, the prognostic importance of SAM and related gradients in cats with HCM is unknown and the therapeutic importance of abolishing dynamic gradients can therefore be debated.

19. What treatment should be used for asymptomatic cats?

Whether asymptomatic cats should receive any treatment is arguable. Currently, there are no data to verify that medical intervention will either delay or prevent the onset of clinical signs or sudden death. Furthermore, there is no indication that treatment with either diltiazem or a beta-blocker is needed to arrest progression of the hypertrophy in adult cats. Diltiazem and enalapril are agents shown to induce regression of hypertrophy in some cats. Therefore, it may be reasonable to administer one of these agents to asymptomatic cats with moderate to severe hypertrophy for 3 to 6 months to determine whether regression occurs.

20. Do angiotensin-converting enzyme (ACE) inhibitors have a role in treatment of cats with HCM?

The role of ACE inhibitors in the management of feline HCM is a somewhat controversial topic. ACE inhibitors have been shown to have antihypertrophy and antifibrotic effects on the myocardium in some laboratory species with induced heart disease. In addition, administration of ACE inhibitors reduces plasma aldosterone concentration, thereby helping to alleviate circulatory congestion. One study of cats with HCM showed that patients treated with enalapril had greater regression of hypertrophy than a control group receiving either beta-adrenergic antagonists or calcium channel antagonists. However, a specific comparison between enalapril-treated and diltiazem-treated cats was not made. Moreover, the effect of enalapril on diastolic function, clinical signs, and survival was not addressed. It is important to point out that ACE inhibitors are vasodilating agents and therefore have the potential of causing hypotension in cats with reduced ventricular end-diastolic volume.

For these reasons, the ACE inhibitors are generally not considered to be first-line or sole agents for management of feline HCM. Usually, the ACE inhibitors are used in addition to calcium channel antagonists and diuretics in refractory cases or in cats with biventricular failure. When used, ACE inhibitors should be dosed modestly and not used in combination with aspirin. Enalapril, benazepril, or quinapril are usually given orally at a dose of 0.25–0.50 mg/kg once daily.

21. Are there any drugs or interventions that should be avoided in cats with HCM?

Certain drugs and interventions are potentially harmful to cats with hypertrophic cardiomyopathy. These include positive inotropic agents and arteriolar-dilating agents. Positive inotropic agents, including digitalis, catecholamines, and phosphodiesterase inhibitors, increase the myocardial oxygen demand, thereby exacerbating myocardial ischemia. In addition, positive inotropic agents may cause systolic pressure gradients resulting in asynchrony of contraction and relaxation. Arteriolar-dilating agents may cause severe hypotension due to inadequate preload reserve in cats with this disease. Arteriolar dilation also exacerbates intraventricular gradients.

Dissociative anesthetic agents, such as ketamine hydrochloride, are also potentially deleterious because of the positive chronotropic and negative lusitropic effects of these agents. Similarly, acepromazine maleate is potentially harmful because of its peripheral vasodilating effect. Sodium-containing medications and fluids and sodium-enriched diets should be used cautiously or avoided. Similarly, rapid administration of intravenous fluids can precipitate congestive failure. Finally, it is wise to avoid stressing cats with HCM since stress usually produces an increase in heart rate and contractility. Judicious use of sedative agents such as the benzodiazepines, the narcotics, and etomidate may impose less risk than performing diagnostic procedures without sedation.

22. What is the most effective way to prevent systemic arterial thromboembolism in cats with HCM?

At this time there is no universally and consistently effective method of preventing thromboembolism in cats with HCM. The most appropriate approach to prevention of thromboembolic complications is to improve cardiac function. Although aspirin inhibits platelet aggregation in normal cats and improves collateral circulation in cats with experimentally induced aortic thrombosis, this drug does not prevent systemic arterial thromboembolism in cardiomyopathic cats. Furthermore, aspirin administration may have a significant adverse effect on the renal and circulatory status of cats with congestive heart failure. Warfarin is an alternative to aspirin in cats that are believed to be at high risk for embolic events. Anticoagulation using warfarin is not without adverse effects and necessitates careful monitoring of blood coagulation times.

23. What is the prognosis for cats with HCM?

The prognosis for cats with HCM is quite variable and may be difficult to determine for some patients. Different forms of the disease may carry a different prognosis. For example, Maine coon cats with heritable HCM often have progressive, severe disease, whereas heritable HCM in American shorthair cats is usually more benign. Asymptomatic adult cats with mild to moderate LVH, normal LV diastolic dimension, and minimal left atrial enlargement probably have a good long-term prognosis, although the disease may progress in severity in some of these cats. Asymptomatic cats with moderate to severe hypertrophy and left atrial enlargement are probably at risk of developing heart failure, thromboembolism, or sudden death. However, in human HCM patients reduced LV diastolic dimension is the only morphologic abnormality associated with functional limitation and an unfavorable prognosis. Although cats with congestive heart failure had a median survival time of 3 months in one retrospective study, suggesting a poor prognosis for this group of patients, treatment was not considered in this study. Some cats with congestive heart failure will stabilize on medication and do well for a very long time. Cats with atrial fibrillation, biventricular failure, or systemic thromboembolism have a poor prognosis.

CONTROVERSY

24. Does outflow tract obstruction exist in patients with HCM?

Human patients with HCM often have significant pressure gradients across the left ventricular outflow tract (LVOT) during systole. However, the true physiologic meaning of these gradients is uncertain. LVOT pressure gradients have not been definitively demonstrated in feline HCM patients. Continuous Doppler and color Doppler recordings from some cats with HCM reveal high-velocity turbulent flow in the LVOT, and these Doppler-derived velocity measurements have been used in the modified Bernoulli equation to obtain measurements of gradients. Yet because HCM patients do not have a fixed, discrete obstruction, the validity of the modified Bernoulli equation, which neglects the viscous resistance component and the flow acceleration component of blood flow, is doubtful.

While one can argue over the existence of LVOT gradients in feline HCM patients, a more intriguing controversy is whether such gradients in feline patients or in human patients represent true mechanical obstruction (i.e., a true impediment to flow) or whether these gradients are simply the result of a powerful and rapidly ejecting ventricle. Pressure gradients are produced by acceleration and blood flow, and large gradients can be generated when blood flows at high velocity with little volumetric mass transfer, as is generally the situation during systole in patients with HCM.

Gradients in HCM were initially assumed to represent a mechanical, albeit dynamic, impediment to LV ejection due to a symmetrically hypertrophied interventricular septum. Later, with development of improved radiographic and echocardiographic resolution, anterior displacement of the mitral valve against the septum was noted and this systolic anterior motion (SAM) has become a widely accepted explanation for the outflow tract obstruction that is believed to exist.

However, it is known that pressure gradients can exist in the absence of obstruction. Data discrediting the theory of obstruction in human HCM patients include the fact that there are no differences in the clinical manifestations or in the severity of symptoms between those patients with and those without pressure gradients. This observation appears to be true in feline HCM patients also.

In summary, it is probably accurate to say that subaortic pressure gradients exist in some cats with HCM, particularly those with asymmetric septal hypertrophy. Yet there is little evidence that cats with gradients have LV outflow obstruction. When gradients occur, therapeutic interventions should be directed toward decreasing their magnitude in order to reduce oxygen demand and to improve the synchrony of relaxation and contraction. Gradient reduction may be achieved through the use of either calcium channel blockers or beta-adrenergic blocking agents.

BIBLIOGRAPHY

1. Atkins CE, Gallo AM, Kurzman ID, et al: Risk factors, clinical signs, and survival in cats with a clinical diagnosis of idiopathic hypertrophic cardiomyopathy: 74 cases (1985–1989). JAMA 201:613–618, 1992.
2. Bonagura JD, Stepien RL, Lehmkuhl LB: Acute effects of esmolol on left ventricular outflow obstruction in cats with hypertrophic cardiomyopathy: A Doppler-echocardiographic study. Proc Am Coll Vet Intern Med 9:878, 1991.
3. Bright JM, Golden AL: Evidence for or against the efficacy of calcium channel blockers for management of hypertrophic cardiomyopathy in cats. Vet Clin North Am Small Anim Pract 21:1023–1034, 1991.
4. Bright JM, Golden AL, Daniel GB: Feline hypertrophic cardiomyopathy—variations on a theme. J Small Anim Pract 33:266–274, 1992.
5. Bright JM, Herrtage ME, Schneider JF: Pulsed Doppler assessment of left ventricular diastolic function in normal and cardiomyopathic cats. J Am Anim Hosp Assoc (in press).
6. Johnson LM, Atkins CE, Keene BW, et al: Pharmacokinetic and pharmacodynamic properties of conventional and CD-formulated diltiazem in cats. J Vet Intern Med 10:316–320, 1996.
7. Kittleson MD: Hypertrophic cardiomyopathy In Kittleson MD, Kienle RD (eds): Small Animal Cardiovascular Medicine. St. Louis, Mosby, 1998, pp 347–362.
8. Manganelli F, Betocchi S, Losi MA, et al: Influence of left ventricular cavity size on clinical presentation in hypertrophic cardiomyopathy. Am J Cardiol 83:547–552, 1999.
9. Murgo JP: The hemodynamic evaluation in hypertrophic cardiomyopathy: Systolic and diastolic dysfunction. Cardiovasc Clin 19:193–220, 1988.
10. Murgo JP: Systolic ejection murmurs in the era of modern cardiology—what do we really know? J Am Coll Cardiol 32:1596–1602, 1998.
11. Murgo JP, Miller JW: Hemodynamic, angiographic and echocardiographic evidence against impeded ejection in hypertrophic cardiomyopathy. In Goodwin JF (ed): Heart Muscle Disease. Lancaster, UK, 1985, p 187.
12. Pasipoularides A, Murgo JP, Miller JW, et al: Nonobstructive left ventricular ejection pressure gradients in man. Circ Res 61:220–227, 1987.
13. Peterson EN, Moise NS, Brown CA, et al: Heterogeneity of hypertrophy in feline hypertrophic heart disease. J Vet Intern Med 7:183–189, 1993.
14. Rush JE, Freeman LM, Brown DJ, et al: The use of enalapril in the treatment of feline hypertrophic cardiomyopathy. J Am Anim Hosp Assoc 34:38–41. 1998.
15. Sugrue DD, McKenna WJ, Dickie S, et al: Relation between left ventricular gradient and relative stroke volume ejected in early and late systole in hypertrophic cardiomyopathy. Assessment with radionuclide cineangiography. Br Heart J 52:602–609, 1984.
16. Wilson W, Criley JM, Ross RS: Dynamics of left ventricular emptying in hypertrophic subaortic stenosis. A cineangiographic and hemodynamic study. Am Heart J 73:4–16, 1967.

39. FELINE RESTRICTIVE CARDIOMYOPATHY

Rebecca L. Stepien, D.V.M., M.S.

1. What is the difference between restrictive myocardial diseases and restrictive cardiomyopathy?

Restrictive myocardial diseases are diseases in which diastolic filling of the ventricle is limited by poor relaxation of the ventricular myocardium (a functional abnormality) or poor ventricular compliance (related to the mechanical properties of the myocardium). Restrictive myocardial diseases may occur as a result of systemic disorders (e.g., infiltrative neoplasia or myocardial damage as a result of myocardial infarction) or be primary (idiopathic). The idiopathic form of restrictive myocardial disease is termed restrictive cardiomyopathy (RCM). Idiopathic RCM may involve changes in the myocardium (termed myocardial RCM) or endomyocardium (termed endomyocardial RCM). The etiologies and echocardiographic findings of these two forms of RCM may differ.

2. What is known about the etiologies of the two forms of RCM?

Not enough. In cats, endomyocardial RCM is usually manifest as endomyocarditis (i.e., inflammatory infiltrates are present) or endomyocardial fibrosis. These pathologic findings may result from viral infection, inflammatory, or immune-mediated processes, but clear cause-and-effect relationships have not been documented. In the case of myocardial RCM, myocardial infiltrates are seldom present, and evidence of amyloid or other metabolic storage material within the myocytes (a common finding in human RCM) is also absent. At this point, the etiology of feline myocardial RCM remains obscure. In any case, the end result in most clinical cases is diastolic dysfunction.

3. What is the prevalence of restrictive myocardial disease in cats?

The exact prevalence of feline restrictive myocardial disease is unknown. There are no historical or physical findings that are unique to restrictive myocardial disease in the cat; echocardiography is the only noninvasive means by which a definitive diagnosis may be made. Restrictive myocardial diseases appear to be less common than hypertrophic myocardial disease, but the clinical similarities between these two conditions suggests that echocardiographic evaluation of all cats with clinical evidence of cardiac disease is warranted.

4. Explain the pathophysiology of congestive heart failure due to diastolic dysfunction.

The inability of the myocardium to relax rapidly and/or completely can result in high end-diastolic pressures in the ventricle, even when ventricular volume is normal or small. Atrial pressures rise to overcome the increase in resistance to ventricular filling. Atrial emptying is impaired due to decreased ventricular compliance, further increasing atrial pressures. The inability of the ventricle to relax completely is compounded when tachycardia or tachyarrhythmias are present, because less time is available in diastole for ventricular filling. Lastly, tachycardia in conjunction with ventricular hypertrophy limits the perfusion of the myocardium and resulting ischemia further decreases myocardial compliance. These processes result in elevated atrial pressures and resulting signs of fluid accumulation (e.g., pulmonary edema or pleural effusion) in the presence of reduced stroke volume.

5. What is the clinical presentation of RCM?

Clinical presentation of cats with RCM differs depending on the stage of disease and presence of complications, but it is generally similar to other types of cardiomyopathies. RCM may be diagnosed in animals presented for (1) investigation of a murmur or gallop rhythm noted in an asymptomatic animal; (2) signs of congestive heart failure (i.e., dyspnea, lethargy, weight loss, collapse); or (3) aortic thromboembolism (ATE).

6. How do the clinical findings of this disease differ from those of the other cardiomyopathies?

There is seldom enough information in the history and physical examination findings to differentiate RCM from other cardiomyopathies of cats. Similar to many idiopathic cardiomyopathies, cats with RCM are typically middle-aged to older. RCM cats appear to have ascites as a manifestation of CHF more frequently and may be more prone to develop atrial fibrillation and other arrhythmias than cats with other cardiomyopathies, but the presence of these findings does not rule out other causes of congestive heart failure (CHF). In cases of CHF of any cause, radiographic findings may reveal varying amounts of pulmonary infiltrates with concurrent pulmonary venous and arterial enlargement consistent with cardiogenic edema. The cardiac silhouette is typically enlarged with marked left and right atrial enlargement in cats with RCM; these findings are similar to those of hypertrophic cardiomyopathy (HCM).

7. How is restrictive myocardial disease diagnosed as the cause of a cat's clinical signs?

Echocardiographic findings form the basis of differentiation of restrictive myocardial diseases from other feline cardiomyopathies, including hypertrophic and dilated myocardial diseases.

8. What echocardiographic findings indicate restrictive myocardial disease?

The echocardiographic diagnosis of restrictive myocardial disease is considered if evidence of diastolic dysfunction is present and HCM has been excluded. The diagnosis of idiopathic RCM relies on documentation of the presence of certain anatomic and functional changes and the exclusion of other diagnoses likely to produce similar symptoms. Diastolic dysfunction can be documented by Doppler echocardiography or by inference after evaluating two-dimensional and M-mode echocardiographic findings. Doppler documentation of diastolic function is usually sought through evaluation of the mitral inflow velocity patterns.

9. What does a normal mitral inflow velocity pattern look like, and which patterns indicate diastolic dysfunction?

At normal heart rates, Doppler interrogation of mitral valve inflow usually reveals a biphasic pattern. In early diastole, ventricular pressure is lower than atrial pressure and blood enters the ventricle, resulting in the Doppler E wave on a spectral Doppler tracing. During diastasis, blood flow velocities gradually decrease from the peak pressure of the E wave, then peak again when atrial contraction occurs (the A wave). When heart rates exceed 150 bpm, the E and A waves may merge. This is one factor that can limit the diagnostic utility of Doppler evaluation of diastolic function in small animals. Mitral valve inflow dynamics are highly heart rate– and preload-dependent, but in some circumstances inspection of the E and A waves of mitral inflow can provide useful information with respect to left ventricular diastolic function.

Inflow patterns seen in cases of RCM (when abnormal) are usually typical of a relaxation abnormality or display a restrictive pattern. Relaxation abnormality patterns have decreased E wave amplitude with a decreased acceleration and prolonged deceleration time, increased A wave amplitude and prolonged isovolumetric relaxation time (IVRT). In contrast, restrictive filling patterns have markedly high E wave velocities with shortened deceleration time and low-velocity A waves. Isovolumetric relaxation time is reduced.

10. What two-dimensional or M-mode findings are supportive of diastolic dysfunction?

Diastolic dysfunction is suspected when significant atrial enlargement is present in the absence of valvular disease or systolic dysfunction. Valvular abnormalities are commonly diagnosed as changes in the thickness, length, or motion of the valves or of the supporting structures (e.g., papillary muscles or chordae tendineae). Systolic dysfunction may be ruled out if global measures of contractile function appear to be normal (i.e., normal fractional shortening). It is important to recognize, however, that segmental wall motion abnormalities may occur in cases of RCM or any other cardiomyopathy; in these cases, the measured fractional shortening must be evaluated in context with other echocardiographic and Doppler findings.

11. Differentiate between the echocardiographic appearance of myocardial RCM vs. endomyocardial RCM.
Typical findings of **myocardial RCM** include:
• Severe left or biatrial enlargement
• Normal left ventricular cavity size
• Normal to slightly thickened left ventricular free wall and interventricular septal measurements
• Normal to mildly decreased fractional shortening values
• No evidence of valvular disease (normal-appearing leaflets and supporting structures, minimal or no regurgitation documented by Doppler)
• Atrial "smoke" (spontaneous echo contrast) or an organized thrombus in the atrium
Typical findings of **endomyocardial RCM** include:
• Severe left atrial dilatation and variable right atrial dilatation
• Normal to small left ventricular cavity size
• Normal to slightly thickened left ventricular free wall and interventricular septal measurements
• An echogenic "bridge" across the left ventricular cavity (free wall to septum), often resulting in visible narrowing of the cavity just below the mitral valve. A mid-ventricular systolic velocity gradient may be identified by Doppler examination. This "bridge" represents a fibrous scar of the endocardium (see figure).
• Normal contractile function (usually assessed using fractional shortening)
• Variable right ventricular thickening or dilation
• Atrial "smoke" (spontaneous echo contrast) or an organized thrombus in the atrium
• Other findings may be present in any combination: regional thickening or thinning of the left ventricular walls, variability in the echodensity of the walls ("speckling"), and mild atrioventricular valvular regurgitation.

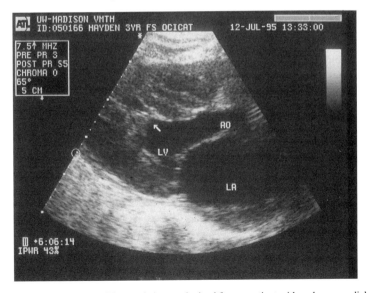

Echocardiographic right parasternal long-axis image obtained from a patient with endomyocardial restrictive cardiomyopathy. Fibrous tissue *(arrow)* bridges the left ventricular lumen; the left atrium (LA) is enlarged.

Occasionally, the echocardiogram of cats with suspected RCM will reveal convincing evidence of diastolic dysfunction but findings do not fit easily into a single category of cardiomyopathy (e.g., ventricular wall thickening is slightly increased or fractional shortening is slightly decreased). These animals are often diagnosed as having "unclassified cardiomyopathy."

12. What therapy is recommended for treatment of RCM with CHF?

Regardless of the type of RCM diagnosed, the primary physiologic abnormality is diastolic dysfunction. The challenge of treating RCM lies in the management of any CHF or arrhythmias that may be present while simultaneously avoiding over-reduction of ventricular filling pressure (i.e., atrial pressure), which can further compromise ventricular filling and limit cardiac output.

Treatment of CHF manifest as pulmonary edema consists of acute administration of oxygen and furosemide. If pleural effusion is present, therapeutic thoracocentesis may be necessary. Chronically, administration of an angiotensin-converting enzyme inhibitor such as enalapril may limit neurohormonal activation and reduce the need for large doses of diuretics. Spironolactone may be helpful in limiting fluid accumulation in animals with ascites. In some cases, administration of digoxin is helpful in controlling heart failure, especially when accompanied by supraventricular arrhythmias such as atrial fibrillation.

13. What antiarrhythmic therapy is recommended for cats with RCM and arrhythmias?

Arrhythmias associated with RCM are often supraventricular in origin (i.e., atrial tachycardia or atrial fibrillation), but ventricular arrhythmias may also occur. Supraventricular arrhythmias can often be controlled with digoxin therapy, but in the case of atrial fibrillation, diltiazem (a calcium channel blocker) or a beta blocker (e.g., atenolol) may be needed to provide additional slowing of the ventricular response rate. One of these drugs is usually added to digoxin if the ventricular response rate to atrial fibrillation remains > 200–220 bpm. Ventricular arrhythmias are most effectively treated with beta blockers such as atenolol, but it is important to note that due to their negative inotropic effects, beta blockers should not be administered until signs of CHF are resolved. In many cases, frequent single ventricular ectopics will resolve with effective therapy of CHF, and do not require direct antiarrhythmic therapy.

14. How can arterial thromboembolism be prevented?

At present, there is no consistently effective and safe therapy for the prevention of aortic thromboembolism (ATE). Aspirin or coumarin are the agents most frequently administered in hopes of preventing ATE but the efficacy of administration of these medications prior to the occurrence of thromboembolism is unknown. Both drugs are associated with side effects, some of which can be life-threatening. Some clinicians base decisions regarding prophylactic use of such agents on the degree of left atrial enlargement or the presence or absence of left atrial "smoke" or an already existing atrial thrombus. At this time, the decision to administer antithrombotic drugs prophylactically is based on clinical experience, tolerance of the drug by the animal, and the willingness and ability of the owner to administer and, in the case of coumarin, participate in chronic monitoring of the drug effects.

15. What is the prognosis for cats with RCM?

Prior to the occurrence of CHF or severe arrhythmias, cats diagnosed with RCM may remain asymptomatic for years, but once CHF has occurred, the prognosis is guarded. Most animals that respond well to therapy for CHF and avoid thromboembolic complications can live comfortably for 3–6 months. Animals with severe recurrent pleural effusions and/or atrial fibrillation may have a worse prognosis.

CONTROVERSY

16. Should asymptomatic cats with RCM receive any treatment?

For: The ventricular dysfunction observed in cats with restrictive myocardial disease of any type is diastolic in nature. Incomplete relaxation of the ventricular muscle in diastole restricts ventricular filling, limiting cardiac output. In addition, incomplete diastolic relaxation of the myocardium may limit myocardial perfusion and lead to the development of myocardial fibrosis and arrhythmias. Medications known to improve diastolic function may lead to faster and more complete ventricular relaxation, improving myocardial perfusion and cardiac output.

Calcium channel blockers (e.g., diltiazem) have been recommended to improve diastolic function in animals with restrictive myocardial diseases. Both beta blockers and calcium channel blockers have been advocated as medications to slow the heart rate and lengthen the time available for ventricular filling and myocardial perfusion. Theoretically, chronic administration of diltiazem would improve diastolic function, improving quality of life and prolonging the period of time before an animal with RCM develops clinical heart failure. Administration of calcium channel blockers or beta blockers would slow the heart rate and improve cardiac output by allowing more time for ventricular filling.

Against: Although the ability of both calcium channel blockers and beta blockers to reduce heart rate is well-accepted, it is unknown whether the theoretic therapeutic properties of these drugs translate into recognizable clinical benefit. There is no evidence at this time that administration of any medications prior to the onset of clinical signs of cardiac disease (e.g., arrhythmias or CHF) in cats with RCM has a beneficial effect. Clinical trials regarding efficacy of these drugs in this setting have not been performed, so the correct dose to achieve the intended effect is unknown.

BIBLIOGRAPHY

1. Fox PR: Feline cardiomyopathies. In Fox PR, Sisson D, Moise NS (eds): Textbook of Canine and Feline Cardiology, 2nd ed. Philadelphia, W.B. Saunders, 1999, pp 621–678.
2. Harpster NK, Baty CJ: Warfarin therapy of the cat at risk of thromboembolism. In Bonagura JD(ed): Kirk's Current Veterinary Therapy XII: Small Animal Practice. Philadelphia, W.B. Saunders, 1995, pp 868–873.
3. International Small Animal Cardiac Health Council: Recommendations for diagnosis of heart disease and treatment of heart failure in small animals. In Fox PR, Sisson D, Moise NS (eds): Textbook of Canine and Feline Cardiology, 2nd ed. Philadelphia, W.B. Saunders, 1999, pp 883–901.
4. Kittleson MD, Kienle RD: Feline unclassified and restrictive cardiomyopathy. In Kittleson MD, Kienle RD (eds): Small Animal Cardiovascular Medicine. St. Louis, Mosby, 1998, pp 363–369.
5. Liu S-K, Fox PR: Cardiovascular pathology. In Fox PR, Sisson D, Moise NS (eds): Textbook of Canine and Feline Cardiology, 2nd ed. Philadelphia, W.B. Saunders, 1999, pp 817–844.
6. Miller MW: Restrictive cardiomyopathy. In August JR (ed): Consultations in Feline Internal Medicine, 3rd ed. Philadelphia, W.B. Saunders, 1997, pp 286–291.
7. Stalis IH, Bossbaly MJ, Van Winkle TJ: Feline endomyocarditis and left ventricular endocardial fibrosis. Vet Pathol 32:122–126, 1995.
8. Stepien RL: Specific feline cardiopulmonary conditions. In Luis Fuentes V, Swift S (eds): BSAVA Manual of Small Animal Cardiorespiratory Medicine and Surgery. Shurdington, UK, British Small Animal Veterinary Association, 1998, pp 244–261.

40. FELINE DILATED CARDIOMYOPATHY

Rebecca L. Stepien, D.V.M., M.S.

1. Differentiate between a dilated heart and dilated cardiomyopathy.

Diseases leading to ventricular dilatation include diseases that lead to myocardial dysfunction (e.g., taurine deficiency), high-output metabolic diseases (e.g., anemia or thyrotoxicosis), intra- and extracardiac shunts, and diseases of the heart valves (e.g., mitral or aortic regurgitation). Ventricular dilatation and decreased systolic function in the absence of an identifiable cause is termed idiopathic dilated cardiomyopathy (DCM). DCM was the second most common clinical cardiomyopathy in cats prior to 1987, but after the relationship between taurine deficiency and DCM in cats had been recognized, most cat foods have been supplemented with taurine. Taurine-deficient DCM, once prevalent, is now diagnosed much less frequently. At present, cats with echocardiographic evidence of cardiac dilatation and decreased systolic function in the absence of systemic or nutritional causes are considered to have idiopathic DCM.

2. What is the pathophysiology of taurine deficiency?

The activity of cysteinesulfinic acid decarboxylase, an enzyme necessary for endogenous taurine synthesis, is low in cats. In addition, conjugation of bile acids with taurine is obligatory in cats. Therefore, if taurine intake is inadequate, taurine body stores are gradually depleted. The myocardium requires taurine for normal structure and function; chronic taurine deficiency results in myocardial failure.

3. How can taurine deficiency be ruled out as a cause of DCM?

At present, a small number of pet cats with DCM are taurine-deficient. Cats at risk include cats eating unusual diets or receiving urinary acidifiers while they are potassium-depleted. Diagnosis of taurine-deficient DCM is established when compatible clinical and echocardiographic signs are present and the whole blood taurine concentration is < 100 nmol/ml. Normal whole blood taurine concentration in cats is > 200 nmol/ml. Whole blood taurine measurement is preferred to plasma taurine measurements due to the daily fluctuations of plasma taurine concentrations that may be seen in normal cats. Central retinal degeneration may be identified in taurine-deficient cats, and usually persists even after taurine repletion.

4. Explain the pathophysiology of congestive heart failure due to systolic dysfunction.

When myocardial contractile function is reduced, the amount of blood remaining in the ventricle at the end of systole (end-systolic volume) is increased. This leads to a volume load on the ventricle and subsequent dilatation. In addition, the increased end-diastolic volume of the ventricle prevents adequate emptying of the atrium during diastole, leading to elevations in atrial pressures and, eventually, signs of heart failure. When dilatation of the ventricle leads to changes in the atrioventricular valve apparatus, mitral or tricuspid regurgitation may increase atrial pressures. Lastly, decreased contractile function decreases cardiac output, resulting in low-output signs, such as exercise intolerance or lethargy.

5. What is the typical clinical presentation of DCM?

Clinical presentation of cats with DCM is similar to other types of cardiomyopathies. DCM may be diagnosed in animals presented for (1) investigation of a murmur or gallop rhythm noted in an asymptomatic animal; (2) signs of congestive heart failure (i.e., dyspnea, lethargy, weight loss, collapse); or (3) aortic thromboembolism (ATE).

6. How do the clinical findings of this disease differ from those of the other cardiomyopathies?

History and physical examination findings in cats with DCM are similar to those of cats with other types of cardiomyopathies. Cats with DCM due to taurine deficiency may have retinal lesions typical of central retinal degeneration, or a history of an unusual diet. Most cases of idiopathic DCM are presented with signs of congestive heart failure (CHF), including dyspnea, pulmonary crackles, muffled heart sounds due to pleural effusion, and hypothermia. Thromboembolism is the presenting sign in about 20% of cases. Radiographic signs of CHF (e.g., pulmonary infiltrates and/or pleural effusion) are similar those to other cardiomyopathies. The cardiac silhouette is typically generally enlarged and may be globoid in appearance. Electrocardiographic abnormalities such as evidence of left atrial or ventricular enlargement are common, as are arrhythmias. Ventricular arrhythmias, especially ventricular tachycardia, may be more frequently seen in DCM than other cardiomyopathies, but the presence of ventricular arrhythmias does not exclude other diagnoses. With the exception of central retinal degeneration, none of these clinical findings or diagnostic test results are specific for idiopathic or taurine-deficient DCM.

7. What is the basis of the arrhythmias that may be seen in cats with DCM?

Atrial premature depolarizations, atrial tachycardia, or atrial fibrillation may occur in cats with DCM due to atrial stretch and fibrosis. Ventricular arrhythmias, including ventricular tachycardia, may occur due to myocardial damage or secondary to hypoxia related to CHF.

8. How is idiopathic DCM diagnosed as the cause of a cat's clinical signs?

Echocardiographic findings form the basis of differentiation of DCM from other feline cardiomyopathies. Once echocardiographic evidence of DCM is documented, taurine deficiency should be ruled out based on whole blood taurine concentration measurement. If taurine concentrations are normal, idiopathic DCM is diagnosed. Therapy of DCM presumptively includes taurine supplementation until taurine deficiency has been ruled out, or lack of response to supplementation has been documented.

9. What echocardiographic findings are diagnostic of DCM?

The echocardiographic criteria for diagnosis of DCM include ventricular dilatation in the presence of reduced systolic function, and in the absence of evidence of valvular or vascular abnormalities. Typical echocardiographic findings in cats with DCM include:
- Severe left or biatrial enlargement
- Left or biventricular dilatation
- Normal to thinned left ventricular free wall and interventricular septal measurements
- Evidence of decreased systolic function
- No evidence of valvular disease (normal-appearing leaflets and supporting structures, minimal or no regurgitation documented by Doppler)
- Atrial "smoke" (spontaneous echo contrast) or an organized thrombus in the atrium

Mitral and/or tricuspid regurgitation may be documented by Doppler, but are usually secondary to distortion of the valvular apparatus related to ventricular dilatation and valve leaflets are normal in appearance.

10. What echocardiographic findings are supportive of systolic dysfunction?

Systolic dysfunction is diagnosed when indices of ventricular contractile function (e.g., fractional shortening, ejection fraction) are decreased in the absence of any other cause of decreased performance (e.g., elevated afterload). Echocardiographic criteria for myocardial failure in cats include a fractional shortening less than 30% and a left ventricular end-systolic measurement of > 12 mm.

11. What therapy is recommended for treatment of DCM with CHF?

Regardless of the cause of DCM, emergency medical therapy of CHF is the same. Treatment focus is on relieving life-threatening dyspnea, support of cardiac output and supportive care of the distressed patient. Relief of dyspnea is accomplished through oxygen administration, tho-racocentesis if significant pleural effusion is present, and administration of injectable furosemide. Dermal nitroglycerin ointment (2%) may be used as an adjunctive therapy. While administration of adequate doses of furosemide may be life-saving, the patient should be closely monitored for dehydration and evidence of decreased cardiac output (e.g., progressive azotemia).

12. What can be done acutely to treat signs of hypotension and low cardiac output, and what are the possible side effects of therapy?

Cardiac output support is provided acutely by administration of intravenous inotropic agents. Dobutamine is preferred to dopamine because it is associated with fewer arrhythmias in the clin-ical setting. Dopamine is administered as a continuous-rate infusion starting at a very low dose (~ 2 µg/kg/min) and titrated to effect (i.e., stronger pulses, better mucous membrane perfusion, increased body temperature) up to 10 µg/kg/min. The most common side effect at higher doses is seizure activity, either focal or generalized. These effects disappear when the drug administration is acutely stopped, and many animals that exhibit seizures during administration of dobutamine can tolerate lower doses when the drug is reintroduced.

13. What supportive measures should be provided for cats with DCM and acute CHF?

Supportive measures include provision of a low-stress environment, minimal handling, and support of body temperature in the form of heating pads. A less common presentation of DCM appears as low cardiac output signs in the absence of congestive signs. These cats are usually significantly dehydrated, and their signs of collapse, lethargy, and hypothermia are fre-quently accompanied by relative bradycardia (heart rates 120–150 bpm). These animals usually respond to judicious administration of intravenous fluids at submaintenance to maintenance rates, with close monitoring for the development of congestive signs. Half-strength saline or half-strength lactated Ringer's solution with potassium supplementation is usually used to limit sodium load.

14. What are the recommendations for chronic therapy of DCM?

Once acute congestive heart failure signs are controlled, chronic therapy for DCM is similar to that recommended for therapy of canine DCM, with the exception of taurine supplementation in taurine-deficient animals. All cats with DCM should receive taurine supplementation until re-sults of taurine concentration measurement are available. Because oral taurine supplementation is generally very safe, taurine should be administered chronically if DCM is diagnosed and mea-sured taurine concentrations are not available.

Chronic therapy of systolic dysfunction consists of furosemide (if CHF is present) and oral digoxin. Angiotensin-converting enzyme inhibitor administration is recommended to decrease afterload and reduce sodium and water retention. Spironolactone may be effective to limit fluid accumulation in animals with refractory heart failure, and prevents further potassium loss. Potassium depletion may occur as a side effect of furosemide administration and inappetence; oral potassium supplements may be administered based on serum electrolyte monitoring.

15. What is the recommended therapy for atrial arrhythmias in cats with DCM?

In most cases of DCM accompanied by atrial arrhythmias, digoxin is the drug of choice for therapy due to its supraventricular antiarrhythmic and positive inotropic effects. Occasional atrial premature complexes (< 40/min) need not be treated primarily and may resolve with resolution of CHF signs. The goal of therapy when atrial tachycardia or atrial fibrillation is present is to de-crease the ventricular rate to < 200–220 bpm. If digoxin administration and resolution of CHF does not resolve the arrhythmia, oral diltiazem (a calcium channel blocker) or an oral beta blocker (e.g., atenolol) may be added to the digoxin therapy. Calcium channel blockers and beta blockers should not be used simultaneously, and beta blockers should not be used until CHF is resolved.

16. How are ventricular arrhythmias treated in cats with DCM?

Acutely, ventricular tachycardia may be treated with lidocaine (0.25–1.0 mg/kg IV bolus over 5 minutes). In many cases, acute oxygen administration or thoracocentesis leads to resolution of hypoxia and related arrhythmias. If ventricular arrhythmias are chronic after resolution of acute CHF, beta blockers (e.g., atenolol) may be used for chronic antiarrhythmic therapy.

17. How does the prognosis for cats with idiopathic DCM differ from those with taurine-deficient DCM?

The prognosis for cats with taurine-deficient DCM is markedly different from that of cats with idiopathic DCM. In both cases, however, the highest mortality occurs during the first few days of congestive heart failure. If acute signs of heart failure can be controlled, cats with idiopathic DCM may survive up to several months, but may not survive more than a few weeks post-CHF. In contrast, cats with taurine-deficient DCM who survive the initial bout of CHF may eventually require no medication at all, as their myocardial function improves in response to taurine supplementation. Traditional therapy for DCM is necessary until systolic function improves; in most cases, echocardiographic improvement can be seen in 6–12 weeks. Decreased left ventricular cavity size and improved fractional shortening are usually seen, but these values may not return to normal. Nonetheless, clinical stability can usually be achieved and cardiac medications may be discontinued. Taurine supplementation should be lifelong in these animals. In any case of DCM, the occurrence of arterial thromboembolism as a complication is a poor prognostic sign.

BIBLIOGRAPHY

1. Atkins CE, Snyder PS, Keene BW, et al: Efficacy of digoxin for treatment of cats with dilated cardiomyopathy. J Am Vet Med Assoc 196:1463–1469, 1990.
2. Fox PR: Feline cardiomyopathies. In Fox PR, Sisson D, Moise NS (eds): Textbook of Canine and Feline Cardiology, 2nd ed. Philadelphia, W.B. Saunders, 1999, pp 621–678.
3. Moise NS, Dietze AE, Mezza LE, et al: Echocardiography, electrocardiography, and radiography of cats with dilatation cardiomyopathy, hypertrophic cardiomyopathy and hyperthyroidism. Am J Vet Res 47:1476–1486, 1986
4. Pion PD, Kittleson MD, Rogers QR, et al: Myocardial failure in cats associated with low plasma taurine: A reversible cardiomyopathy. Science 237:764–768, 1987.
5. Pion PD, Kittleson MD, Thomas WP, et al: Response of cats with dilated cardiomyopathy to taurine supplementation. J Am Vet Med Assoc 201:275–284, 1992.
6. Pion PD, Kittleson MD, Thomas WP, et al: Clinical findings in cats with dilated cardiomyopathy and relationship of findings to taurine deficiency. J Am Vet Med Assoc 201:267–274, 1992.
7. Sisson DD, Knight DH, Helinski C, et al: Plasma taurine concentrations and M-mode echocardiographic measures in healthy cats and in cats with dilated cardiomyopathy. J Vet Intern Med 5:232–2381, 991.
8. Stepien RL, Miller MW: Cardiovascular disease. In Wills JM, Simpson KW (eds): The Waltham Book of Clinical Nutrition of the Dog and Cat. Oxford, Pergamon, 1994, pp 353–371.

41. FELINE ENDOMYOCARDITIS

Maribeth J. Bossbaly, V.M.D.

1. What is endomyocarditis (EMC)?

Endomyocarditis (EMC) is an acute cardiopulmonary disease of cats that may be associated with a recent stressful event (such as neutering, declawing, anesthesia, relocation, or vaccination). The primary pathologic findings are an acute interstitial pneumonia in combination with variable degrees of endomyocardial inflammation.

2. What is the history of EMC?

Liu first described endomyocarditis in 1974. The histopathology was well defined; however, the risk factors and diagnostic criteria were not described until 1994.

3. What is the cause of EMC?

The underlying cause of EMC has not been identified. There also is no evidence to date to prove or disprove that the trigger agent for the lesions in the heart and lungs is the same. Special stains for bacteria and fungi have been negative.

4. Suggest a typical signalment including risk factors that would suggest a diagnosis of EMC.

Cats presenting with EMC are predominantly neutered males between the ages of 1–4. These cats present with an acute onset of dyspnea often following a recent stressful event (5–21 days prior). A seasonal incidence appears to exist for the fall months.

5. What are the physical examination findings of this disease?

Vital signs. Cats with EMC are commonly presented for emergency evaluation of marked dyspnea with increased respiratory rate and effort. The patient may be anxious and distressed. Heart rates are often elevated on physical exam of a patient with EMC. However, tachycardia is not that uncommon in healthy cats in the clinic due to elevated adrenergic tone, which is thought to be related to anxiety. Therefore, tachycardia is a nonspecific finding and may be solely physiologic.

Auscultation. Auscultation often reveals bilateral crackles and an exaggerated respiratory effort. A murmur or gallop may be present and the murmur may vary in quality and intensity. Variable intensity heart sounds may be appreciated due to the extreme effort of breathing. An irregular rhythm is auscultated in cases presenting with an arrhythmia.

Other signs. Evidence for thromboembolic disease may occasionally be present. Generally, these cats have no history of any abnormalities prior to the onset of their acute dyspnea. Signs referable to the thrombosed area would be noted. The aorta and iliac bifurcation are the most common sites in cats with sites such as the forelimbs, kidney, brain, and gastrointestinal tract less common.

6. What abnormalities are detected on the electrocardiogram?

The electrocardiogram (ECG) provides information about the heart rate, rhythm, size, and position in the thorax. The findings are varied and nonspecific for this disease. Sinus tachycardia is commonly seen solely or in combination with other arrhythmias including ventricular premature complexes, atrial premature complexes, bundle branch blocks, and complete atrioventricular block.

7. Describe the radiographic findings in EMC.

The cardiac silhouette may be enlarged with radiographic evidence of minimal left atrial enlargement. Because of the presence of an interstitial pneumonia, pulmonary infiltrates are not uncommon and may be bilateral and severe. In general, the pulmonary changes exceed the degree of cardiomegaly and should make one suspicious of a diagnosis of EMC.

8. What echocardiographic findings typify EMC?

In EMC, the echocardiographic evaluation may reveal changes within the endomyocardium (hyperechogenicity). The incidence of this finding varies and can be very subjective. Diastolic left ventricular wall thickness can be normal to mildly increased (0.6–0.7 cm) with a normal to mild increase in left atrial size (1.5–1.7 cm). Occasionally, Doppler echocardiographic studies of mitral valve inflow suggest diastolic dysfunction, which may result from hypertrophy or endocardial inflammation/fibrosis.

9. How do I make a definitive diagnosis of EMC if most of the findings are nonspecific?

Currently, a definitive diagnosis of EMC can only be made on postmortem examination and requires extensive evaluation of the heart. Clinically, there are no pathognomonic signs but there should be a strong index of suspicion when a young, previously healthy male cat presents with an acute onset of respiratory distress, especially if there is a history of a stressful event occurring days to weeks prior to the onset of clinical signs.

10. Does EMC occur in dogs as well?

EMC is unique to cats. No other disease in any other species is similar; histologically, no other cardiac disease has the distribution of lesions like EMC. EMC is considered by some to be a form of left ventricular endocardial fibrosis (restrictive cardiomyopathy) and to represent temporally different manifestations of a single disease entity.

11. What are the pathologic findings in EMC?

Gross. Typically, at necropsy, cats with EMC have enlarged hearts. The left atrium may be dilated. Opacity of the endocardium within the left ventricle may be quite striking and occasionally red foci of hemorrhage are present.

Histologic. Varying degrees of endocardial inflammation with infiltrates of neutrophils, macrophages, plasma cells, and lymphocytes are seen. Fibroplasia of the endocardium has been the most striking feature reported. These lesions involve predominantly the left side and are typically most severe in the dorsal septal wall of the left ventricle. The interstitial pneumonia produces early lesions characterized by eosinophilic fibrillar material and histiocytes within alveolar spaces. There are various histologic stages identified and the older lesions tend to have type II alveolar cell hyperplasia and interstitial fibrosis (scarring).

12. What are the goals in the treatment of EMC?

Providing an oxygen-rich environment and decreasing stress are of primary importance. Cats that are dyspneic tolerate handling and manipulation poorly. If the cat is anxious due to the severity of the dyspnea, light sedation may be attempted with butorphanol, 0.5 mg/kg subcutaneously or intramuscularly. Because the dyspnea is likely due to the presence of an interstitial pneumonia and not cardiogenic pulmonary edema, judicious use of diuretics is advised to avoid volume depletion and dehydration.

13. Are there any other therapies that are recommended?

The use of steroids, diuretics, and vasodilators has been attempted, but the efficacy of these therapies is unknown. The author has had variable success with initial high-flow oxygen (FiO_2 60–70%) and light sedation in combination with low-dose diuretics, particularly furosemide (0.25–0.5 mg/kg IV q 6–8 hrs). Any specific structural and functional disturbances that are diagnosed via echocardiography and Doppler should be addressed with appropriate therapy. For example, if unequivocal left ventricular hypertrophy is present, diltiazem may be utilized. Arrhythmias should also be addressed in terms of specific therapy.

14. What is the prognosis for a cat that presents with EMC?

Because the etiology of this disease is unknown and very little literature is published, prognosis is unknown. The author has obtained long-term follow-up from the owners of a small number of cats diagnosed with EMC; they reported that the cats were apparently healthy and were not receiving cardiac medications. The author has observed several cats that presented with severe dyspnea that required high-flow oxygen for several days (about 72 hours) before being weaned onto room air. A few cases even required ventilatory support through the critical period.

The difficulty in definitively diagnosing this disease also poses a challenge to appropriate support and treatment implementation. Once a diagnosis of EMC is suspected, it is essential to avoid extensive manipulation and reduce stress. Supportive care with oxygen and other therapies as deemed appropriate should be considered. Overzealous use of diuretics should be avoided. Because of the proposed temporal relationship between EMC and left ventricular fibrosis, owners should be educated and counseled accordingly.

BIBLIOGRAPHY

1. Abbott JA: Feline myocardial disease. In Wingfield WE (ed): Veterinary Emergency Medicine Secrets. Philadelphia, Hanley & Belfus, 1997, pp 194–200.
2. Atkins CE, Gallo AK, Kurzmann ID, Cowen P: Risk factors, clinical signs, and survival in cats with a clinical diagnosis of idiopathic hypertrophic cardiomyopathy: 74 cases (1985–1989). J Am Vet Med Assoc 201:613–618, 1992.
3. Bossbaly MJ, Stalis I, Knight DK, Van Winkle TJ: Feline endomyocarditis: A clinical/pathological study of 44 cases [abstract]. J Vet Intern Med 8:144, 1994.
4. Liu SK: Pathology of feline heart disease. In Kirk RW (ed): Current Veterinary Therapy V. Philadelphia, W.B. Saunders, 1974, pp 341–344.
5. Sammarco CD, Bossbaly MJ: Cardiomyopathy and endomyocardial disease in cats. In Smith FWK Jr, Tilley LP (eds): The 5-Minute Veterinary Consult, 2nd ed. Philadelphia, Lippincott Williams & Wilkins, in press.
6. Stalis IH, Bossbaly MJ, Van Winkle TJ: Feline endomyocarditis and left ventricular endocardial fibrosis. Vet Pathol 32:122–126, 1995.

42. FELINE SECONDARY MYOCARDIAL DISEASES

Betsy R. Bond, D.V.M.

1. What is secondary myocardial disease?

Secondary myocardial disease is a disease of the cardiac muscle rather than the valves, coronary vessels, great vessels, or pericardium and is therefore similar to primary myocardial disease. However, primary myocardial disease has no known initiating cause, whereas secondary myocardial disease occurs secondary to systemic or metabolic abnormalities.

2. What are some examples of secondary myocardial disease in cats?

The two most common examples are thyrotoxic heart disease and hypertensive heart disease. Two rare causes are acromegaly (excessive production of growth hormone) and taurine deficiency.

3. I thought taurine deficiency as a cause of cardiomyopathy was eliminated with additional supplementation of all cat foods since the late 1980s. How could a cat develop taurine deficiency now?

Taurine deficiency can develop in cats that are fed poorly formulated home-made diets, such as vegetarian diets. However, any cat that has an inability to absorb nutrients because of gastrointestinal disease (e.g., infiltrative bowel disease or lymphosarcoma) could also become taurine-deficient.

4. How does hyperthyroidism affect the heart?

Thyroid hormone seems to affect the heart in three ways: (1) directly at the cellular level; (2) indirectly through the sympathetic nervous system; and (3) through derangements of energy metabolism and the peripheral circulation. **Directly**, thyroid hormones stimulate cardiac hypertrophy and increase contractility and heart rate. The indirect effects of the **sympathetic nervous system** are suspected because (1) there are positive inotropic and chronotropic responses that mimic adrenergic stimulation, and (2) hyperthyroid cats respond positively to β-adrenergic blockers. However, this mechanism may be due to increased sensitivity to epinephrine rather than to stimulation of the sympathetic nervous system. **Increased tissue metabolism** causes peripheral dilation and increased blood volume. The resulting increase in stroke volume can elevate blood pressure, but hypertension may be offset by the peripheral dilation. The net effect is a high-output, volume-overloaded state in which the heart is in danger of failing even though cardiac output is maintained.

5. What are typical symptoms and physical findings in a cat with hyperthyroidism?

The most common clinical symptom of a cat with hyperthyroidism is weight loss in spite of a good appetite. Other common symptoms include hyperactivity, vomiting and diarrhea, polyuria and polydypsia, and increased fecal volume. Most cats will also have a palpable nodule in the cervical area on either side of the trachea. Tachycardia (heart rate ≥ 240 beats/minute) and a cardiac murmur are often present on auscultation. Weight loss may or may not be evident.

6. What are the differences between thyrotoxic heart disease and hypertrophic cardiomyopathy?

Hypertrophic cardiomyopathy most properly refers to an idiopathic myocardial disease that is most common in young and middle-aged cats. It is characterized echocardiographically by hypertrophy of a nondilated ventricle in the absence of known cause. Confusion arises occasionally because some cats with cardiac disease secondary to hyperthyroidism have similar echcoardiographic features. Based upon the hemodynamic abnormalities expected in hyperthyroidism, biventricular dilation and hypertrophy would be predicted. However, some cats with hyperthyroidism develop an apparently disproportionate degree of left ventricular hypertrophy and as a result have echocardiographic features that closely resemble diopathic hypretrophic cardiomyopathy. Evaluation of a serum T_4 level is recommended for cats older than 6 years of age that have clinical evidence of cardiovascular disease.

7. How often does congestive heart failure develop in cats with hyperthyroidism?

This complication of hyperthyroidism is currently rare because feline hyperthyroidism is now a well-recognized disorder. The diagnosis is often made early in the course of the disease and complications of severe and unrelenting hyperthyroidism are now uncommon. In fact, when congestive heart failure is observed in hyperthyroid cats, the possibility that pre-existing cardiac disease predisposed the patient to failure should probably be considered.

Because the nature of cardiac dysfunction in hyperthyroid animals with heart failure is not necessarily predictable, diagnostic evaluation should include echocardiographic examination. In fact, congestive heart failure has been documented in hyperthrryoid cats that had echocardiographic findings of ventricular dilation and hypokinesis—features that are typical of dilated cardiomyopathy. Presumably, this echocardioraphic appearance reflected systolic myocardial dysfunction that was a consequence of a chronic, high cardiac-output state. Because systolic myocardial dysfunction resulting from chronic hyperthyroidism may be irreversible, echocardiographic evaluation of animals with heart failure is necessary for the prognostic information that it provides.

8. What cardiovascular changes should I expect to see in cats with thyrotoxic disease and when should a full cardiac work-up (radiographs, ECG, and echocardiogram) be performed?

Cardiomegaly (especially left ventricular enlargement) is often seen on thoracic radiographs. In more advanced stages some cats will also have radiographic evidence of pulmonary edema and/or pleural effusion. Electrocardography reveals tall R-waves with sinus tachycardia. Echocardiographic changes include left ventricular hypertrophy and dilation of the left atrium and ventricle. These changes are much less common now than they were 10 years ago because of increased frequency and earlier screening for hyperthyroidism.

It is usually sufficient to obtain only a thoracic radiograph when the disease is first diagnosed. In specific cases, other tests may be indicated. For example, electrocardiographic evaluation is recommended when physical examination suggests the presence of arrhythmia. Additionally, in those cases in which there is radiographic evidence of congestive heart failure, echocardiographic examination is recommended. In uncomplicated cases, an echocardiogram is indicated if cardiovascular changes remain 2 months after appropriate antithyroid therapy.

9. What is the best method of diagnosing thyrotoxicosis and when should the test be performed?

An elevated serum T_4 concentration is diagnostic for hyperthyroidism in cats, although serum T_4 concentrations can fluctuate in and out of the normal range in some cats. Occasionally, a cat that suffers from another disease may have a falsely low serum T_4 concentration. If there is a strong degree of suspicion that hyperthyroidism is present, the test should be repeated at a later time (i.e., 1–3 months). T_3 suppression and thyrotropin-releasing hormone stimulation tests are also available for cats with suspected hyperthyroidism and a normal T_4. Currently, free T_4 is measured to diagnose occult hyperthyroidism. Any cat older than 6 years of age showing typical symptoms should be tested.

10. Are radionuclide scans useful in evaluating thyroid dysfunction?

Radionuclide scans have the advantages of indicating whether one or both lobes of the thyroid gland are involved and showing whether ectopic thyroid tissue is present. The drawbacks include expense, scarcity of facilities that can perform the scan, and the need for general anesthesia.

11. Are there any other laboratory findings besides an elevated T_4 concentration that are consistent with the diagnosis of hyperthyroidism?

Common serum biochemical abnormalities include high alkaline phosphatase, lactate dehydrogenase, aspartate transaminase, and alanine transaminase.

12. Is there one best treatment for thyroid disease?

There are three basic treatments and each has its advantages and disadvantages.

Surgery. Surgery to remove the affected lobe or lobes has the major advantage of being curative with very little follow-up required. However, surgery is costly and its success depends on the experience of the surgeon. The major problems that can be encountered are failure to remove all diseased tissue and postoperative hypocalcemia that occurs because of inadvertent removal of the parathyroid glands. In addition, if only one lobe is removed, the tumor may reoccur in the remaining lobe at a later time.

Radioactive iodine (^{131}I). This treatment is safe and relatively simple. Its advantages are that it avoids the potential side effects and inconvenience of daily administration of oral medications, as well as the risks associated with surgery. Its two major drawbacks are: (1) it requires a nuclear medicine isolation ward, and (2) it requires boarding at a facility that can properly dispose of radioactive waste.

Medical therapy. The two most common oral medications used to treat hyperthyroidism are methimazole (Tapazole) and propylthiouracil (PTU). Most cats tolerate methimazole better than PTU. The disadvantages of methimazole are that it does not cure the disease, it can cause side effects such as vomiting, anorexia, and lethargy, and it requires frequent monitoring. Serious side effects (anemia, leukopenia, thrombocytopenia) are rare but should they occur, the medication must be discontinued.

One additional concern for all elderly cats regardless of the type of therapy is inducing azotemia as a result of lowering serum T_4 concentrations. Thyroid hormone raises cardiac output, which increases glomerular filtration rate and renal plasma flow. When that stimulation is removed, azotemia or renal failure can result. Therefore, therapy with methimazole should be instituted and renal function followed prior to irreversible treatments (surgery or radioactive iodine).

13. What adjunctive therapy should be administered for cats that are in congestive heart failure or extremely tachycardic (heart rates persistently > 240 bpm)?

Furosemide should be administered for pulmonary edema or pleural effusion, and beta-adrenergic blockers for tachyarrhythmias. The dose of furosemide should be tailored to the need of the cat in balancing dehydration while preventing heart failure. Atenolol is a beta-adrenergic blocker that is effective in lowering the heart rate. I usually start at a dose of 6.25 mg per cat ($\frac{1}{4}$ of a 25 mg tablet) and adjust it gradually upward until a target heart rate of < 180 bpm is achieved. These medications can usually be discontinued once antithyroid medications bring serum T_4 concentrations back to normal levels. Therapy of congestive heart failure due to thyrotoxic heart disease is ideally based upon radiographic and echocardiographic findings. In selected cases, afterload-reducing agents and even digoxin may be indicated.

14. How is methimazole administered and what kind of monitoring does it require?

Methimazole is initially administered at a dose of 5–15 mg/day divided twice daily. After 2–3 weeks, follow-up examination and serum T_4, CBC, platelet count, and serum chemistry profile are performed. The dose of methimazole is adjusted according to serum T_4 levels; repeat levels are drawn every 2–3 weeks until serum T_4 concentrations are in the normal range. Methimazole should be discontinued if agranulocytosis, thrombocytopenia, anemia, or azotemia occur. Since adverse effects usually occur within the first 3 months of therapy, recheck examinations should be scheduled every 2–3 weeks during that time and every 2–3 months thereafter.

15. Are there alternative medications if severe adverse effects occur?

Sodium ipodate may be used in cats at a dose of 100 mg once daily, that cats seem to tolerate well with few side effects. Its major disadvantage is that it must be specially formulated.

One important distinction is that serum T_4 concentrations remain elevated during treatment with ipodate, so efficacy of the drug is monitored using serum T_3 concentrations.

16. Why do I need to be worried about hypertension in cats?

Hypertension has been shown to be common in cats with chronic renal disease, and occasionally hyperthyroidism. It can cause retinal detachment and acute blindness, cardiac hypertrophy, and vascular disease, among other things. These conditions are potentially reversible with therapy.

17. What is a good therapy for hypertension?

Several drugs have been tried and found lacking as single agents. They include beta-adrenergic blockers, short-acting calcium channel blockers, and angiotensin-converting enzyme inhibitors. The best single agent so far is amlodipine (Norvasc), a long-acting calcium channel blocker that affects the blood vessels but has very little effect on the heart. The dosage is ¼ of a 2.5 mg tablet once daily. The blood pressure is rechecked in 1–2 weeks, and the dosage adjusted according to response. The dosage can be adjusted upward by increasing to ½ tablet once daily or ¼ tablet twice daily. Because the tablets crumble easily, administering ½ tablet is often the better option.

18. What is the effect of systemic hypertension on the heart?

Systemic hypertension that results from elevated vascular resistance imposes a pressure overload on the left ventricle. Compensatory concentric hypertrophy, i.e., hypertrophy without chamber dilation, is the expected result. The hypertrophied ventricle is stiffer than normal, which can impair ventricular filling and lead to atrial dilation. The echocardiographic appearance of hypertensive heart disease is therefore characterized by left ventricular hypertrophy and sometimes atrial dilation. In most cases, the cardiac abnormalities are relatively mild and congestive heart failure due to hypertensive heart disease is uncommmon.

19. Is it feasible for a small practice to own a blood pressure machine?

It is very feasible, although the technique of obtaining blood pressure measurements in cats requires some expertise. A good unit unit for a small practice is an ultrasonic (Doppler) unit model 811-BL from Parks Medical Electronics Inc., Aloha, OR. It is relatively inexpensive, about $600 per unit. It does not measure diastolic pressure, but this is not a major drawback in animals.

20. What is acromegaly and how does it affect the heart?

Acromegaly is a rare condition in cats in which there is chronic hypersecretion of growth hormone by a pituitary tumor. In addition to causing insulin-resistant diabetes mellitus, it can cause cardiomegaly, left ventricular hypertrophy, and congestive heart failure. Treatment consists of surgery, radiotherapy, or medical therapy. Surgery is not an option for most cats because of the location of the tumor, and many hospitals do not have access to radiotherapy. Further investigation into medical therapy is needed. In addition, elevated serum growth hormone concentrations has been reported to be elevated in cats with hypertrophic cardiomyopathy compared with normal cats and cats with other cardiac disease, but the connection is unknown.

21. What is doxorubicin and why should we be concerned about it?

Doxorubicin is an anthracycline antibiotic used as chemotherapeutic agent against certain neoplasias. In dogs it causes dose-related atrial and ventricular arrhythmias, dilated cardiomyopathy, and congestive heart failure.

22. Does doxorubicin cause the same degree of cardiotoxicity in cats as it does in dogs?

Cats seem to be relatively resistant to adverse effects of doxorubicin, but electrocardiograms and radiographs should be closely monitored during and after therapy. Some symptoms of toxicity may only become apparent months after completion of therapy.

BIBLIOGRAPY

 1. Binns SH, Sisson DD, Buoscio DA, et al: Doppler ultrasonographic, oscillometric sphygmomanometric, and photoplethysmographic techniques for noninvasive blood pressure measurement in anesthetized cats. J Vet Intern Med 9:405–414, 1995.
 2. Birchard SJ, Peterson ME, Jacobson A: Surgical treatment of feline hyperthyroidism: Results of 85 cases. J Am An Hosp Assoc 20:705–709, 1984.
 3. Bond BR, Fox PR, Peterson ME, et al: Echocardiographic findings in 103 cats with hyperthyroidism. J Am Vet Med Assoc 192:1546–1549, 1988.
 4. DiBartola SP, Broome MR, Stein BS, et al: Effect of treatment of hyperthyroidism on renal function in cats. J Am Vet Med Assoc 208:875–878, 1996.
 5. Ferguson DC: Free thyroid hormone measurements in the diagnosis of thyroid disease. In Kirk RW, Bonagura JD (ed): Current Veterinary Therapy XII: Small Animal Practice. Philadelphia, W.B. Saunders, 1995, pp 360–364.
 6. Fox PR, Peterson ME, Broussard JD: Electrocardiographic and radiographic changes in cats with hyperthyroidsm: Comparison of populations evaluated during 1992–1993 vs. 1979–1982. J Am Anim Hosp Assoc 35:27–31, 1999.
 7. Grandy JL, Dunlop CI, Hodgson DS, et al: Evaluation of the Doppler ultrasonic method of measuring systolic arterial blood pressure in cats. Am J Vet Res 53:1166–1169, 1992.
 8. Graves TK, Peterson ME: Occult hyperthyroidism in cats. In Kirk RW, Bonagura JD (ed): Current Veterinary Therapy XI: Small Animal Practice. Philadelphia, W.B. Saunders, 1992, pp 334–337.
 9. Hansen B: Blood pressure measurement. In Kirk RW, Bonagura JD (ed): Current Veterinary Therapy XII: Small Animal Practice. Philadelphia, W.B. Saunders, 1995, pp 110–112.
10. Henik RA, Snyder PS, Volk LM: Treatment of systemic hypertension in cats with amlodipine besylate. J Am An Hosp Assoc 33:226–234, 1997.
11. Jacobs G, Panciera D: Cardiovascular complications of feline hyperthyroidism. In Kirk RW, Bonagura JD (ed): Current Veterinary Therapy XI: Small Animal Practice. Philadelphia, W.B. Saunders, 1992, pp 756–759.
12. Kittleson MD, Pion PD, DeLellis LA, et al: Increased serum growth hormone concentration in feline hypertrophic cardiomyopathy. J Vet Int Med 6:320–324, 1992.
13. Kobayashi DL, Peterson ME, Graves TK, et al: Hypertension in cats with chronic renal failure or hyperthyroidism. J Vet Int Med 4:58–62, 1990.
14. Lesser M, Fox PR, Bond BR: Assessment of hypertension in 40 cats with left ventricular hypertrophy by Doppler-shift sphygmomanometry. J Small Anim Pract 33:55–58, 1992.
15. Littman MP: Spontaneous systemic hypertension in 24 cats. J Vet Intern Med 8:79–86, 1994.
16. Moise NS, Dietze AE: Echocardiographic, electrocardiographic, and radiographic detection of cardiomegaly in hyperthyroid cats. J Am Vet Res 47:1487–1494, 1986.
17. Murray LAS, Peterson ME: Ipodate treatment of hyperthyroidism in cats. J Am Vet Med Assoc 211:63–67, 1997.
18. Peterson ME: Propylthiouracil in the treatment of feline hyperthyroidism. J Am Vet Med Assoc 179:485–487, 1981.
19. Peterson ME, Keene B, Ferguson DC, et al: Electrocardiographic findings in 45 cats with hyperthyroidism. J Am Vet Med Assoc 179:934–937, 1982.
20. Peterson ME, Kintzer PP, Cavanagh PG, et al: Feline hyperthyroidism: Pretreatment clinical and laboratory evaluation of 131 cases. J Am Vet Med Assoc 183:103–110, 1983.
21. Peterson ME, Hurvitz AI, Leib MS, et al: Propylthiouracil-associated hemolytic anemia, thrombocytopenia, and antinuclear antibodies in cats with hyperthyroidism. J Am Vet Med Assoc 184:806–808, 1984.
22. Peterson ME, Becker DV: Radionuclide thyroid imaging in 135 cats with hyperthyroidism. Vet Radiol 25:23–27, 1984.
23. Peterson ME, Kintzer PP, Hurvitz AI: Methimazole treatment of 262 cats with hyperthyroidism. J Vet Int Med 2:150–157, 1988.
24. Peterson ME, Taylor RS, Greco DS, et al: Acromegaly in 14 cats. J Vet Int Med 4:192–201, 1990.
25. Peterson ME, Gamble DA: Effect of nonthyroidal illness on serum thyroxine concentrations in cats: 494 cases (1988). J Am Vet Med Assoc 197:1203–1208, 1990.
26. Turrel JM, Feldman EC, Hays M, et al: Radioactive iodine therapy in cats with hyperthyroidism. J Am Vet Med Assoc 184:554–559, 1984.
27. Thoday KL, Mooney CT: Medical management of feline hyperthyroidism. In Kirk RW, Bonagura JD (ed): Current Veterinary Therapy XI: Small Animal Practice. Philadelphia, W.B. Saunders, 1992, pp 338–345.

43. MYOCARDITIS

Michael B. Lesser, D.V.M.

1. What is myocarditis?

Myocarditis is inflammation of the heart muscle. It is most often caused by infectious agents affecting the myocytes, cardiac vascular structures, and interstitium. Viral, bacterial, rickettsial, fungal, and protozoal infections have all been associated with myocardial inflammation.

2. What causes the myocardial inflammation?

Direct invasion of the myocardial tissue, toxin production, and immune-mediated myocardial damage can all be involved in myocardial inflammation. *Trypanosoma cruzi* leads to granulomatous changes, while viral disease is associated with immune-mediated changes. Systemic vasculitis may affect the vascular structures of the heart (i.e., coronary structures).

3. Who is affected by myocarditis?

Dogs and cats are both susceptible to myocardial inflammation. Young dogs in the southeastern U.S. have been reported with myocarditis caused by *Trypanosoma cruzi* (Chagas' disease), while dogs from Texas have been reported with myocarditis caused by *Hepatozoon canis*. Cats may develop myocarditis associated with *Toxoplasma gondii* or feline infectious peritonitis (FIP). Very young dogs may develop myocarditis associated with parvovirus, distemper virus, and herpesvirus. Parvoviral infection within the first few weeks of life has been associated with dilated cardiomyopathy at 5–6 months of age. Systemic fungal illnesses such as coccidioidomycosis, cryptococcosis, and aspergillosis may lead to fungal myocarditis. Lyme disease may also be associated with myocarditis. Any animal with severe systemic sepsis may develop myocardial involvement and myocarditis. Immunosuppressed patients, such as those on chemotherapy and FELV/FIV–positive cats, may be particularly susceptible to myocardial inflammation secondary to systemic illness.

4. When should I suspect myocarditis?

Any time an animal has the onset of a cardiovascular abnormality associated with a systemic illness, myocarditis should be suspected. Exercise intolerance, weakness, labored breathing, and coughing are all signs associated with myocardial dysfunction. Arrhythmias with or without concurrent myocardial dysfunction can be seen with myocarditis. Young dogs with a history of severe viral illness, in particular parvovirus, and those living in the southeastern U.S. that develop heart disease should be suspect of having myocarditis. Cats with systemic signs of FIP or toxoplasmosis may develop cardiac dysfunction secondary to myocardial involvement. Idiopathic acute nonsuppurative myocarditis has been described in young cats in association with sudden death.

5. What diagnostic tests should be performed if myocarditis is suspected?

1. **Auscultation** may reveal a systolic or diastolic murmur or a gallop rhythm (usually S_3). Auscultation may reveal no abnormalities if there is limited myocardial dysfunction.

2. **Electrocardiography** may detect ventricular and supraventricular tachyarrhythmias as well as various degrees of AV block in patients with myocarditis. Patterns associated with chamber enlargement may be seen with cardiomegaly.

3. **Thoracic radiographs** may show signs associated with congestive heart failure, such as pulmonary edema, pleural effusion, and cardiomegaly. Pulmonary granulomas may be visible in fungal or other granulomatous diseases. The cardiac silhouette may be normal if the damage to the myocardium is limited.

4. **Echocardiography:** With severe myocardial inflammation the myocardium may become hyokinetic. Patchy areas of inflammation may lead to regional dyskinesis. Grossly the myocardium has mottled echogenicity with both hypoechoic and hyperechoic areas. These changes in myocardial echogenicity may be subtle and difficult to appreciate.

5. **Endomyocardial biopsy** is the most definitive way of documenting myocardial inflammation. Inflammatory cells, fungal elements, protozoa, and other infectious agents may all be seen within the endomyocardial biopsy specimen. The tissues should be evaluated by a pathologist experienced in reading heart muscle samples.

6. **Laboratory tests:** CBC, complete biochemical profile, and urinalysis should be performed in all patients suspected of having myocarditis. Appropriate serology should be performed based on the index of suspicion for involvement of infectious agents.

6. How should I treat myocarditis?

The treatment of myocarditis should be twofold. First, the underlying cardiac abnormalities must be addressed. Arrhythmias should be treated with appropriate antiarrhythmic therapy. Congestive heart failure is treated with a combination of furosemide, ACE inhibitors, and digoxin based on the degree of myocardial dysfunction. Second, the underlying inciting cause of the myocardial inflammation needs to be addressed. If an infectious agent is diagnosed, appropriate antimicrobial or antifungal treatment should be instituted. In the case of doxorubicin myocarditis, the therapy should be discontinued. In the case of systemic immune-mediated disease associated with myocarditis, appropriate immunosuppressive therapy is indicated.

7. What is the prognosis in cases of myocarditis?

The extent of myocardial damage present at the time of the diagnosis often determines the long-term outcome. Severe myocardial dysfunction has a guarded prognosis. Severe arrhythmias that are difficult to control also have a guarded prognosis. If the underlying inciting agent related to the myocardial inflammation is determined, there is a better chance of reducing further damage to the myocardium. Unfortunately, the cause for many cases of suspected myocarditis cannot be definitively diagnosed. The extent of damage can be severe and irreversible by the time some patients are first seen. However, early diagnosis and treatment may significantly improve the survival of patients with myocarditis when detected prior to significant myocardial damage.

BIBLIOGRAPHY

1. Lesser MB: Myocarditis. In Tilley LP, Smith FP (eds): The 5-Minute Veterinary Consult. Baltimore, Williams & Wilkins, 1997, pp 850-851.
2. Fox PR: Myocardial diseases. In Ettinger SJ (ed): Textbook on Veterinary Internal Medicine, 3rd ed. Philadelphia, W.B. Saunders, 1989.
3. Liu SK: Cardiovascular pathology. In Fox PR (ed): Canine and Feline Cardiology. New York, Churchill-Livingstone, 1988.

44. TRAUMATIC MYOCARDITIS

Jonathan A. Abbott, D.V.M.

1. What is traumatic myocarditis?

Traumatic myocarditis is a syndrome of arrhythmias associated with blunt trauma. By definition, myocarditis is inflammation of the myocardium, which is unlikely to be present in typical cases; in fact, direct trauma to the heart, which is probably unnecessary for the development of this syndrome, is more likely to result in contusion or necrosis than inflammation. However, despite its limitations, the term traumatic myocarditis has become accepted; it is generally used to denote the electrocardiographic abnormalities that can be associated with blunt trauma in the dog. Usually, the trauma is the result of the animal being hit by a car.

2. How can the heart be harmed by blunt trauma?

Blunt trauma can harm the heart through any of the following mechanisms: (1) unidirectional forces (a "blow" to the heart); (2) bidirectional or compressive forces; (3) decelerative forces; and (4) concussive forces—forces that are sufficient to result in the development of arrhythmias but not in structural damage of the heart.

The role of direct trauma to the heart should not be overemphasized. It is unlikely that thoracic trauma is required to produce the syndrome of traumatic myocarditis. In the author's experience the syndrome is produced as readily by abdominal or pelvic trauma as it is by thoracic injury.

3. What is the typical signalment of patients with traumatic myocarditis? Do cats suffer from traumatic myocarditis?

Traumatic myocarditis is most commonly observed in medium- and large-breed dogs that have sustained trauma in road accidents. Small dogs may also develop this syndrome although this seems to be less common. Possibly this is because larger dogs are more likely than small dogs to survive a traffic accident even after sustaining substantive trauma. Cats seem less subject to the development of arrhythmias in association with extracardiac disease than dogs; the syndrome of traumatic myocarditis is not generally recognized in the cat.

4. What type of arrhythmias are most commonly encountered in patients that have sustained blunt trauma?

All manner of arrhythmias have been associated with blunt trauma in the dog. Ventricular tachyarrhythmias develop most commonly, but supraventricular tachyarrhythmias and even bradyarrhythmias, including AV block, have been observed in association with trauma. Most often, the arrhythmias of traumatic myocarditis take the form of premature ventricular complexes, paroxysmal ventricular tachycardia, or runs of accelerated idioventricular rhythm.

5. What is an accelerated idioventricular rhythm and how is it different from ventricular tachycardia? Why is it important to distinguish them?

Electrocardiographically, ventricular rhythms are recognized by QRS morphology. While supraventricular complexes are narrow or of short duration, ventricular complexes are wide and typically have a bizarre configuration. Cardiac rhythms that originate from the ventricles are common in patients that have sustained blunt trauma. Often, however, these ventricular rhythms are relatively slow. The terminology of slow ventricular rhythms is confusing. Idioventricular tachycardia (or accelerated idioventricular rhythm) is used to refer to cardiac rhythms that arise from the ventricles but are not so fast as to constitute a tachycardia. These rhythms might arise from subsidiary pacemakers within the ventricles. When ventricular pacemaker tissue is responsible for the cardiac rhythm, the term idioventricular rhythm is used. For example, the slow ventricular escape rhythm that is observed in patients with third-degree AV block is referred to as an idioventricular rhythm. Typically, the intrinsic rate of the idioventricular rhythm in the dog is about 40 bpm. It is possible that the slow ventricular rhythms that are observed in patients that have sustained trauma are rapid idioventricular rhythms, thus the terms idioventricular tachycardia or accelerated idioventricular rhythm are used. The intuitively comprehensible oxymoron "slow ventricular tachycardia" has also been applied to these arrhythmias.

Idioventricular tachycardias are distinct from true ventricular tachycardias in that they are relatively slow; often, the rate is similar to that of the sinus node. Unlike ventricular tachycardia, idioventricular tachycardias are usually initiated by late diastolic complexes rather than by truly premature ventricular complexes. In other words, the first complex of a run of idioventricular tachycardia follows a short pause in the rhythm. Because the ventricular rhythm begins after a pause and has a rate that is similar to that of the sinus node, fusion complexes are common. The ventricular rhythm often begins and ends with a fusion complex (see figure on following page).

Idioventricular tachycardia is slower than ventricular tachycardia although the rate that distinguishes these rhythms is not clear. It has been suggested that idioventricular tachycardias are those ventricular rhythms that have rates that are between 60 and 100 bpm; ventricular tachycardias have rates greater than 100 bpm. These limits were likely extrapolated from criteria used to classify similar rhythms in people. In dogs, heart rates less than 160 bpm are considered to be normal. Therefore, using a similar conceptual basis, it is probably appropriate to consider ventricular tachycardias in the dog to be those rhythms that originate from the ventricles and have rates greater 160 bpm; accelerated idioventricular rhythm have rates between 80 and 160 bpm.

There is certainly overlap between ventricular tachycardia and idioventricular tachycardia. Idioventricular tachycardias are perhaps best typified by their behavior. The rate is usually slow and similar to that of the sinus node; fusion complexes are common, and may begin and end the ventricular rhythm. The rate that the idioventricular tachycardia adopts often seems depend on autonomic influences; in a single patient, ventricular rhythms with similar or identical QRS morphology may accelerate or decelerate. In contrast, ventricular tachycardias are typically rapid, regular, and are initiated by premature ventricular complexes.

The distinction between the two is important because idioventricular tachycardias are usually benign; they cause little in the way of hemodynamic compromise and seldom seem to degenerate to lethal arrhythmias such as ventricular fibrillation. Thus the recognition of idioventricular rhythms as distinct from ventricular tachycardia has important therapeutic implications.

6. What is the etiopathogenesis of traumatic myocarditis? Is cardiac injury necessary for the development of arrhythmias?

The cause of traumatic cardiac arrhythmias is not known. It is unlikely that direct trauma to the heart is required. Extracardiac factors including electrolyte derangements, acid-base disturbance, and hypoxia may play a role. Additionally, disordered autonomic traffic might contribute to the development of traumatic arrhythmias; for example, adrenergic stimulation of Purkinje fibers at a time when the sinus node is restrained by parasympathetic influence could explain the electrocardiographic appearance of some traumatic arrhythmias.

7. What kind of monitoring is suggested for patients with traumatic myocarditis?

Careful monitoring of the vital signs through the physical examination is advisable for all patients that have sustained trauma. When arrhythmias are detected, it is recommended that they be elucidated electrocardiographically. Many of the ventricular arryhthmias observed in association with trauma are slow and presumably benign. However, it is important to recognize that potentially dangerous ventricular tachycardias can also develop in the setting of blunt trauma. For some patients, conscientious neglect is appropriate; for others, therapy and continuous electrocardiographic monitoring is indicated.

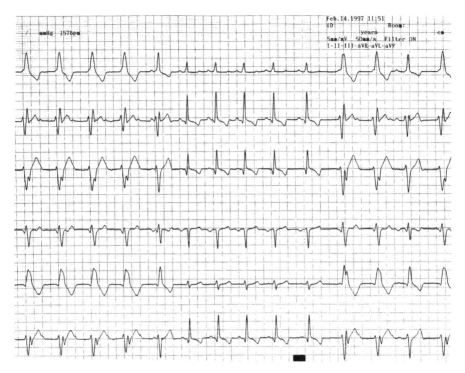

Multichannel electrocardiographic recording obtained from a Labrador retriever that had been hit by a car 36 hours previously. Following a short period of accelerated idioventricular rhythm (AIVR), the sinoatrial node "captures" the rhythm for the space of five complexes after which the ventricular rhythm is again evident. The rate of the ventricular rhythm is about 150 bpm. Particularly in leads I, III, and aVF, the final complex of the first period of AIVR differs from the others and careful inspection reveals that it is preceded by a P wave—it is a fusion complex. The second period of AIVR begins following a short pause in the sinus rhythm; the third and possibly the second complex of this ventricular rhythm are fusion complexes. Note that the rate of AIVR is actually slower that the sinus rate. (Recorded at 50 mm/sec; leads I, II, III, aVR, aVL, and aVF are shown from top to bottom, 5 mm = 1 mV.)

8. What is the time course of development of arrhythmias associated with trauma?

Although the natural history of traumatic myocarditis is not well described, the arrhythmias typically develop 24 hours or more after the accident. Electrocardiograms recorded on presentation of dogs that have sustained blunt trauma are usually normal or demonstrate sinus tachycardia associated with shock.

9. How is traumatic myocarditis treated?

When the patient's clinical status allows, initial efforts are directed toward alleviating extracardiac abnormalities that can contribute to the development of arrhythmias. For example, hypoxia associated with pneumothorax can be reduced or eliminated through thoracocentesis. Pain management is also important and the judicious use of narcotics can have indirect, beneficial effects on the cardiac rhythm. Electrolyte derangements, acid-base disturbances and other extracardiac abnormalities should also be addressed.

10. What about antiarrhythmic drug therapy?

The therapy of ventricular arrhythmias is a controversial topic and poses a challenging problem of risk vs. benefit assessment. Antiarrhythmic agents are not completely benign; many are negatively inotropic and all can occasionally worsen arrhythmias. The latter phenomenon is known as proarrhythmia.

An accurate electrocardiographic diagnosis is crucial to the reasoned approach to arrhythmia management. In the author's opinion, the need to pharmacologically treat single ventricular ectopic complexes is questionable and the author never does so unless there is compelling evidence that the premature complexes are impairing systemic perfusion. Slow ventricular tachycardia with a rate less than 180 bpm is usually well tolerated. Pharmacologic antiarrhythmic therapy is indicated when there are clinical signs of poor perfusion or when clinical signs can reasonably be anticipated based upon the electrocardiographic character of the arrhythmia. For example, it is reasonable to assume that a sustained ventricular tachycardia with a rate of 240 bpm will ultimately lead to hemodynamic decompensation, if not death; in this case, antiarrhythmic therapy is reasonable even in the absence of clinical signs.

When rapid ventricular tachycardia is observed, the intravenous administration of lidocaine is the initial treatment of choice. When the administration of lidocaine fails to effect conversion to sinus rhythm or slow the ventricular rate adequately, alternative antiarrhythmic agents such as procainamide, esmolol, or even bretyllium should be considered.

11. What is the prognosis for patients with traumatic myocarditis?
The prognosis for traumatic myocarditis is generally good. While it is not to say that the syndrome is completely benign, most dogs recover within 5–7 days of trauma and this is probably true irrespective of whether or not antiarrhythmic therapy is initiated.

BIBLIOGRAPHY

1. Abbott JA: Traumatic myocarditis. In Bonagura JD (ed): Current Veterinary Therapy XII: Small Animal Practice. Philadelphia, W.B. Saunders, 1995, pp 846–850.
2. Abbott JA, King RR: Third-degree atrioventricular block following nonpenetrating chest trauma in a dog. J Small Anim Pract 34:377–380, 1993.
3. Alexander JW, Bolton GR, Koslow GL: Electrocardiographic changes in nonpenetrating trauma to the chest. J Am Anim Hosp Assoc 11:160, 1975.
4. Macintire DK, Theron TG: Cardiac arrhythmias associated with multiple trauma in dogs. J Am Vet Med Assoc 184:541–545, 1984.
5. Madewell BR, Nelson DT, Hill K: Paroxysmal atrial fibrillation associated with trauma (traffic accident) in a dog. J Am Vet Med Assoc 171:273–275, 1977.

45. PERICARDIAL DISEASE

Wendy A. Ware, D.V.M., M.S.

1. What is the normal structure and function of the pericardium?

The pericardium is a double-layered sac that encases the heart and is attached to the great vessels at the heartbase. It consists of an outer fibrous layer (parietal pericardium) and an inner serous membrane covering the heart (visceral pericardium or epicardium). A small amount of clear, serous fluid is normally present between these layers and acts to reduce friction. The pericardium limits acute distention of the heart and maintains normal cardiac position, geometry, and ventricular compliance. The pericardium also forms a barrier to inflammation or infection of surrounding structures.

2. Do congenital pericardial malformations often cause clinical problems?

Peritoneopericardial diaphragmatic hernia (PPDH) is the most common pericardial malformation in dogs and cats. Abnormal embryonic development (probably of the septum transversum) allows persistent communication between the pericardial and peritoneal cavities at the ventral midline. The pleural space is not involved. Other congenital defects, such as umbilical hernia, sternal malformations, and cardiac anomalies also may be present. Males appear to be affected more frequently than females. The malformation is common in cats as well. Clinical signs are variable and result from herniation of abdominal contents into the pericardial space.

Pericardial cysts are rare anomalies thought to originate from abnormal fetal mesenchymal tissue or from incarcerated omental or falciform fat from a small PPDH. Other congenital defects of the pericardium itself are extremely rare in dogs and cats; most are discovered incidentally on postmortem examination. Both partial (usually on the left side) and complete absence of the pericardium have been reported.

3. How is PPDH diagnosed?

Clinical signs associated with PPDH usually develop within the first year or so of life, but can appear at any age (cases have been diagnosed between 4 weeks and 15 years of age). Some animals never develop clinical signs and are diagnosed fortuitously. Clinical signs are usually gastrointestinal or respiratory. Vomiting, diarrhea, anorexia, weight loss, abdominal pain, cough, dyspnea, and wheezing are most often reported; shock and collapse can also occur. The physical examination may indicate muffled heart sounds on one or both sides of the chest, displacement or attenuation of the apical precordial impulse, an "empty" feel on abdominal palpation (with herniation of many organs), and rarely, signs of cardiac tamponade.

Thoracic radiography is often diagnostic or highly suggestive of PPDH. Characteristic findings include enlargement of the cardiac silhouette with dorsal tracheal displacement, overlap of the diaphragmatic and caudal heart borders, and abnormal fat and/or gas densities within the cardiac silhouette. On lateral view, a pleural fold is usually evident, extending between the caudal heart shadow and the diaphragm ventral to the caudal vena cava. Gas-filled loops of bowel crossing the diaphragm into the pericardial sac, a small liver, or few organs within the abdominal cavity may also be observed. Echocardiography is useful in confirming the diagnosis in cases in which the diagnosis is equivocal. A gastrointestinal barium series is diagnostic if stomach and/or intestines are in the pericardial cavity. Fluoroscopy, nonselective angiography (especially if only falciform fat or liver has herniated), celiography, or pneumopericardiography also have been used in diagnosis. Electrocardiographic changes are inconsistent; decreased amplitude complexes and axis deviations caused by cardiac position changes sometimes occur.

4. What is the recommended treatment for PPDH?

In symptomatic animals, therapy involves surgical closure of the peritoneal-pericardial defect after returning viable organs to their normal location. The presence of other congenital abnormalities and the animal's clinical signs may influence the decision to operate. The prognosis in uncomplicated cases is excellent. Older animals without clinical signs may do well without surgery. Trauma to organs chronically adhered to the heart or pericardium during attempted repositioning is a potential concern in older animals.

5. In what ways can a structurally normal pericardium become diseased?

The accumulation of excess or abnormal fluid is the most common pericardial disorder. Pericardial effusion occurs more commonly in dogs compared to cats. Constrictive pericardial disease is recognized occasionally in dogs, but rarely in cats.

6. What types of fluid accumulate in the pericardium?

In dogs, most pericardial effusions are serosanguinous or sanguinous. The fluid usually appears dark red, with a packed cell volume of over 7%, a specific gravity over 1.015, and a protein concentration between 3–6 g/dl. Mostly red blood cells are found on cytology, but reactive mesothelial, neoplastic, or other cells may be seen. The fluid does not clot unless the effusion resulted from very recent hemorrhage.

Transudates, modified transudates, and exudates are found occasionally in both dogs and cats. Pure transudates are clear, with a low cell count (less than 2500 cells/µl), specific gravity (less than 1.012), and protein content (less than 1 g/dl). Modified transudates may appear slightly cloudy or pink-tinged; cellularity is low but the specific gravity (1.015–1.030) and total protein concentration (2–5 g/dl) are higher than in a pure transudate. Exudates appear cloudy to opaque, or serofibrinous to serosanguinous. The white cell count (over 15,000/µl), specific gravity (over 1.015), and protein concentration (over 3 g/dl) are high. Cytologic findings are related to the etiology.

7. Most pericardal effusions in dogs are hemorrhagic. What are the typical causes?

Dogs older than 7 years are likely to have neoplastic hemorrhagic effusion. Hemangiosarcoma is by far the most common neoplasm causing hemorrhagic pericardial effusion in dogs. Hemorrhagic pericardial effusion also results from various heartbase tumors and pericardial mesotheliomas. Hemangiosarcomas usually arise from the right atrial wall, especially in the auricular area. Chemodectoma, arising from chemoreceptor cells at the base of the aorta, is the most common heartbase tumor. Other heartbase tumors also can occur, including thyroid, parathyroid, lymphoid, or connective tissue neoplasms. Pericardial mesotheliomas are uncommon but have been reported in dogs and cats.

Idiopathic (so-called "benign") pericardial effusion has been described most frequently in medium-to-large breeds of dogs. The German shepherd, golden retriever, Great Dane, and Saint Bernard may be predisposed. Although dogs of any age can be affected, most are 6 years old or younger. Evidence of mild inflammation is common and pericardial fibrosis can result with time.

Other causes of intrapericardial hemorrhage include left atrial rupture secondary to severe mitral insufficiency, coagulopathy (e.g., warfarin-type rodenticides), and penetrating trauma (including iatrogenic laceration of a coronary artery during pericardiocentesis).

8. What conditions cause pericardial transudates and exudates?

Transudative effusions can be caused by congestive heart failure, pericardioperitoneal diaphragmatic hernias, hypoalbuminemia, pericardial cysts, or toxemias that increase vascular permeability (including uremia). Usually these conditions are associated with small volumes of pericardial effusion and cardiac tamponade is uncommon.

Exudates are rarely found in small animals. Pericarditis is unusual in association with systemic infections; but infectious pericarditis has been reported with actinomycosis, disseminated tuberculosis, *Pasturella multocida* and other bacterial infections, coccidioidomycosis, and rarely systemic protozoal infections. Sterile exudative effusions have occurred with leptospirosis, canine distemper, and idiopathic benign pericardial effusion in dogs, and with feline infectious peritonitis and toxoplasmosis in cats. Chronic uremia occasionally causes a sterile, serofibrinous or hemorrhagic effusion in animals.

9. How does pericardial disease in cats differ from that in dogs?

Cases of acquired pericardial disease are uncommon in cats; of these, pericardial effusion from feline infectious peritonitis is most often identified. Effusions secondary to congestive heart failure (especially hypertrophic cardiomyopathy), lymphoma, systemic infections, and rarely, renal failure are also found in cats. Hemangiosarcoma involving the heart is uncommon.

10. Does pericardial effusion always cause problems?

Unless intrapericardial fluid pressure rises to meet or exceed normal cardiac filling pressure, the accumulation of fluid within the pericardial space has little to no clinical consequence. When fluid accumulates slowly, the pericardium can distend to accommodate the increased volume and still maintain low intrapericardial pressure. As long as intrapericardial pressure is low, cardiac filling and output remain relatively normal. However, pericardial tissue is relatively noncompliant; therefore, rapid fluid accumulation or very large effusions cause intrapericardial pressure to rise quickly. Pericardial fibrosis and thickening further limit the compliance of this tissue. When intrapericardial pressure rises toward and above normal atrial and venous pressures cardiac filling is compromised resulting in a syndrome known as cardiac tamponade. Aside from the hemodynamic consequences, very large pericardial effusions occasionally cause clinical signs from lung and/or tracheal compression (dyspnea and cough) or esophageal compression (dysphagia or regurgitation).

11. When is cardiac tamponade present?

The relatively inelastic pericardium causes a steep intrapericardial pressure–volume relationship when effusion accumulates quickly. Cardiac tamponade develops when the presence of pericardial fluid raises intrapericardial pressure toward and above cardiac diastolic pressure. This externally compresses the heart and progressively limits filling, causing a fall in cardiac output. Eventually, the pressures in all cardiac chambers and great veins equilibrate during diastole.

12. What are the main consequences of cardiac tamponade?

As tamponade develops and cardiac output decreases, neurohumoral compensatory mechanisms of heart failure are activated. Signs of systemic venous congestion become especially prominent with time. Low cardiac output, arterial hypotension, and poor perfusion of other organs as well as the heart can ultimately lead to cardiogenic shock and death. The rate of pericardial fluid accumulation and the distensibility of the pericardial sac determine whether and how quickly cardiac tamponade develops. Rapid accumulation of even small volumes can markedly raise intrapericardial pressure, since the pericardium can stretch only slowly. The presence of a large volume of pericardial fluid implies a gradual process. Although cardiac contractility is not directly affected by pericardial effusion, reduced coronary perfusion during tamponade can impair both systolic and diastolic function.

13. Are there characteristic clinical manifestations of cardiac tamponade?

Clinical findings in animals with cardiac tamponade reflect poor cardiac output and right-sided (most commonly) congestive heart failure. Congestive failure arises from compensatory volume retention, as well as the direct effects of impaired cardiac filling. Right-sided signs predominate because of the right heart's thinner walls and low pressures, although signs of biventricular failure may occur. Nonspecific clinical signs, such as lethargy, weakness, poor exercise tolerance, or inappetence may be noted before obvious ascites develops. However, rapid accumulation of even small volumes of fluid (50–100 ml) can cause acute tamponade, shock, and death. In such cases, pulmonary edema, jugular venous distention, and hypotension may be evident without signs of pleural and peritoneal effusions or enlargement of the cardiac silhouette.

Historical findings of weakness, exercise intolerance, abdominal enlargement, tachypnea, syncope, and cough are typical. Significant loss of lean body mass occurs in some chronic cases. Jugular vein distention and/or positive hepatojugular reflux, hepatomegaly, ascites, labored respiration, and weakened femoral pulses are common physical examination findings. A palpable decrease in arterial pulse strength during inspiration (pulsus paradoxus) might be discernable in some cases. High sympathetic tone commonly produces sinus tachycardia, pale mucous membranes, and prolonged capillary refill time. The precordial impulse is palpably weak with a large pericardial fluid volume. Heart sounds are muffled in animals with moderate-to-large pericardial effusions. Lung sounds are muffled ventrally with pleural effusion. Pleural effusion and ascites are also common signs in cats with cardiac tamponade. Although pericardial effusion does not cause a murmur, concurrent cardiac disease may do so. Fever may be associated with infectious pericarditis.

14. What is pulsus paradoxus?

Cardiac tamponade exaggerates the normal respiratory variation in arterial blood pressure; this phenomenon is known as pulsus paradoxus and is recognized clinically as an inspiratory decrease in the strength of the arterial pulse. Inspiration reduces intrapericardial and right atrial pressures relative to pressures within the great veins; this facilitates right heart filling and therefore, right ventricular output. Simultaneously, the reduction in pleural pressure decreases the pulmonary vein–left atrial pressure gradient and impedes left ventricular filling. The interventricular septum bulges leftward because of the inspiratory increase in right ventricular filling; consequently, left heart output and systemic arterial pressures decrease during inspiration. The variation in systolic arterial pressure is greater than 10 mmHg in animals with cardiac tamponade and pulsus paradoxus.

15. What is the role of radiography in the diagnosis of pericardial disease?

Thoracic radiography is useful for detecting the enlarged cardiac silhouette resulting from pericardial fluid accumulation. Massive pericardial effusion causes the "classic" round, globoid-shaped cardiac shadow ("basketball heart") seen on both views. Other findings associated with tamponade include pleural effusion, caudal vena cava distension, hepatomegaly, and ascites. Pulmonary opacities compatible with edema and distended pulmonary veins are unusual; in fact, the reduced right ventricular output usually results in pulmonary hypoperfusion. Some heartbase tumors cause deviation of the trachea or a soft tissue mass effect. Metastatic lung lesions are common in dogs with hemangiosarcoma.

16. What is the role of echocardiography in the diagnosis of pericardial disease?

Echocardiography allows rapid detection of pericardial fluid and may document an underlying neoplasm or other cardiac condition. Therefore, it is the diagnostic test of choice when it is available.

17. What other diagnostic techniques are available?

Other radiographic techniques are less commonly used. Fluoroscopy demonstrates diminished-to-absent motion of the cardiac shadow, since the heart is surrounded by fluid. Angiocardiography is currently used only rarely for the diagnosis of pericardial effusion and cardiac tumors because of the wide availability of echocardiography; however, it typically reveals increased endocardial-to-pericardial distance. Cardiac neoplasms can cause displacement of normal structures, filling defects, and angiographic vascular "blushing". Echocardiography has also essentially replaced the use of pneumopericardiography in the evaluation of animals with pericardial effusion. For pneumopericardiography, CO_2 or air is injected into the drained pericardial sac to outline the heart. Radiographs are taken from different orientations, but the left lateral and dorsoventral views are most helpful because they allow the injected gas to outline the right atrial and heart base areas, respectively, where tumors are most common.

Central venous pressure (CVP) measurement may be useful in some cases, especially if jugular veins are difficult to assess or it is unclear whether right heart filling pressures are elevated. A CVP above 10–12 cm H_2O is common with pericardial disease; normally CVP is < 8 cm H_2O.

18. Is a large, round cardiac silhouette on radiographs pathognomonic for pericardial effusion?

While a large "globoid" cardiac silhouette is often seen, this totally round heart shape is not observed in many cases. Smaller volumes of pericardial fluid accumulation allow various cardiac contours to be identified, especially those associated with the atria. Conversely, other cardiac diseases besides large volume pericardial effusion can cause the cardiac silhouette to become very large and rounded, for example, dilated cardiomyopathy or tricuspid valve dysplasia.

19. Are there typical electrocardiographic changes that occur with pericardial disease?

Although there are no pathognomonic ECG findings, the following abnormalities are suggestive of pericardial effusion: diminished amplitude QRS complexes (less than 1 mV in dogs), electrical alternans, and ST segment elevation (suggesting an epicardial injury current). Sinus tachycardia is common in association with cardiac tamponade. Atrial and/or ventricular tachyarrhythmias may also occur.

20. So, what is electrical alternans?

Electrical alternans is a recurring alteration in the size of the QRS complex (or sometimes the T wave) with every beat. It results from the heart physically swinging back and forth within the pericardium and is most often associated with a large volume of pericardial fluid. Electrical alternans may be most evident at heart rates between 90 and 140 bpm or in certain body positions (e.g., standing rather than lateral recumbency).

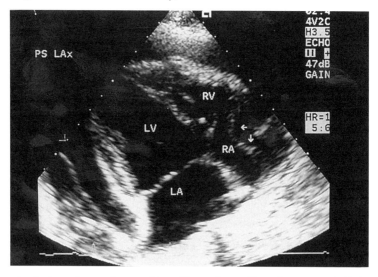

Two-dimensional echocardiogram from an older golden retriever with cardiac tamponade. Pericardial fluid surrounds the heart and collapse of the right atrial wall is apparent (arrows). Right ventricular size is also compromised. Right parasternal long axis view; LA, left atrium; LV, left ventricle; RA, right atrium; RV, right ventricle.

21. What's so great about echocardiography?

Echocardiography is highly sensitive for detecting even small volumes of pericardial fluid. Since fluid is sonolucent, pericardial effusion appears as an echo-free space between the bright parietal pericardium and the epicardium (see figure above). Abnormal cardiac wall motion and chamber shape, and intrapericardial or intracardiac mass lesions can also be imaged (see figure below). Diastolic compression or collapse of the right atrium and sometimes right ventricle, is consistent with cardiac tamponade. It is important to remember that the volume of the effusion is not the main determinant of hemodynamic compromise, but rather how fast it has accumulated.

The right ventricular and atrial walls are often well visualized and may appear hyperechoic due to the surrounding fluid. Better visualization of the heartbase and mass lesions is generally obtained before pericardiocentesis is performed.

Identification of the parietal pericardium in relation to the echo-free fluid helps differentiate pleural from pericardial effusion. Most pericardial fluid accumulates near the cardiac apex, since the pericardium adheres more tightly to the heartbase; there is usually little fluid behind the left atrium. Furthermore, evidence of collapsed lung lobes or pleural folds can often be seen within pleural effusion. Sometimes pleural effusion, a markedly enlarged left atrium, a dilated coronary sinus, or persistent left cranial vena cava can be confused with pericardial effusion. Careful scanning from several positions helps differentiate these conditions.

A complete two-dimensional echo examination is important to screen for mass lesions. All portions of the right atrium and auricle, right ventricle, ascending aorta, and pericardium itself should be carefully evaluated. The left cranial transducer position is especially useful for examining the right atrium and auricle. Transesophageal echocardiography is a sensitive technique that is well suited to the detection of intrapericardial mass lesions.

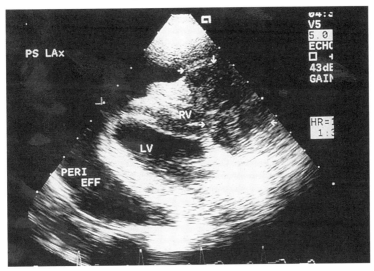

Echocardiogram from a 10-year-old Schnauzer/poodle mix (right parasternal long axis view). A large volume of pericardial effusion (peri eff) is seen around the heart. A 3 × 4.5 cm tumor mass (small arrows) arising from the right atrium is seen adjacent and dorsal to the compressed right ventricle. LV, left ventricle; RV, right ventricle.

22. What if I don't have access to echocardiography?

In most cases, the presence of cardiac tamponade is strongly suggested by the clinical history and physical examination. Radiographic findings usually support the clinical suspicion. Suggestive ECG findings may also be present. If the patient's condition appears stable and referral for echocardiography is feasible, then that can be pursued for definitive diagnosis. However, if the patient with suspected tamponade has severe signs, pericardiocentesis should be done immediately. If a catheter system is used for this, pneumopericardiography can be done after initial drainage if desired.

23. Since cardiac tamponade causes ascites and other signs of right heart failure, isn't treatment with furosemide, a vasodilator, and digoxin appropriate?

It is important to differentiate cardiac tamponade from other causes of right-sided heart failure since the treatment is very different. Diuretics and vasodilators, by reducing cardiac filling pressure, can further diminish cardiac output and exacerbate hypotension and shock. Digoxin and other positive inotropic drugs do not improve cardiac output or ameliorate the signs of tampon-ade, since the underlying pathophysiology is impaired cardiac filling, not poor contractility. Pericardiocentesis is the therapeutic procedure of choice. It also provides diagnostic information. Signs of congestive heart failure usually resolve quickly after intrapericardial pressure is reduced by fluid removal. In some animals a diuretic may be of limited value after pericardiocentesis. Pericardial effusions secondary to other diseases causing congestive heart failure, congenital malformations, or hypoalbuminemia do not usually cause tamponade and often resolve with management of the underlying condition.

24. What is the best initial treatment for cardiac tamponade?
Pericardiocentesis!

25. How can I safely drain the pericardial space?
Pericardiocentesis is a relatively safe procedure when carefully performed. Local anesthesia is used. Sedation may be helpful depending on the clinical status and temperament of the animal; struggling or moving by the patient is to be avoided. An ECG monitor should be attached for the procedure, since needle/catheter contact with the heart commonly causes ventricular arrhythmias.

A variety of equipment can be used for pericardiocentesis. A butterfly needle or appropri-ately long hypodermic or spinal needle attached to extension tubing is adequate in emergency sit-uations. A safer alternative, which reduces the risk of cardiopulmonary laceration during fluid aspiration, is an over-the-needle catheter system (e.g., Angiocath). An 18–20-gauge (1.5–2" long) needle (depending on patient size) is easy to use as long as the needle-catheter unit is advanced well into the pericardial space so that the catheter is not deflected out of the pericardium as the needle is removed. Larger over-the-needle catheter systems (e.g., 12–16-g, 4–6") allow for faster fluid removal in large dogs; a few additional small side holes can be cut (smoothly) near the tip of the catheter to facilitate flow. During initial catheter placement the extension tubing is attached to the needle stylet; after the catheter is advanced into the pericardial space and needle removed, the extension tubing is attached directly to the catheter. For all methods a three-way stopcock is placed between the tubing and a collection syringe.

26. How should the animal be positioned?
Pericardiocentesis is usually done from the right side of the chest to minimize risk of trauma to the lungs (by using the area of the cardiac notch) and major coronary vessels (which are lo-cated mostly on left).The patient is usually placed in left lateral or sternal recumbency to allow more stable restraint, especially if the animal is weak or excitable. Good success can also be had using an elevated echocardiography table with a large cut-out; the animal is placed in right lateral recumbency and the tap is performed from underneath. The advantage with this method is that gravity pulls fluid down to the right side; but, if adequate space is not available for wide sterile skin preparation or needle/catheter manipulation, this approach is not advised. Echo guidance can be used, but is not necessary unless the effusion is of very small volume or appears com-partmentalized. Sometimes needle pericardiocentesis can be successfully performed while the animal is standing or in sternal recumbency, but the risk of injury is increased if the animal sud-denly moves.

27. How is the pericardial tap performed?
Shave and surgically prepare the skin over a wide area of the right precordium (from about the third to seventh intercostal spaces and from sternum to costochondral junction). Using sterile gloves and aseptic technique, locate the puncture site by palpating for where the cardiac impulse is strongest (usually between the fourth and sixth ribs just lateral to the sternum). The lateral tho-racic radiograph can be helpful in making an initial determination of an appropriate site for peri-cardiocentesis. Local anesthesia is necessary when using larger catheters and recommended for needle pericardiocentesis. Infiltrate 2% lidocaine (with sterile technique) at the skin puncture site, underlying intercostal muscles, and into the underlying pleura. A small stab incision is made

in the skin to allow catheter entry. Remember to avoid the intercostal vessels just caudal to each rib when entering the chest.

Once the needle has penetrated the skin, the operator's assistant should gently apply negative pressure to the attached syringe as the operator slowly advances the needle toward the heart. It sometimes helps to aim the tip of the needle toward the patient's opposite elbow. Be sure to observe the tubing so that fluid will be seen as soon as it is aspirated. Pleural fluid (usually straw-colored) may enter the tubing first. The pericardium creates increased resistance to needle advancement and may produce a subtle scratching sensation. With gentle pressure, advance the needle through the pericardium; a loss of resistance may be noted with needle penetration and pericardial fluid (usually dark red) will appear in the tubing. If the needle contacts the heart a scratching or tapping sensation is usually felt, the needle may move with the heartbeat, and ventricular premature complexes are provoked; the needle should be retracted slightly. Avoid excessive needle movement within the chest. If a catheter system is used, after the needle/stylet is well within the pericardial space advance the catheter, remove the stylet, and attach the extension tubing to the catheter. Remember to save initial fluid samples for cytology and microbiologic culture, then aspirate as much fluid as possible.

28. Oh, oh... This fluid looks like blood—is it from inside the heart?

Pericardial effusion usually looks quite hemorrhagic, especially in dogs, and it may be disconcerting to see dark, bloody fluid being aspirated from so near the heart. But, pericardial fluid can be differentiated from intracardiac blood in several ways. Unless there was very recent hemorrhage into the pericardium, the fluid will not clot. If the clinical status of the patient allows, it is sometimes helpful to place a small aliquot of the effusion, 3 or 4 ml, into a serum tube and then wait a short time. If a clot does not develop in the serum tube, it is safe to continue aspirating from the pericardium. In addition, the PCV of the pericardial fluid is usually less than that of peripheral blood, and when spun in a hematocrit tube the supernatant is xanthochromic (yellow-tinged). Furthermore, as pericardial fluid is drained, the patient's ECG complexes increase in amplitude, tachycardia diminishes, and the animal often takes a deep breath and appears more comfortable.

29. What complications can occur from pericardiocentesis?

Complications of pericardiocentesis include ventricular tachyarrhythmias from direct myocardial injury or puncture; these are usually self-limiting when the needle is withdrawn. Coronary artery laceration with myocardial infarction or further bleeding into the pericardial space can occur but is uncommon, especially when pericardiocentesis is done from the right side. Lung laceration causing pneumothorax and/or hemorrhage is also a potential complication during the procedure. In some cases, dissemination of infection or neoplastic cells into the pleural space may occur.

30. Can I tell from the pericardial fluid what the underlying cause is?

Pericardiocentesis usually yields a hemorrhagic effusion; less frequently the fluid is suppurative or transudative. Samples should be submitted for cytologic analysis and saved for possible bacterial (or fungal) culture. However, differentiation of sanguinous neoplastic effusions from benign hemorrhagic pericarditis is usually impossible on the basis of cytology alone. Reactive mesothelial cells within the effusion may closely resemble neoplastic cells; furthermore, chemodectomas and hemangiosarcomas may not shed cells into the effusion.

Analysis of pericardial fluid pH can be helpful in differentiating benign inflammatory pericarditis from neoplastic and other noninflammatory causes of pericardial effusion. Neoplastic effusions tend to have a pH of 7.0 or greater, while in non-neoplastic, inflammatory disease (usually benign idiopathic pericarditis) pH values are often less than 7.0. Dogs with pericardial effusion secondary to congestive heart failure or atrial rupture also have pericardial fluid pH values similar to arterial blood (> 7.0). If cytology and fluid pH suggest an infectious/inflammatory cause, the pericardial fluid should be cultured. Fungal titers (e.g., coccidioidomycosis) or other serologic tests may be helpful in some cases.

31. How should a dog with idiopathic, "benign" pericardial effusion be managed after initial pericardiocentesis?

Dogs with idiopathic pericarditis are initially treated conservatively. Medical therapy may consist of a glucocorticoid (e.g., prednisone, 1 mg/kg/day PO tapering over 2–4 weeks) after ruling out infectious causes by pericardial fluid culture or cytology. The efficacy of this therapy in preventing recurrent idiopathic pericardial effusion is not known, however.

Periodic reevaluation of animals using radiography or echocardiography is advised to detect recurrence. Apparent recovery occurs after one or two pericardial taps in about half of affected dogs. Cardiac tamponade recurs after a variable time (days to years) in other cases. Effusion that recurs after 2 or 3 pericardiocenteses and antiinflammatory therapy is treated by surgical subtotal pericardiectomy. Removal of the pericardium ventral to the phrenic nerves allows drainage to the larger absorptive surface of the pleural space. In general, creation of only a small pericardial window is not recommended.

32. For neoplastic pericardial effusions, what are the treatment options?

Neoplastic effusions are also initially drained to relieve cardiac tamponade. Therapy may involve attempted surgical resection or surgical biopsy, chemotherapy, or conservative therapy until episodes of cardiac tamponade become unmanageable. Surgical resection of hemangiosarcoma is often not possible because of the size and extent of the tumor, although small tumors involving only the tip of the right auricle have been successfully removed. If hemangiosarcoma is diagnosed or strongly suspected on the basis of clinicopathologic and echocardiographic findings, chemotherapy (e.g., doxorubicin, cyclophosphamide, with or without vincristine) may provide some palliation. Partial pericardiectomy may avert recurrence of tamponade; however, metastatic dissemination throughout the thoracic cavity may be facilitated by this procedure. Pericardial mesothelioma also disseminates widely throughout the pleural space after pericardiectomy. Prognosis is generally poor in dogs with hemangiosarcoma or mesothelioma.

Heartbase tumors (e.g., chemodectoma) tend to be slow-growing and locally invasive, with low metastatic potential. Partial pericardiectomy may prolong the life of affected dogs for months to years. Because of local invasion, complete surgical resection is rarely possible, but biopsy is indicated if chemotherapy is contemplated. Effusion secondary to myocardial lymphoma often responds to pericardiocentesis and chemotherapy.

33. What is constrictive pericardial disease?

Constrictive pericardial disease occurs when visceral and/or parietal pericardial thickening and scarring restrict ventricular diastolic filling. Fusion of the parietal and visceral pericardial layers can occur and obliterate the pericardial space, or the visceral layer (epicardium) alone can be involved. Sometimes a small amount of pericardial effusion is present (constrictive-effusive pericarditis). Histologically there is usually increased fibrous connective tissue and variable amounts of inflammatory and reactive infiltrates. The etiology of constrictive pericardial disease is often unknown. Acute inflammation with fibrin deposition and perhaps varying degrees of pericardial effusion are thought to precede the development of constrictive disease. Specific causes identified in some dogs include recurrent idiopathic hemorrhagic effusion, infectious pericarditis (e.g., actinomycosis, mycobacteriosis, coccidioidomycoses), metallic foreign bodies in the pericardium, tumors, and idiopathic osseous metaplasia and/or fibrosis of the pericardium.

With advanced constrictive disease, ventricular filling is essentially limited to early diastole before ventricular expansion is abruptly curtailed. Any further ventricular filling is accomplished only at high venous pressures. Compromised filling reduces cardiac output. Compensatory mechanisms of heart failure cause fluid retention, tachycardia, and vasoconstriction.

34. How do I diagnose constrictive pericardial disease?

Diagnosis of constrictive pericardial disease can be difficult. Clinical signs of right-sided congestive heart failure predominate and abdominal distention (ascites), dyspnea or tachypnea, tiring, syncope, weakness, and weight loss are common owner complaints. Occasionally there is a history of pericardial effusion. As with cardiac tamponade, ascites and jugular venous distention are the most consistent clinical findings. Weakened femoral pulses and muffled heart sounds are also found. An audible, diastolic pericardial knock, resulting from the abrupt deceleration of ventricular filling in early diastole has been described, but has not been commonly identified in dogs. A systolic murmur or click, probably caused by concurrent valvular disease, or a diastolic gallop sound may be heard.

Radiographic findings include mild-to-moderate cardiomegaly, pleural effusion, and caudal vena cava distension. Reduced cardiac motion may be evident on fluoroscopy. Constrictive pericardial disease can produce subtle but suggestive echocardiographic changes, such as flattening of the left ventricular freewall in diastole and abnormal septal motion. The pericardium may appear thickened and intensely echogenic, but differentiation of this from normal pericardial echogenicity may be difficult. ECG abnormalities have included sinus tachycardia, P-wave prolongation, and small QRS complexes.

Invasive hemodynamic studies are the most diagnostic. Central venous pressures of over 15 mmHg and high mean atrial and diastolic ventricular pressures are common. The classic early diastolic dip in ventricular pressure, followed by a middiastolic plateau, is not consistently seen in dogs with constrictive pericardial disease, however. Angiocardiography can be normal or it may reveal atrial and vena caval enlargement, and increased endocardial-pericardial distance.

35. How is constrictive pericardial disease treated?
Constrictive pericardial disease is treated by surgical pericardiectomy. The procedure is more likely to be successful if only the parietal pericardium is involved. Visceral pericardial involvement requires epicardial stripping which increases the difficulty and associated complications of surgery. Pulmonary thrombosis (sometimes massive) is reported to be a relatively common postoperative complication. Tachyarrhythmias are another complication of surgery. Moderate doses of diuretics may be helpful in the postoperative period, but positive inotropic and vasodilating drugs are not indicated. Without surgical intervention the disease is progressive and ultimately fatal.

BIBLIOGRAPHY

1. Aronsohn M: Cardiac hemangiosarcoma in the dog: A review of 38 cases. J Am Vet Med Assoc 187:922–926, 1985.
2. Berg J: Pericardial disease and cardiac neoplasia. Semin Vet Med Surg 9:185–191, 1994.
3. Berry CR, Lombarde CW, Hager DA, et al: Echocardiographic evaluation of cardiac tamponade in dogs before and after pericardiocentesis: Four cases (1984–1986). J Am Vet Med Assoc 192:1597–1603, 1988.
4. Bouvy BM, Bjorling DE: Pericardial effusion in dogs and cats. Part I. Normal pericardium and causes and pathophysiology of pericardial effusion. Compend Contin Educ 13:417–424, 1991.
5. Bouvy BM, Bjorling DE: Pericardial effusion in dogs and cats. Part II. Diagnostic approach and treatment. Compend Contin Educ 13:633–641, 1991.
6. Edwards NJ: The diagnostic value of pericardial fluid pH determination. J Am Anim Hosp Assoc 32:63–67, 1996.
7. Kerstetter KK, Krahwinkel DJ, Millis DL, et al: Pericardiectomy in dogs: 22 cases (1978–1994). J Am Vet Med Assoc 211:736–740, 1997.
8. Miller MW, Sisson DD: Pericardial disorders. In Ettinger SJ, Feldman EC (eds): Textbook of Veterinary Internal Medicine, 5th ed. Philadelphia, W.B. Saunders, 2000, pp 923–936.
9. Rush JE, Keene BW, Fox PR: Pericardial disease in the cat: A retrospective evaluation of 66 cases. J Am Anim Hosp Assoc 26:39–46, 1990.
10. Sisson D, Thomas WP, Ruehl WW, et al: Diagnostic value of pericardial fluid analysis in the dog. J Am Vet Med Assoc 184:51–55, 1984.
11. Thomas WP, Reed JR, Bauer TG, et al: Constrictive pericardial disease in the dog. J Am Vet Med Assoc 184:546–553, 1984.
12. Thomas WP, Reed JR, Gomez JA: Diagnostic pneumopericardiography in dogs with spontaneous pericardial effusion. Vet Radiol 25:2–16, 1984.
13. Thomas WP, Sisson D, Bauer TG, et al: Detection of cardiac masses in dogs by two-dimensional echocardiography. Vet Radiol 25:65–72, 1984.
14. Wallace J, Mullen HS, Lesser MB: A technique for surgical correction of peritoneal pericardial diaphragmatic hernia in dogs and cats. J Am Anim Hosp Assoc 28:503–510, 1992.
15. Ware WA: Cardiac neoplasia. In Bonagura JD (ed): Kirk's Current Veterinary Therapy XII. Philadelphia, W.B. Saunders, 1995, pp 873–876.
16. Wright KN, DeNovo RC, Patton CS, et al: Effusive-constrictive pericardial disease secondary to osseous metaplasia of the pericardium in a dog. J Am Vet Med Assoc 209:2091–2095, 1996.

46. COR PULMONALE

Steven L. Marks, B.V.Sc., M.S., MRCVS

1. What is cor pulmonale?

Cor pulmonale is the term used to describe right-sided heart disease that results from lung or pulmonary vessel pathology; in either case, it is the consequence of abnormally high pulmonary artery pressures. The right heart disease takes the form of dilation and/or hypertrophy of the right-sided cardiac chambers.

2. Describe the pathophysiology of cor pulmonale.

Cor pulmonale is the sequel of pulmonary vasoconstriction or obstruction causing increased pulmonary vascular resistance. Alveolar hypoxia appears to be the most potent stimulus of pulmonary vasoconstriction in most species. Alveolar hypoxia leads to regional hypoxemia, hypercapnia, and acidosis, which lead to the vasoconstriction. Pulmonary thromboembolism is the most common cause of pulmonary artery obstructive disease (see Chapters 47 and 48).

3. What are the normal pulmonary arterial pressures in the dog and cat?

Normal pulmonary arterial pressures range between 15–30 mmHg in systole and 5–15 mmHg in diastole, with a mean of 8–20 mmHg.

4. Define pulmonary hypertension.

Pulmonary hypertension is an increase in pulmonary arterial pressure. Systolic pulmonary artery pressures that exceed 30 mmHg are considered abnormal.

5. How do we measure pulmonary arterial pressures?

Direct measurement of pulmonary arterial pressure requires the placement of a pulmonary arterial catheter. A flow-directed balloon catheter (Swan-Ganz) is commonly used. This catheter has multiple lumens and ports and can be used to measure pulmonary arterial pressure, central venous pressure, cardiac output, and capillary wedge pressure. Indirect measurement of pulmonary arterial pressure can be accomplished by Doppler echocardiography.

6. How is Doppler echocardiography used in the diagnosis of cor pulmonale?

Doppler echocardiography is a form of cardiac ultrasound that provides information regarding blood flow direction, velocity, and character. The detection and quantification of pressure differences within the circulation is one of the primary uses of Doppler echocardiography. A clinically valid simplification of the Bernoulli equation states that blood flow velocity is related to the pressure difference (or gradient), across a discrete narrowing in a vessel or cardiac chamber:

$$\Delta P = 4\ v^2$$

where DP is the pressure gradient and v is the post-obstructive velocity measured by Doppler. This principle is applied most often to the assessment of patients with pulmonic or aortic stenosis. However, it is equally valid when used to calculate the pressure difference across a regurgitant valve. In this way, it can be used to determine the systolic right atrial/right ventricular pressure difference in patients with tricuspid valve regurgitation:

$$RV_S - RA_S = 4\ v_{TR}^2$$

where RVS is the right ventricular pressure during systole, RA_S is the right atrial pressure during systole and v_{TR} is the peak velocity of the tricuspid valve regurgitant jet. In the absence of pulmonic stenosis, which can be readily excluded by Doppler study, pulmonary artery and right ventricular pressures are equal during systole. The right atrial pressure can be estimated from physical findings; in the absence of jugular distention or ascites, it is likely to be less than 5 mmHg. Therefore, the v_{TR} obtained by Doppler allows estimation of the systolic pulmonary artery pressure:

$$RV_S = PA_S$$

where PA_S is the systolic pulmonary artery pressure, so that

$$PA_S = 4 \, v_{TR}^2 + RA_S$$

When pulmonic valve regurgitation is present, an analogous method can be used to determine the diastolic pulmonary artery pressure. Tricuspid valve incompetence can be detected by Doppler study in many healthy animals and is very common in patients with cor pulmonale; this technique is a practical and noninvasive means of evaluating patients with cor pulmonale.

7. List causes of cor pulmonale.

Any disease that leads to pulmonary hypertension can lead to cor pulmonale. Cor pulmonale may be chronic or acute in nature. The most common cause of acute cor pulmonale is pulmonary thromboembolism. Below is a list of disorders that can cause cor pulmonale.

- Heartworm disease
- Pulmonary thromboembolism
- Chronic obstructive pulmonary disease
- Bronchitis
- Bronchiectasis
- Asthma
- Infiltrative pulmonary disease
- Chronic hypoxemia

8. How is cor pulmonale diagnosed?

The diagnosis of cor pulmonale is based on history, clinical signs, and diagnostic evaluation. The history and clinical signs will vary depending on the etiology of the underlying disease; however, most signs refer to the respiratory system. The history associated with cor pulmonale may be chronic, acute, or acute exacerbation of chronic disease. Clinical signs related to right-sided congestive heart failure also may be present.

Diagnostic evaluation may include, but is not limited to, thoracic radiographs, ECG, echocardiography, and blood gas analysis. A complete database should include a CBC, biochemistry panel, and urinalysis to evaluate for the presence of concurrent systemic disease.

9. List the common clinical signs of pulmonary hypertension.

- Exercise intolerance
- Cyanosis
- Hemoptysis
- Tachypnea
- Dyspnea
- Abnormal heart sounds, including split S_2 and tricuspid murmur

10. What are the clinical signs associated with right-sided heart failure?

- Jugular venous distention
- Hepatosplenomegaly
- Ascites
- Murmur of tricuspid regurgitation
- Split second heart sound on auscultation

11. What ECG abnormalities may be seen with cor pulmonale?

(1) Right axis deviation and (2) deep S waves in leads I, II, III, and aVF.

12. How is cor pulmonale treated?

Treatment of cor pulmonale is directed toward the underlying disease. The goals of therapy are to eliminate or palliate the pulmonary hypertension. Specific therapy may include (1) oxygen; (2) vasodilators; and (3) bronchodilators. Additional therapy may include treatment of right-sided heart failure with angiotensin-converting enzyme (ACE) inhibitors, salt-restrictive diets, and diuretics. Control of inflammatory or infectious diseases with anti-inflammatory or antimicrobial agents may lead to decreased pulmonary vascular resistance.

13. What is the prognosis of pulmonary hypertension?

The prognosis for pulmonary hypertension depends on the underlying disease. For the most part, the prognosis is guarded to poor when significant pulmonary hypertension or right-sided congestive heart failure is present.

14. What is the most common cause of cor pulmonale in the dog?

Heartworm disease.

15. Can cats have cor pulmonale?

Cats can have cor pulmonale and the etiology and pathogenesis are similar to the dog.

BIBLIOGRAPHY

1. Allen DG, Mackin A: Cor pulmonale. In Tilley L (ed): Handbook of Canine and Feline Cardiology. Philadelphia, W.B. Saunders, 1995, pp 211–223.
2. Atkins CE: The role of non-cardiac disease in the development and precipitation of heart failure. Vet Clin North Am Small Anim Pract 21:1035–1080, 1991.
3. Atkins CE: Cardiac manifestation of systemic and metabolic disease. In Fox PR, Sisson D, Moise NS (eds): Textbook of Canine and Feline Cardiology. Philadelphia, W.B. Saunders, 1999, pp 759–762.
4. Darke P, Bonagura JD, Kelly DF: Color Atlas of Veterinary Cardiology. London, Mosby-Wolfe, 1996, pp 147–153.
5. Dennis JS: The pathophysiologic sequelae of pulmonary thromboembolism. Compend Cont Ed Small Anim Pract 13:1811–1818, 1991.
6. Fox PR: Cor pulmonale. In Kirk RW (ed): Current Veterinary Therapy IX. Philadelphia, W.B. Saunders, 1986, pp 313–317.
7. Johnson LR, Hamlin RL: Recognition and treatment of pulmonary hypertension. In Bonagura JD (ed): Kirk's Current Veterinary Therapy XII. Philadelphia, W.B. Saunders, 1995, pp 887–892.
8. Perry LA, Dillon AR, Bowers TL: Pulmonary hypertension. Compend Cont Ed Small Anim Pract 13:226–233, 1991.
9. Wiedman HP, Matthay RA: Cor pulmonale. In Braunwald E (ed): Heart Disease: A Textbook of Cardiovascular Medicine. Philadelphia, W.B. Saunders, 1997, pp 1604–1625.

47. PULMONARY THROMBOEMBOLISM

Steven L. Marks, B.V.Sc., M.S., MRCVS

1. Define pulmonary thromboembolism (PTE).

The term thromboembolism is derived from the roots thrombus and embolism. A thrombus is an intravascular deposit of fibrin and formed blood elements. Embolism is the blocking of an artery with a clot or foreign material that has been brought to this site by blood flow. Pulmonary thromboembolism occurs when the entire thrombus or part of the thrombus formed at one location travels via the vascular system and lodges in the pulmonary artery.

2. What is Virchow's triad?

Virchow's triad refers to the pathophysiologic conditions that may lead to thromboembolism: (1) hypercoagulability; (2) endothelial injury; and (3) blood stasis.

3. List the disorders associated with PTE in the dog and cat.

- Immune-mediated hemolytic anemia
- Neoplasia
- Pancreatitis
- Hypothyroidism
- Hyperlipidemia
- Trauma
- Sepsis
- Heart disease
- Hyperadrenocorticism
- Nephrotic syndrome
- Heartworm disease
- Disseminated intravascular coagulation (DIC)
- PTE can also be an idiopathic disorder

4. What other anatomic regions can be affected by thromboembolism?

Any artery theoretically can have an embolism. Other common areas include the aorta, internal iliac arteries, cerebral arteries, brachial arteries, renal arteries, arteries supplying the gastrointestinal tract, and femoral arteries.

5. What clinical signs can be associated with PTE?

- Tachypnea
- Dyspnea
- Depression
- Tachycardia

6. What are the pathophysiologic consequences of PTE?

PTE can lead to pulmonary hypertension. With significant PTE, ventilation perfusion mismatch occurs leading to bronchoconstriction and vasoconstriction. Vasoactive substances released from the emboli lead to increased vascular resistance. This leads to increases in pulmonary arterial pressures and right ventricular pressures.

7. What are the basic pathophysiologic mechanisms that can lead to hypoxemia?

- Hypoventilation
- Diffusion barrier impairment
- Decreased available oxygen
- Ventilation perfusion mismatch/intrapulmonary shunting
- Anatomical right-to-left shunt, such as tetralogy of Fallot

8. Which of these processes is responsible for the hypoxemia seen with PTE?

PTE generally leads to ventilation perfusion mismatch.

9. What diagnostic procedures can be performed to confirm PTE?

It is difficult to reach a definitive antemortem diagnosis of PTE. Information provided by echocardiography, radiography, ventilation/perfusion radionuclide studies, and arterial blood gas analysis can be used to support a presumptive diagnosis. However, selective pulmonary arteriography remains the gold standard in the diagnosis of this challenging disorder.

If possible, diagnostic procedures should also be directed toward identifying the underlying disease process. Most commonly used procedures are CBC, biochemical profile, urinalysis, prothrombin time, partial thromboplastin time, and activated clotting time.

10. Describe the radiographic findings that suggest PTE.

Initially thoracic radiographs may be normal and this finding, seemingly inconsistent with the presentation of respiratory distress, may be suggestive of PTE. The caudal lung lobes are most commonly affected and blunted pulmonary arteries with wedge-shaped areas of interstitial or alveolar opacities may be present.

11. What echocardiographic findings suggest PTE?

The arrival of a large thrombus in a pulmonary artery increases total pulmonary vascular resistance and imposes a pressure overload on the right ventricle. Abnormalities of septal motion and increases in right atrial or ventricular size can be observed in some cases of PTE. Additionally, Doppler assessment of tricuspid valve regurgitation velocities can lead to a noninvasive diagnosis of pulmonary hypertension, which, in association with other clinical findings, can support a diagnosis of PTE.

12. What is the cardinal sign of PTE on blood gas analysis?

There are no findings on blood gas analysis that are pathognomonic for PTE; however, hypoxemia is the most common abnormality.

13. How is the A–a gradient calculated and why is it increased in animals with PTE?

The alveolar to arterial (A–a) gradient is calculated using the following formulas:

$$PAO_2 = (BP - 47) FIO_2 - PCO_2 \times 1.2$$

BP = barometric pressure (760 mmHg at sea level)
47 = the vaporization pressure of water
FIO_2 = fraction inspired oxygen (0.21 at room air)
PCO_2 and PaO_2 are obtained from arterial blood gas analysis. At sea level, the formula can be simplified to:

$$PAO_2 = 150 - PCO_2 \times 1.2$$
$$\text{A–a gradient} = PAO_2 - PaO_2 \text{ (normal} < 10 \text{ mmHg)}$$

The A–a gradient becomes elevated due to the decrease in PaO_2.

14. Why are animals with PTE responsive to oxygen?

The ventilation perfusion mismatch leads to the hypoxemia and pulmonary arterial blood is diverted to other areas of the lung. Supplemental oxygen allows the diverted blood to become oxygenated and may increase PaO_2.

15. How is PTE treated?

The treatment for PTE should be directed toward the underlying disease process, if identified. Emergency management of PTE is supportive and should include oxygen supplementation, fluid therapy, and bronchodilator therapy. The use of corticosteroids is of questionable benefit and thrombolytic agents have not been commonly used.

16. What drugs can be used as prophylaxis for PTE?
- Heparin
- Warfarin

17. How can oxygen be supplied to veterinary patients?
- Face mask
- Flow-by
- Nasal cannula
- Oxygen canopy
- Oxygen cage

18. What is the prognosis for PTE?

In general, the prognosis for PTE is guarded and somewhat dependent on the underlying disease.

CONTROVERSY

19. Are thrombolytic agents beneficial in the management of PTE?

Thrombolytic agents, such as streptokinase and tissue plasminogen activator, have been used on a limited basis for thromboembolism in the dog and cat.

BIBLIOGRAPHY

1. Baty CJ, Hardie EM: Pulmonary thromboembolism: Diagnosis and treatment. In Bonagura JD (ed): Current Veterinary Therapy XI. Philadelphia, W.B. Saunders, 1992, pp 137–142.
2. Camps-Palau MA, Marks SL, Cornick JL: Small animal oxygen therapy. Comp Cont Educ Pract Vet 21:587–598, 1999.
3. Dennis JS: Clinical features of canine pulmonary thromboembolism. Comp Cont Educ Pract Vet 15:1595–1603, 1993.
4. Johnson LR, Lappin MR, Baker DC: Pulmonary thromboembolism in 29 dogs: 1985–1995. J Vet Intern Med 13:338–345, 1999.
5. LaRue MJ, Murtaugh RJ: Pulmonary thromboembolism in dogs: 47 cases (1986–1987). J Am Vet Med Assoc 197:1368–1372, 1990.

48. PATENT DUCTUS ARTERIOSUS

Jonathan A. Abbot, D.V.M.

1. What is the ductus arteriosus (DA)? What is its function?

The ductus arteriosus, or arterial duct, is a blood vessel that provides a communication be-tween the systemic and pulmonary circulations. It arises from the proximal descending aorta and courses cranioventrally, where it joins the dorsal aspect of the main pulmonary artery. In utero, the duct provides a means for fetal blood to skirt the pulmonary capillary bed. In the fetal circu-lation, oxygenation of blood occurs in the placenta. Of the blood that leaves the right ventricle, the greatest proportion traverses the DA and is conveyed to caudal sites in the body through the descending aorta.

2. What is a patent ductus arteriosus (PDA)?

Although the precise mechanisms are incompletely understood, postnatal increases in oxygen tension result in a prostaglandin cascade that causes contraction of the muscular layer of the DA and closure of the duct. The process begins immediately after birth and in most species is complete within 3 to 4 days. Subintimal necrosis of the DA and scarring contribute to complete anatomic closure.

In some individuals, closure of the duct does not occur or is incomplete, and the vessel is then known as a patent ductus arteriosus (PDA). A duct is simply a tube and is therefore by defi-nition patent. For this reason, some prefer the term "persistently patent duct" in order to empha-size the pathologic nature of failed postnatal ductal closure.

3. How does the fetal circulation change in the immediate postnatal period?

Resistance is the hydraulic force that must be overcome in order to achieve or maintain flow through a vessel. Vascular resistance is related, in an approximate fashion, to flow and pressure by Ohm's law ($BP = R \times Q$, where BP is blood pressure, R is vascular resistance, and Q is flow, or cardiac output). In the fetal circulation, pulmonary vascular resistance is much greater than systemic vascular resistance. This is why systemic blood flow greatly exceeds pulmonary blood flow despite the fact that the pressures in the two circulations are similar. Very shortly after birth, pulmonary vascular resistance falls and the increase in pulmonary blood flow is accompanied by a decrease in pulmonary artery pressure. If the duct is patent, blood flow across the ductus fol-lows the path of least resistance, and moves from the aorta to the pulmonary artery.

4. Trace the pattern of blood flow in a patient with a PDA; what are the pathophysiologic consequences of the PDA?

If the ductus is patent and pulmonary vascular resistance falls appropriately following birth, blood can cross the duct from the high-pressure/high-resistance systemic circulation to enter the low-resistance pulmonary circulation. Therefore, a proportion of the left ventricular stroke volume will leave the aorta through the PDA and enter the main pulmonary artery. From here, the shunt volume together with the systemic venous return is conveyed to the lungs and then, through the pulmonary veins, to the left atrium and ventricle. Thus, the shunt volume that leaves the aorta augments the pulmonary venous return, increasing the volume of the left atrium and left ventricle. So, despite the fact that the shunt direction is "left-to-right," a PDA imposes a volume overload on the *left atrium and left ventricle*.

5. What is the pathogenesis of heart failure due to PDA?

When pulmonary vascular resistance is normal, the direction of ductal shunt is from left to right. The increase in pulmonary venous return results in left ventricular dilation and hypertrophy;

the degree of cardiac enlargement is roughly proportional to the size of the shunt. The volume load on the left heart can cause diastolic pressures within the left ventricle to rise, and this pressure elevation is reflected back upon the pulmonary venous circulation. If pulmonary venous pressures become sufficiently high, fluid is forced out of the pulmonary capillaries and edema results. Thus, *left-sided congestive heart failure* is the potential consequence of a *left-to-right* PDA.

6. Why are signs of heart failure not usually observed until the patient is months or, rarely, years old?

An overwhelming volume overload can result in the syndrome of congestive heart failure when myocardial function is normal; this is apparently the case in many dogs with heart failure due to mitral valve regurgitation. However, myocardial dysfunction or failure, sometimes known as cardiomyopathy of overload, is a potential consequence of a longstanding PDA, and this is an additional factor that can contribute to the development of congestive signs. Heart failure due to a PDA is usually associated with the development of myocardial dysfunction or the development of mitral valve regurgitation resulting from ventricular dilation; this may explain the age of onset of congestive signs.

7. What determines the amount of blood that flows through the PDA and back to the lungs?

The size of the shunt is determined by three main factors: (1) the diameter of the DA; (2) length of the DA; and (3) the relationship between the pulmonary and systemic vascular resistance.

When pulmonary vascular resistance is low and the duct has a wide bore, the shunt is large. In contrast, if the duct is large but vascular pathology has resulted in an increase in pulmonary vascular resistance, the shunt is small. In fact, if pulmonary vascular resistance exceeds systemic vascular resistance, the shunt may be bidirectional or in a right-to-left direction. This is sometimes referred to as a "right-to-left PDA" or "reversed PDA"; this presentation of the patent ductus is uncommon and discussed further in the section that addresses cyanotic heart disease.

8. What causes PDA in the dog?

A hereditary basis for PDA has been confirmed in miniature and toy poodles. In these breeds the pattern of inheritance is complex, suggesting that it is a quasicontinuous or threshold trait. In other breeds of dogs, genetic transmission has not been proven. However, PDA demonstrates clear breed predispositions and a genetic basis is likely or should probably be assumed in most cases.

9. Why does the duct fail to close in dogs with PDA?

In 1971, Buchanan observed that failure of ductal closure in a colony of miniature poodles with hereditary PDA resulted from abnormal development of ductal tunica media. Affected dogs had muscular hypoplasia and the arrangement of the muscle fibers that were present was abnormal so that the histologic appearance of the duct resembled the aorta. The histopathology extended a variable distance from the aortic aspect of the duct towards the pulmonary artery so that severely affected dogs had a tubular duct and less severely affected dogs had a duct that narrowed as it joined the pulmonary artery. Similarities of ductal morphology in dogs of other affected breeds suggest that this is the pathogenesis of PDA in most, if not all, cases.

10. What is the prevalence of PDA in dogs?

Although there may be geographical differences, PDA is one of the most common congenital cardiovascular malformations in the dog. In the United States, PDA is the most common congenital cardiovascular malformation.

11. What signalment is typical for small animals with PDA?

PDA is observed most commonly in small-breed dogs. Miniature poodles, Maltese, bichon frise, Pomeranians, and others are predisposed to ductal patency. Females are affected more often than males, with a ratio of about 2.5 to 1. The lesion is usually detected early in life, often during the first routine veterinary visit. A three-month-old, female small-breed dog (such as a Pomeranian) is a fairly typical signalment for affected dogs.

PDA is uncommon in the cat.

12. What abnormalities does the patient history reveal in patients with PDA?

PDA is usually first identified when a cardiac murmur is detected during routine veterinary examination of a seemingly healthy puppy. Clinical signs of left-sided congestive heart failure, such as cough, dyspnea, and exercise intolerance, are occasionally reported by the owner. However, the owner is seldom aware that the pet has cardiac disease. In fact, the patient history is unremarkable in many, if not most, *puppies* with congenital heart disease, and this can be the case even when the lesion is sufficiently severe that it will shorten the patient's life. Occasionally, adult dogs are presented for veterinary evaluation of clinical signs of heart failure that are the result of a previously undetected and uncorrected PDA.

13. What findings are expected on auscultation?

A continuous murmur heard over the left craniodorsal aspect of the heart base is the auscultatory hallmark of the PDA. The murmur is often but not always loud and is usually relatively coarse; it peaks in intensity at or about the second heart sound and then fades during diastole. This murmur is sometimes referred to as a "machinery" murmur. It is important to recognize that a continuous murmur is one that begins during systole and continues without interruption into diastole. That is to say, a murmur that fades to inaudibility during diastole is still described as continuous provided that it begins before the second heart sound. Continuous murmurs must be distinguished from to-and-fro or "bellows" murmurs, which consist of separate systolic and diastolic murmurs. In dogs, to-and-fro murmurs most commonly result from endocarditis of the aortic valve or ventricular septal defects that are complicated by aortic valve regurgitation.

Most dogs with a subclinical PDA have a murmur that can be heard throughout diastole; however, those dogs with pulmonary hypertension related to left-sided congestive heart failure may have a continuous murmur that is noticeably abbreviated.

Careful auscultation of the patient with a PDA may also reveal a systolic murmur over the left cardiac apex. This murmur is due to functional mitral valve regurgitation, that is, mitral valve regurgitation that results from dilation of the left ventricle and mitral annulus rather than a structurally abnormality of the mitral valve leaflets. In dogs with a large ductus, a third heart sound that reflects high transmitral flow rates and probably reduced ventricular compliance results in a gallop rhythm.

14. What is the differential diagnosis for a continuous murmur in a young dog?

As previously stated, a continuous murmur is a single murmur that begins before and ends after the second heart sound. A pressure gradient that persists throughout the cardiac cycle is required to generate a continuous murmur. Most often, this gradient is explained by a communication between the systemic and pulmonary vasculature, although an arteriovenous fistula or severe peripheral pulmonary artery stenosis can also result in a continuous murmur. The pressure difference between the left and right ventricles drops to nearly zero during diastole; because of this, a ventricular septal defect does not explain a continuous murmur. Occasionally, a murmur that is continuous will be heard in cases of left-to-right aorticopulmonary window; however, that defect is uncommon and usually results in a "silent" right-to-left shunt due to high pulmonary vascular resistance. Additionally, a fistula resulting from an aortic sinus rupture or even truncus arteriosus with pulmonary ostial stenosis can also result in a continuous murmur.

To-and-fro murmurs resulting from ventricular septal defect and concurrent aortic valve regurgitation, pulmonary stenosis with audible pulmonary valve regurgitation, and subaortic stenosis with audible aortic valve regurgitation can be difficult to distinguish from continuous murmurs. However, provided that a murmur is truly continuous, the probability that the murmur results from a PDA is overwhelming.

15. Describe the femoral arterial pulse in PDA.

When the DA is patent, the resulting femoral arterial pulse is brisk or bounding and is some-times described as a "water-hammer" pulse. The amplitude or strength of the arterial pulse reflects the difference between systolic and diastolic pressures, which is called the pulse pressure. When the DA is patent, the low-resistance pulmonary circulation provides a sink for diastolic "run-off." As a result, diastolic pressures tend to be abnormally low and the pulse pressure is wide.

16. What radiographic findings are expected in cases of ductal patency?

Plain thoracic radiographs demonstrate enlargement of the cardiac silhouette that is com-mensurate with shunt volume. Radiography has limited ability to distinguish the specific cham-bers of the heart and this is often demonstrated by the PDA. Despite a radiographic appearance that suggests generalized cardiomegaly, echocardiographic studies in left-to-right PDA confirm that the left atrium and ventricle are enlarged and the right ventricle is normal or even small. Enlargement of the left atrium can be quite obvious and result in a bulge at the 3-o'clock position of the cardiac silhouette in the ventrodorsal projection. Aneurysmal dilation of the proximal aorta and main pulmonary artery may also deform the ventrodorsal cardiac silhouette. In some cases, this results in an appearance of three bulges at the 1-, 2-, and 3-o'clock positions.

In most cases, the pulmonary vessels are enlarged and appear to be increased in number. This appearance of pulmonary hyperemia or pulmonary hyperperfusion can be difficult to distin-guish from the presence of interstitial pulmonary edema. Left atrial enlargement together with pulmonary opacities indicates left-sided congestive heart failure. It should be recognized that the size of the duct and of the shunt is variable; some patients have a small ductus and relatively subtle radiographic findings although a large and radiographically apparent shunt is more common.

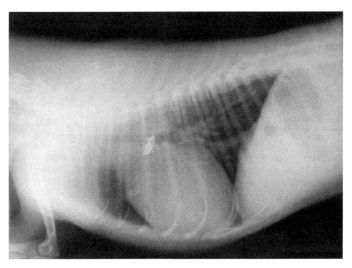

Lateral thoracic radiograph obtained from a 16-month-old female Maltese dog. Two metallic coils have been placed in the ductus arteriosus.

17. What electrocardiographic abnormalities are associated with PDA?

The electrocardiogram (ECG) can be normal although there is often a left ventricular hyper-trophy pattern characterized by R waves that exceed 2.5 mV in lead II. Evidence of left atrial en-largement in the form of wide P waves may also be seen. Additionally, arrhythmias can complicate the presentation of the PDA. Atrial premature complexes or atrial fibrillation are oc-casionally evident. A critical mass of atrial myocardium is required to sustain the arrhythmia of fibrillation and the finding of atrial fibrillation in a puppy reflects marked left atrial enlargement.

18. What echocardiographic findings are associated with patency of the ductus arteriosus?

Dilation and hypertrophy of the left ventricle is evident echocardiographically in patients that have moderate and large left-to-right shunts. Echocardiographic examination also demonstrates left atrial enlargement. Left ventricular systolic performance may be normal or in some cases a low shortening fraction suggests myocardial dysfunction. Direct visualization of the PDA is usually possible when the study is performed by an experienced echocardiographer. The ductus extends from the descending aorta to the bifurcation of the main pulmonary artery. It is best demonstrated by a cranial left parasternal image of the pulmonary artery bifurcation.

Doppler flow studies are used to confirm that blood flows into the main pulmonary artery. Color-flow Doppler studies demonstrate a diastolic color mosaic that originates near the pulmonary artery bifurcation and extends retrograde toward the pulmonic valve. In many cases, the jet extends beyond the pulmonic valve and results in mild pulmonic regurgitation. Spectral Doppler shows continuous disturbed flow within the pulmonary artery (see figure below). Direct visualization of the duct is unnecessary when the typical Doppler findings of a continuous flow disturbance originating at the pulmonary artery bifurcation findings are present.

Additional findings detected by Doppler study include functional mitral regurgitation resulting from dilation of the valve annulus. When a substantial shunt is present, aortic flow velocities are often higher than normal. This does not necessarily reflect aortic obstruction but rather the ejection of a large left ventricular stroke volume.

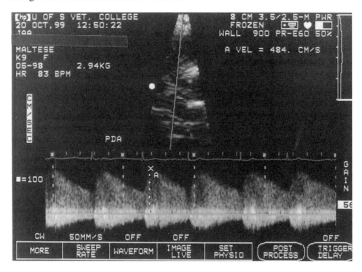

Continuous-wave Doppler echocardiographic study performed with the ultrasound beam directed through the patent duct of a 16-month-old female Maltese dog. There is a high-velocity jet directed toward the transducer and into the main pulmonary artery. The signal is continuous, but the velocity peak occurs at about the T-wave of the electrocardiogram; this event corresponds to the second heart sound and the Doppler profile provides a graphic depiction of the patient's continuous murmur.

19. Is echocardiography required for the diagnosis of PDA?

PDA is essentially a physical diagnosis. When a continuous murmur is present in a puppy of typical signalment, the cause is almost always a PDA. However, Doppler echocardiographic examination is recommended as a noninvasive means of confirming the diagnosis. The echocardiographic evaluation of systolic function may also provide prognostic information that can influence therapy (see figure top of next page). Additionally, echocardiography provides a noninvasive means of detecting concurrent cardiac defects that might have an impact on prognosis and management.

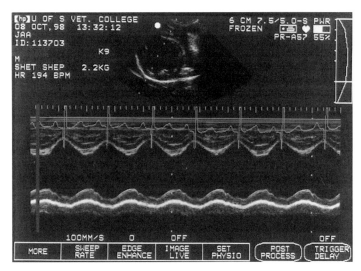

M-mode echocardiographic image obtained from an 8-week-old male Shetland sheepdog. M-mode echocardiography provides a one-dimensional view of the heart; the ordinate measures distance from the transducer and the abscissa, time. The two-dimensional image from which this M-mode was derived is shown in the inset. The left ventricle is moderately dilated and systolic performance is normal.

20. How is a PDA treated?

Traditionally, PDA has been treated by thoracotomy and surgical ligation of the duct. More recently, the interventional catheterization technique of transcatheter coil occlusion has been used as a minimally invasive alternative to surgery.

21. What is the technique of transcatheter ductal occlusion?

Recently, interventional cardiac catheterization techniques have been employed in the management of patients with PDA. Various methods have been used, usually first in children and then in dogs. Most commonly, the ductus is occluded by the transcatheter placement of thrombogenic Gianturco coils. These coils are available from the manufacturer in various sizes and are supplied in straight, thin, tubular cartridges that facilitate their entry into cardiac catheters. The coils consist of metal with tufts of Dacron that confer thrombogenicity; the coils have "structural memory" and when they are released from the cartridge or catheter, they form a predetermined number of loops.

Many variations of the basic technique for coil placement have been described. However, access to the DA is commonly gained by retrograde approach using the femoral artery. An appropriately sized catheter is placed by fluoroscopic guidance across the ductus. The coil or coils are then deployed through this catheter and the coils are left in place within the ductus. When the procedure is successful, occlusion is rapid and complete (see figure on page 295).

22. What surgical techniques are used to treat PDA?

Surgical techniques involve ligation of the DA following a left lateral thoracotomy. The conventional surgical approach to ductal ligation involves blunt dissection of the medial aspect of the DA. Dissection is performed with forceps that are held parallel to the transverse plane of the DA; the forceps are used to grasp the suture material, which is used to ligate and occlude the PDA. Jackson and Henderson described an alternative surgical technique. Their method involves dissection of the medial aspect of the proximal aorta following a left lateral thoracotomy. A double length of suture material is placed about the DA through the use of blunt hemostats that are placed cranial and caudal to the ductus. This technique requires less blunt dissection of the medial aspect of the DA and might therefore be safer.

23. Is there a role for medical therapy in patients with PDA?

Left ventricular congestive heart failure is a potential consequence of persistent ductal patency. Patients with radiographic evidence of pulmonary edema should be treated medically with diuretics for 1 to 3 days prior to definitive therapy. Attempts are made to clear the lung of edema prior to administration of anesthesia. When atrial fibrillation complicates the presentation, slowing of the ventricular response is suggested prior to attempts at definite repair. Digoxin is appropriate for this purpose although the relatively long elimination half-life of this drug is a potential disadvantage. The cautious use of diltiazem together with digoxin or as a sole agent are possible alternatives. When correction of the PDA cannot be performed for financial or other reasons, medical palliation using an ACE inhibitor, digoxin, and diuretic therapy is reasonable.

24. What is the prognosis of patients with PDA? Do all dogs with PDA require treatment?

Uncorrected, the prognosis for most patients with a PDA is poor. Mortality due to left-sided CHF is high unless the defect is corrected. Given the high mortality associated with uncorrected PDA, it is important to recognize that, of all of the congenital cardiovascular malformations in the dog, PDA is the one most amenable to definitive repair. It must also be emphasized that, as with many other congenital cardiac defects in veterinary medicine, very few patients with PDA have clinical signs at the time of detection. This only serves to emphasize the importance of a definitive diagnosis in all cases of suspected congenital heart disease.

A small number of dogs have a shunt that is small enough that careful monitoring through serial echocardiographic studies can be considered as an alternative to occlusion or ligation of the duct. However, these cases are in the minority and repair is recommended for all but those that have a very small shunt as assessed by a veterinarian with training in the evaluation of canine patients with congenital cardiac disease.

CONTROVERSY

25. What is the best method for correction of PDA?

The transcatheter placement of Gianturco coils is a minimally invasive technique; when successful, it obviates the need for thoracotomy. Morbidity can therefore be expected to be less than that encountered following surgical procedures. The risks associated with the technique are relatively low and relate primarily to failure of ductal occlusion and embolism or "loss" of coils into the pulmonary or systemic vasculature. Embolism of peripheral pulmonary arteries appears to be well tolerated. Coils that migrate to the systemic vasculature should probably be removed by a catheter snare device or, if necessary, surgical exploration.

The procedure must be performed by a practitioner with experience in cardiac catheterization techniques; the need for fluoroscopy might also be considered a disadvantage. Additionally, some patients with PDA are better candidates for ductal occlusion than others and this relates partly to ductal size but probably more importantly to ductal morphology. Unfortunately, angiography or possibly transesophageal echocardiography, both of which require general anesthesia, are necessary to properly characterize ductal size and morphology in the dog. Therefore, coil embolization of the PDA is a viable technique for many dogs with PDA. It is minimally invasive and possibly less expensive than surgical techniques.

Surgical management of the PDA is associated with relatively low risk when it is performed by an experienced surgeon. Clinically complete occlusion is the result in the majority of cases. The procedure requires thoracotomy with its attendant risks and morbidity. However, most young dogs tolerate a left lateral thoracotomy quite well and, with appropriate postoperative analgesia, recovery from the procedure is usually rapid and uneventful. The risks associated with surgical treatment relate primarily to the possibility of intraoperative hemorrhage, which can be severe and fatal.

It is likely then that there will continue to be a role for both surgery and interventional techniques in the management of patients with PDA. There are some patients with very large and tubular ducti that should be treated surgically. However, the relatively new technique of coil embolization is a viable alternative approach to the management of many other patients with PDA.

BIBLIOGRAPHY

1. Bonagura JD, Lehmkuhl LB: Congenital heart disease. In Fox PR, Sisson D, Moise NS (eds): Textbook of Canine and Feline Cardiology: Principles and Clinical Practice, 2nd ed. Philadelphia, W.B. Saunders, 1999, pp 471–535.
2. Fellows CG, Lerche P, King G, Tometzki A: Treatment of patent ductus arteriosus by placement of two intravascular embolisation coils in a puppy. J Small Anim Pract 39:196–199, 1998.
3. Fox PR, Bond BR, Sommer RJ: Nonsurgical transcatheter coil occlusion of patent ductus arteriosus in two dogs using a preformed nitinol snare delivery technique. J Vet Intern Med 12:182–185, 1998.
4. Johnston SA, Eyster GE: Patent ductus arteriosus. In Bonagura JD (ed): Kirk's Current Veterinary Therapy XII: Small Animal Practice. Philadelphia, W.B. Saunders, 1995, pp 780–785.
5. Kittleson MD: Patent ductus arteriosus. In Kittleson MD, Kienle RD (eds): Small Animal Cardiovascular Medicine. St. Louis, Mosby, 1998, pp 218–230.
6. Miller MW: Interventional cardiology: Catheter occlusion of patent ductus arteriosus in dogs. In Bonagura JD (ed): Kirk's Current Veterinary Therapy XIII: Small Animal Practice. Philadelphia, W.B. Saunders, 2000, pp 742–744.
7. Patterson DF: Congenital defects of the cardiovascular system of dogs: Studies in comparative cardiology. Adv Vet Sci Comp Med 20:1–37, 1976.
8. Patterson DF, Pyle RL, Buchanan JW, et al: Hereditary patent ductus arteriosus and its sequelae in the dog. Circ Res 29:1–13, 1971.
9. Patterson DF: Epidemiologic and genetic studies of congenital heart disease in the dog. Circ Res 23:171–202, 1968.

49. AORTIC STENOSIS

Virginia Luis Fuentes, M.A., Vet.M.B., D.V.C., MRCVS

1. What is aortic stenosis? Describe its morphological features.

Stenosis means narrowing; aortic stenosis is a term that refers to various anatomic and functional forms of left ventricular outflow tract obstruction. In small animals, aortic stenosis is most commonly observed as a lesion that is either congenital or develops early in the postnatal period.

The morphologic features of aortic stenosis include the following:

Left ventricular outflow tract. The stenosis may occur at the subvalvular, valvular, or supravalvular level. In dogs, subvalvular lesions are by far the most common, and this type of defect is referred to as subaortic stenosis. In addition to the anatomic site of the lesion, the obstruction may be further described as fixed or dynamic. A fixed obstruction is one that results from a structural or anatomic narrowing of the left ventricular outflow tract. Dynamic obstructions are those in which the narrowing of the left ventricular outflow tract develops during the course of systole. Dynamic obstructions are labile; that is, the severity of the obstruction depends upon physiologic variables such as contractility, afterload, and preload. In subaortic stenosis, fixed lesions range from inconspicuous nodules or linear ridges in the subvalvular area to thick fibrous rings that encircle the left ventricular outflow tract, involving the anterior mitral valve leaflet in the process. Other variations include the fibromuscular tunnel, in which the entire subvalvular outflow tract is narrowed by a collar of fibrous and muscular tissue.

Left ventricular myocardium. When the degree of obstruction is moderate or severe, hypertrophy usually accompanies the left ventricular outflow tract lesions, and the subendocardium may develop fibrotic changes. Intramural coronary lesions have also been reported, consisting of intimal proliferation and medial degeneration.

A **poststenotic dilation** may be present in the ascending aorta.

2. Explain the hemodynamic consequences of aortic stenosis.

AS causes an obstruction to blood flow through the left ventricular outflow tract. This imposes a pressure overload on the left ventricle, which stimulates compensatory hypertrophy. In order to overcome the resistance provided by the narrow outflow tract and maintain systemic arterial pressure, the left ventricle must generate abnormally high systolic pressures. Thus, a pressure gradient develops across the left ventricular outflow tract, and this gradient is proportional to the severity of the stenosis. The combination of high intraventricular pressure and concentric hypertrophy may lead to inadequate myocardial perfusion, especially during exercise. As a consequence, ventricular arrhythmias are comparatively common in AS, and may be responsible for the cause of death in many severely affected dogs. Changes in left ventricular geometry or function may result in mitral regurgitation even when the mitral valve is not involved in the left ventricular outflow tract lesion. Aortic insufficiency is also very common in dogs with AS. Although systolic function is generally preserved in young dogs with AS, older surviving dogs may suffer a progressive decline in myocardial contractility, eventually leading to congestive heart failure.

3. Does the severity of the stenosis progress with time?

The lesions of AS may not even be present at birth; one study in Newfoundlands showed that subvalvular lesions were not present in any pups under 3 weeks of age, but became progressively more severe as the animal reached maturity. It is sometimes disputed whether AS is a true congenital defect for this reason. Although the stenosis develops over the first year, there are only isolated reports of progression after the age of 1 year.

4. How common is AS?

In recent surveys, the incidence of AS appears to have increased. It now generally ranks as the most common or second most common canine congenital cardiac defect.

5. Is AS inherited?

Studies have confirmed that AS is inherited in Newfoundlands, either as a polygenic trait or as an autosomal dominant trait with modifying genes. It is likely that AS is inherited in other breeds that have a high prevalence.

6. List breed predispositions for AS.

The breeds of dog most commonly affected with AS are:
• Newfoundland
• Golden retriever
• Rottweiler
• Boxer
• Samoyed
• Bulldog
• German shepherd
AS does occur in cats, but much less commonly.

7. What are the presenting signs of AS?

Exercise intolerance and exertional syncope are common signs in severely affected dogs. Sudden death may occur in severely affected dogs, sometimes without any premonitory signs. Signs of congestive heart failure (dyspnea, coughing) may develop in older animals with severe AS. Mild lesions may not result in any clinical signs, and may only be detected as an incidental murmur. In fact, patients with AS are usually first identified when a cardiac murmur is detected during routine veterinary examination of a seemingly healthy puppy; most dogs with AS are outwardly normal when the lesion is first detected and this is true even for dogs with severe obstruction. Clinical signs such as exercise intolerance, syncope, or congestive heart failure are most often observed in older animals. This only serves to emphasize the importance of a complete diagnostic evaluation in patients that have congenital cardiac murmurs, because the presence (or absence) of clinical signs in a young puppy with a cardiac murmur is generally a poor indicator of long-term prognosis.

8. Why do dogs with AS faint?

There are several possible mechanisms for syncope in dogs with AS:
• Ventricular arrhythmias
• Inability to increase cardiac output with demand because of a fixed obstruction
• Neurocardiogenic syncope
The latter may occur because of excessive stimulation of ventricular mechanoreceptors, which trigger a reflex bradycardia and peripheral vasodilatation. This causes a profound fall in arterial blood pressure, leading to cerebral hypoperfusion and syncope.

9. What is dynamic left ventricular outflow tract obstruction?

Most dogs with AS have a fixed, or anatomic, obstruction. However, dogs with subaortic AS occasionally develop a dynamic form of obstruction associated with exercise or excitement; this phenomenon has been reported in a series of golden retriever puppies but it is also observed in other breeds afflicted by AS. This dynamic obstruction occurs when the anterior mitral valve leaflet is drawn across into the left ventricular outflow tract during mid- to late systole, causing obstruction to flow (this is called systolic anterior motion of the mitral valve, or SAM). This dynamic obstruction is more likely to occur when contractility is increased, such as with sympathetic adrenergic stimulation, or when afterload is reduced, as can occur with the use of vasodilating drugs.

10. Describe the main findings of AS on physical examination.

The principal abnormality is an ejection-type murmur, which is usually heard best over the aortic valve area at the left heart base, but may be equally loud over the right hemithorax; occasionally, the point of maximal intensity of the murmur is over the right heart base. The murmur often radiates to the left apex, and may be readily heard in the cervical region over the carotid arteries. A soft diastolic murmur may also be heard in dogs with accompanying aortic insufficiency. Other findings on physical examination may be more subtle; in severe cases, the pulses may be weak.

11. What is an ejection-type murmur? What other conditions can give rise to ejection murmurs?

The term ejection-type murmur refers to the phonocardiographic configuration or "shape" of a murmur. Ejection murmurs, also know as crescendo-decrescendo murmurs, have a diamond shape; that is, they increase in intensity in early systole, peak in midsystole and then fade. In general, ejection murmurs result when outflow tract velocities are increased or when blood viscosity is decreased. These factors contribute to the development of turbulence, or disturbed flow, within the outflow tracts. Examples include hemic murmurs, which are associated with anemia, and functional flow murmurs. Truly innocent murmurs develop in the absence of structural or functional cardiac abnormalities. Generally, functional murmurs are of low but variable intensity and are brief in duration. It should be recognized that anatomic or functional pulmonic stenosis can also result in an ejection-type murmur that is heard best over the left cardiac base. In clinical practice, therefore, it can be difficult to distinguish the murmur of AS from one that results from pulmonic stenosis, tetralogy of Fallot, atrial septal defect, or ventricular septal defect. Other clinical findings, including signalment and arterial pulse quality, are helpful in refining the differential diagnosis that is formulated based upon the physical examination.

12. Is the ECG useful in the diagnosis of AS?

Electrocardiography is an insensitive test for AS. Frequently, the resting ECG is completely normal, and increased R wave amplitude or left axis deviation is seen only occasionally, despite concentric left ventricular hypertrophy. ST segment changes may be seen after exercise in severely affected dogs. Holter (24-hour) ambulatory ECG recordings may demonstrate ventricular arrhythmias that are not apparent at rest.

13. What are the expected radiographic changes with AS?

Often radiographic changes are very subtle in AS. Although left ventricular hypertrophy may be present in severe cases, this may produce little change in the cardiac silhouette, as the hypertrophy is concentric. A poststenotic dilatation in the aorta may be the most obvious abnormality. This may be evident as a widening of the cranial mediastinum, or a bulge at the 12- to 1-o'clock position on the dorsoventral view. Occasionally, left atrial enlargement is visible, especially if the animal is developing myocardial failure and pulmonary edema, but this is uncommon.

14. How can two-dimensional echocardiography be used in the assessment of AS?

Two-dimensional (2D) echocardiography is relatively insensitive at detecting mild lesions of AS, although it is helpful for identifying the actual lesions of the stenosis (see figure at top of following page, *left*). Left ventricular hypertrophy may be identified, although this is often subjective in the absence of breed-related normal reference ranges. In severely affected animals, there may be hyperechoic areas in the left ventricular subendocardium caused by fibrosis or even calcific change (secondary to ischemic damage). In animals with depressed myocardial function, echocardiography will demonstrate left ventricular dilation and reduced left ventricular shortening fraction.

15. How can Doppler echocardiography be used in the assessment of AS?

Doppler echocardiography is an invaluable tool for assessing the severity of AS, and is required for the noninvasive diagnosis of AS. Doppler studies allow estimation of the pressure gradient between the left ventricle and the aorta through the measurement of the blood flow velocity

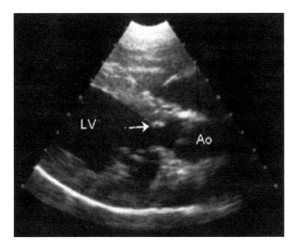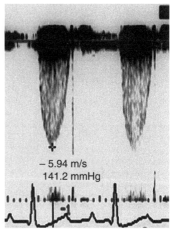

— 5.94 m/s
141.2 mmHg

Echocardiographic images from a boxer dog with severe subaortic stenosis. *Left,* A two-dimensional echocardiographic image, recorded from a right parasternal long axis view. The lesion is visible in the left ventricular outflow tract (arrow), but also includes part of the anterior mitral valve leaflet. *Right,* Spectral Doppler recording of the velocity of blood flow in the aorta. The peak velocity and peak pressure gradient across the stenosis are shown. Aortic blood flow velocities in normal dogs are generally less than 1.7 m/s.

distal to the stenosis (see figure at top of following page, *right*). The modified Bernouilli equation is used to calculate the pressure gradient across the stenosis (in mmHg) using the measured aortic velocity (in m/s):

$$pressure\ gradient = 4 \times aortic\ velocity^2$$

Pressure gradients less than 40 mmHg are generally classed as mild stenosis, pressure gradients from 40–100 mmHg are classed as moderate stenosis, and pressure gradients over 100 mmHg are classed as severe. Doppler echocardiography can also be used to identify mitral regurgitation, mitral stenosis, and aortic insufficiency, all of which may accompany the aortic stenosis.

16. What role does cardiac catheterization currently play in the assessment of AS?
    Cardiac catheterization was traditionally used to diagnose AS and to assess its severity. Doppler echocardiography largely replaces the need for selective catheterization in the diagnosis of AS, and catheterization is most likely to be carried out for interventional procedures such as balloon dilatation of the stenosis.

17. Why are the pressure gradients at cardiac catheterization different from those measured by Doppler?
    The pressure gradient measured directly at cardiac catheterization is generally less than the Doppler-derived gradient. This is partly because the catheter gradient measures the difference between peak left ventricular pressure and peak aortic pressure (peak-to-peak gradient), and these peaks do not occur simultaneously. The Doppler calculation estimates the instantaneous gradient, which is always greater than the peak-to-peak. The other reason is that the pressure gradient depends on *flow* as well as on the narrowness of the stenosis. Cardiac catheterization usually requires general anesthesia, and cardiac output is generally lower than in the conscious dog. Doppler echocardiography can be performed in unsedated dogs, and the higher cardiac output results in a greater pressure gradient.

18. What is the prognosis with AS?
    The prognosis is related to the pressure gradient, with more severe pressure gradients correlating with greater degrees of stenosis and increased risk of complications. There is some variation

in what is reported as a severe gradient; risk of complications based on gradients obtained with catheterization under anesthesia are not necessarily applicable to dogs with gradients measured by Doppler. As a result, figures for severe AS range from > 80 to > 125 mmHg. It is agreed that dogs with severe AS are expected to have shortened survival times, either dying suddenly under the age of 2 or developing congestive failure later in life. Dogs with moderate pressure gradients may remain asymptomatic, or may follow the same clinical course as more severely affected animals. Mildly affected animals were classed as those with a gradient < 35 mmHg in one report, < 75 mmHg in another. These animals are likely to live a normal life span. *All* affected animals are at risk of developing bacterial endocarditis of the aortic valve; this complication is frequently fatal even with aggressive palliative medical care.

19. Why are dogs with AS predisposed to bacterial endocarditis?
Turbulent blood flow striking the aortic valve leaflets can result in endothelial changes on the valve surface that facilitate the adherence of circulating bacteria. In the presence of a bacteremia, dogs with AS are more likely to have bacteria attaching to the aortic valve leaflets than normal dogs. An inflammatory reaction may ensue, which results in the formation of vegetations.

CONTROVERSIES

20. Should AS be treated medically, by balloon dilation, or by surgery?
There is no ideal protocol for the management of AS. Surgical excision of abnormal subaortic tissue is the technique of choice in children, but facilities for this type of surgery in dogs are not widely available, morbidity and mortality rates are high, and there is no evidence of improved survival. Balloon dilatation can be successful in reducing pressure gradients, especially in severe valvular stenosis. Unfortunately, improvement is not always lasting, and the technique is far less successful than in pulmonic stenosis. Medical management is advocated by many, with the primary aim of reducing myocardial oxygen consumption and ventricular arrhythmias. Beta-adrenergic blockers are generally chosen for this purpose. If congestive heart failure develops, management consists of diuretics, with or without the addition of digoxin and ACE inhibitors, providing arterial blood pressure can be monitored. Drugs with vasodilating properties should be used only with caution, if at all, in patients with outflow tract obstruction. When AS is severe, it results in a "fixed cardiac output" in that affected patients can increase cardiac output only through a potentially detrimental increase in left ventricular pressure or heart rate; thus, arterial vasodilation can cause systemic hypotension and reduced coronary perfusion.

21. How can breeders screen their breeding stock for AS?
AS has a genetic basis in the Newfoundland and is almost certainly hereditary in other commonly affected breeds. As has been stated, aortic stenosis exhibits a broad spectrum of severity; some affected animals have a very mild form of the disease while others are severely affected. Unfortunately, mildly affected animals may be capable of transmitting the defect, and the severity of AS observed in the progeny of affected dogs does not always correlate to the severity of obstruction observed in the parents. To further complicate the issue, the detection of mildly affected animals is difficult and opinions differ as to the diagnostic criteria that should be used to identify affected dogs.

However, the most practical means of testing for AS is by auscultation. Examination should be carried out by a board-certified cardiologist when the animal is mature (12 months of age or older). If no murmur is detected, then AS can be effectively ruled out unless there is suspicion of dynamic AS. Some examiners perform auscultation when the dog is at rest and after exercise, to screen for dynamic outflow tract obstruction. Auscultation in puppies can be fraught with difficulties, as AS-affected puppies may not have developed a murmur by 8 weeks, whereas normal puppies of this age can have innocent murmurs that disappear by 16 weeks.

If an ejection murmur is detected, Doppler echocardiography is indicated to identify the source of the murmur. In normal dogs, aortic velocities measured from the left apex are usually less than 1.7 m/s (and often less than 1.5 m/s). Dogs with aortic velocities greater than 2.0 m/s are considered by most to be abnormal, and affected with AS. Dogs with aortic velocities between 1.7 and 2.0 m/s are considered equivocal—AS can neither be diagnosed nor excluded. Whether these dogs have a mild form of AS or physiologic "flow murmurs" is unresolved.

BIBLIOGRAPHY

1. Bonagura JD, Darke PGG: Congenital heart disease. In Ettinger SJ, Feldman EC (eds): Textbook of Veterinary Internal Medicine. Philadelphia, W.B. Saunders, 1995, pp 892–943.
2. Buoscio DA, Sisson D, Zachary JF, Luethy M: Clinical and pathological characterization of an unusual form of subvalvular aortic-stenosis in 4 golden retriever puppies. J Am Anim Hosp Assoc 30:100–110, 1994.
3. DeLellis LA, Thomas WP, Pion PD: Balloon dilation of congenital subaortic stenosis in the dog. J Vet Intern Med 7:153–162, 1993.
4. Dhokarikar P, Caywood DD, Ogburn PN, et al: Closed aortic valvotomy: A retrospective study in 15 dogs. J Am Anim Hosp Assoc 31:402–410, 1995.
5. Kienle RD, Thomas WP, Pion PD: The natural clinical history of canine congenital subaortic stenosis. J Vet Intern Med 8:423–431, 1994.
6. Kittleson MD, Kienle RD: Aortic stenosis. In Kittleson MD, Kienle RD (eds): Small Animal Cardiovascular Medicine. St. Louis, Mosby, 1998, pp 260–272.
7. Komtebedde J, Ilkiw J, Follette DM, et al: Resection of subvalvular aortic stenosis: Surgical and perioperative management in seven dogs. Vet Surg 22:419–430, 1993.
8. Kvart C, French AT, Luis Fuentes V, et al: Analysis of murmur intensity, duration and frequency components in dogs with aortic stenosis. J Small Anim Pract 39:318–324, 1998.
9. Lehmkuhl LB, Bonagura JD: Canine subvalvular aortic stenosis. In Bonagura JD (ed): Kirk's Current Veterinary Therapy XII. Philadelphia, W.B. Saunders, 1995, pp 822–827.
10. Lehmkuhl LB, Bonagura JD, Stepien RL, et al: Comparison of pressure gradients determined by doppler echocardiography and cardiac catheterization in dogs with subaortic stenosis. J Vet Intern Med 6:113–113, 1992.
11. Monnet E, Orton EC, Gaynor JS, et al: Open resection for subvalvular aortic-stenosis in dogs. J Am Vet Med Assoc 209:1255–1261, 1996.
12. Nakayama T, Wakao Y, Ishikawa R, Takahashi M: Progression of subaortic stenosis detected by continuous-wave Doppler: Echocardiography in a dog. J Vet Intern Med 10:97–98, 1996.
13. Pyle RL, Patterson DF, Chacko S: The genetics and pathology of discrete subaortic stenosis in the Newfoundland dog. Am Heart J 92:324–334, 1976.
14. Sisson D: Fixed and dynamic subvalvular aortic stenosis in dogs. In Kirk RW, Bonagura JD (eds): Current Veterinary Therapy XI. Philadelphia, W.B. Saunders, 1992, pp 760–766.
15. Sisson D, Thomas WP: Dynamic subaortic stenosis in a dog with congenital heart disease. J Am Animal Hosp Assoc 20:657–664, 1984.
16. Stepien RL, Bonagura JD: Aortic stenosis clinical findings in six cats. J Small Anim Pract 32:341–350, 1991.

50. PULMONIC STENOSIS

Carroll Loyer, D.V.M.

1. What is pulmonic stenosis?

Pulmonic stenosis is a congenital narrowing of the right ventricular outflow tract. The narrowing can occur just below the pulmonic valve within the right ventricle (subvalvular pulmonic stenosis), at the level of the pulmonic valve (valvular pulmonic stenosis), or above the pulmonic valve in the pulmonary artery (supravalvular pulmonic stenosis). The most common form in dogs is the valvular form.

2. How common is pulmonic stenosis?

Pulmonic stenosis is a frequently observed congenital heart defect in dogs, with only patent ductus arteriosus (PDA) and subaortic stenosis (SAS) being observed more frequently. It accounts for about 11–18% of congenital heart disease diagnoses in dogs. Pulmonic stenosis is very rare in cats.

3. What are dogs with pulmonic stenosis typically presented for?

Typically, pulmonic stenosis is first detected when a cardiac murmur is heard during a routine puppy examination. Many times the pet owner will not notice any signs at all, because very young animals do not exercise for prolonged periods. Some clients will notice some exercise intolerance. Occasionally, an animal may be presented for fainting or ascites (or pleural effusion), but these are generally somewhat older (> 1 year) animals.

4. What will I find on physical examination?

Physical examination reveals a harsh left base systolic murmur that can range from a grade 1/6 to a grade 6/6. Some very astute clinicians and cardiologists can differentiate the pulmonic region from the aortic region, but this is an unrealistic expectation for most veterinarians. Simply differentiating a left heart base murmur from a left apical murmur limits the list of differentials. The two most common causes of left base systolic murmurs in the dog are pulmonic stenosis and subaortic stenosis.

By placing one's hands on both sides of the chest, one can sometimes feel a prominent impulse on the right side. This is called a precordial impulse or "heave," and is normally located at the left apex. There may be a jugular pulse. If the tricuspid valve has begun to leak as a complication of pulmonic stenosis, one may also hear a separate right-sided systolic murmur.

5. What breeds are at higher risk for pulmonic stenosis?

Pulmonic stenosis is often seen in English bulldogs, terriers (West Highland white, Scottish, wire-haired fox, Yorkshire), miniature schnauzers, Chihuahuas, Samoyeds, beagles, keeshonds, mastiffs, and bullmastiffs. Pulmonic stenosis is occasionally seen in other breeds, including German shepherds, spaniels, and retrievers. A hereditary basis for pulmonic stenosis has been proved for beagles and is suspected for other breeds. Note that many of these breeds are smaller breeds, whereas many of the dogs typically affected with subaortic stenosis (another cause of left base murmurs) are larger-breed dogs. This can be a first clue that this animal might have pulmonic stenosis.

6. What causes pulmonic stenosis?

In most dogs, it is abnormal development of the pulmonic valve (valvular dysplasia). In English bulldogs (and boxers), there may be abnormal development of the coronary arteries where the left main coronary artery arises from a single right coronary artery, encircles the pulmonary artery at the level of the pulmonic valve, and contributes to the development of the stenosis. Both supravalvular and true subvalvular (double-chambered right-ventricle) PS are quite uncommon.

7. What is the pathophysiology of pulmonic stenosis?

Pulmonic stenosis causes an obstruction to flow of blood out the right ventricle (see figure below); as a consequence, right ventricular systolic pressure increases in order to maintain flow through the narrowed orifice. This increase in pressure leads to thickening (concentric hypertrophy) of the right ventricle, and this can lead to a "stiff" right ventricle, where diastolic pressure of the right ventricle is also elevated. The degree of these changes is directly related to the degree of obstruction. If the obstruction is very severe, cardiac output across the valve will be limited, especially at exercise (hence the exercise intolerance and the occasional syncope seen in these dogs).

The right ventricular hypertrophy may also cause some secondary obstruction to outflow, produce changes in right ventricular configuration resulting in tricuspid regurgitation, and increase diastolic pressures. These may all lead to the development of high right atrial pressures, right atrial enlargement, and potentially right-sided heart failure (manifest as ascites and pleural effusion). In severe cases coronary artery flow may also be affected, which may contribute to sudden death.

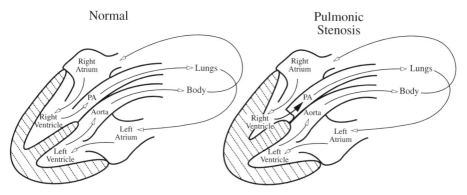

Schematic diagram of normal heart vs. pulmonic stenosis.

8. What does an electrocardiogram show? Will it help me differentiate pulmonic stenosis from subaortic stenosis?

An electrocardiogram of a dog with moderate or severe pulmonic stenosis will often show a right ventricular enlargement pattern. This will be seen as deep S waves in leads I, II, III, and aVF. This can be very useful in differentiating from subaortic stenosis, where one will sometimes see a left ventricular enlargement pattern of large R waves. The electrocardiogram, however, does not provide quantitative information regarding the severity of the disease.

9. Are radiographs helpful in detecting pulmonic stenosis?

Radiographs may show a normal heart since the right ventricular hypertrophy is concentric, and "inside" the heart. There may be some cardiomegaly with right heart enlargement. Sometimes one can see a poststenotic dilatation of the pulmonary artery at the 1:00 position on the DV or VD radiograph. This poststenotic dilation is due to turbulence of blood past the obstruction. There may be right atrial enlargement, seen as elevation of the trachea at the cranial aspect of the heart, and loss of the cranial cardiac waist. Like electrocardiograms, radiographs do not provide quantitative information regarding the severity of the disease.

10. What will an echocardiogram show?

Two-dimensional echocardiography will show the hypertrophy of the right ventricle, right atrial enlargement if present, and can often visualize the poststenotic dilatation. The pulmonic valve can be examined for thickening and "doming" as evidence of valvular pulmonic stenosis (although sometimes the valve is difficult to visualize), and both supravalvular and subvalvular lesions can be appreciated. A muscular component of the stenosis can often be seen just underneath the pulmonic valve and can contribute to "dynamic" (as opposed to fixed) obstruction. The severity of the stenosis can be inferred from the degree of hypertrophy of the right ventricle, but a definitive grading of the stenosis requires Doppler echocardiography. Caution should be used in grading the severity of the stenosis by what the valve looks like.

Spectral Doppler echocardiography provides a reliable, noninvasive method of grading the severity of pulmonic stenosis. Color-flow Doppler is helpful in evaluating for secondary tricuspid stenosis.

11. How does Doppler echocardiography grade the severity of the stenosis?

When pulmonic stenosis is present, the right ventricle must generate abnormally high systolic pressures in order to maintain normal pulmonary artery flow and pressure. Thus, a pressure difference, or gradient, develops across the obstruction. Doppler echocardiography is used to document an increase in velocity of blood flow across the stenotic lesion, and a modification of the Bernoulli equation can be used to convert that velocity to the pressure gradient from right ventricle to pulmonary artery (see Chapter 23). In a normal dog the gradient is zero and there is no pressure difference from the right ventricle to the pulmonary artery during systole. In dogs with mild pulmonic stenosis the pressure gradient is less than 40 mmHg. Dogs with moderate pulmonic stenosis have a pressure gradient of 40–100 mmHg, and dogs with severe pulmonic stenosis have a gradient of > 100 mmHg. Some cardiologists use 80 mmHg as their cutoff between moderate and severe. Doppler echocardiography is recommended for all cases of congenital cardiac disease.

12. What about cardiac catheterization?

Cardiac catheterization is rarely performed with the advent of echocardiography. It shows virtually the same findings as an echocardiogram, but can be quite useful in surgical cases. Cardiac catheterization is also very helpful in determining whether there is an anomalous coronary artery, which can be difficult to assess with echocardiography. If balloon or surgical valvuloplasty is being considered on an English bulldog or boxer, cardiac catheterization beforehand is highly recommended.

13. What is the prognosis for dogs with pulmonic stenosis?

It depends on whether they have mild, moderate, or severe stenosis. It is generally good. Dogs with mild stenosis usually have normal life spans with no signs of exercise intolerance. Dogs with moderate stenosis often have normal life spans, but may be somewhat exercise-intolerant. Dogs with severe pulmonic stenosis are often exercise-intolerant, but may live for surprisingly prolonged periods. They may die suddenly, or may go into right heart failure if tricuspid insufficiency develops.

14. How do I treat pulmonic stenosis?

In cases of mild to moderate pulmonic stenosis, no medical or surgical procedure is indicated, and exercise restriction is generally not necessary (these dogs will usually restrict themselves). If the lesion is severe, either a balloon valvuloplasty or surgical procedure with referral to a cardiologist or institutional surgeon is recommended. Medical therapy with beta-blockers to try to prevent sudden death can be instituted if more aggressive therapy is not an option. In cases of severe pulmonic stenosis without significant subvalvular muscular hypertrophy, most cardiologists will first attempt a balloon valvuloplasty. If this fails, surgery should be considered, but can be fraught with risk. Dogs with pulmonic stenosis should not be bred.

15. What is balloon valvuloplasty and how is the procedure performed?

Balloon valvuloplasty is an interventional cardiac catheterization technique that is used in the management of pulmonic stenosis in the dog. Balloon catheters are equipped with a collapsible balloon that surrounds the catheter near its distal tip. Catheters with a variety of balloon diameter and lengths are available; the appropriate balloon size is typically determined through echocardiographic or angiographic measurement of the valve annulus. Following anesthetic induction, venous access is obtained through the femoral or external jugular vein. Under fluoroscopic guidance, a cardiovascular catheter equipped with an end-hole is guided through the right atrium and ventricle, advanced across the stenotic lesion and into the main pulmonary artery. After direct measurement of the pressure gradient and angiographic assessment of the stenosis, a long, flexible guide-wire, known as an exchange wire, is placed through the catheter and into the pulmonary artery; at this point, the catheter is removed and the exchange wire is left in place. The balloon catheter is then threaded down the wire and the balloon placed across the stenosis. Balloon catheters are rather stiff, which is why they must be introduced over a preplaced guidewire. The balloon is inflated with diluted contrast material two or three times, after which the catheter is removed. When successful, the pressure gradient is immediately reduced by 50% or more. The procedure is minimally invasive and associated with relatively low risk when performed by a veterinarian with experience in cardiac catheterization techniques.

16. What if right heart failure develops?

This is very difficult to manage. The pulmonic stenosis causes "fixed" obstruction, so that arterial dilators are of no use. One can still try diuretics and venodilators (angiotensin-converting enzyme inhibitors are balanced vasodilators and can be used), but the prognosis is poor. Reducing the pulmonic valve gradient with a balloon or surgery would the best option, but carries a high risk at that point.

17. What about concurrent cardiac defects?

Dogs with pulmonic stenosis can also have atrial septal defects, ventricular septal defects, and have tetralogy of Fallot. Depending on the severity of the pulmonic stenosis, they may shunt blood right to left across these other defects, which causes cyanotic cardiac disease (see Chapter 57).

BIBLIOGRAPHY

1. Bonagura JD, Lehmkuhl LB: Congenital heart disease. In Fox PR, Sisson D, Moise NS (eds): Canine and Feline Cardiology. Philadelphia, W.B. Saunders, 1999, pp 471–485.
2. Kittleson MD, Kienle RD: Pulmonic stenosis. In Kittleson MD, Kienle RD (eds): Small Animal Cardiovascular Medicine. St. Louis, Mosby, 1998, pp 248–259.
3. Loyer C: Pulmonic stenosis. In Tilley LP, Smith FWK (eds): The 5-Minute Veterinary Consult. Baltimore, Williams & Wilkins, 1997, pp 990–991.
4. Orton EC: Current indications for cardiac surgery. In Bonagura JD (ed): Kirk's Current Veterinary Therapy XIII. Philadelphia, W.B. Saunders, 1999, pp 745–746.

51. VENTRICULAR SEPTAL DEFECTS

Jonathan A. Abbott, D.V.M.

1. What is a ventricular septal defect?

A ventricular septal defect (VSD) is a deficiency of the interventricular septum that creates a communication between the ventricles. Traumatic acquired ventricular septal defects are occasionally observed in people but have not been reported in animals. In this discussion, VSD will refer to congenital defects of ventricular septation. Failure of embryonic septal components to fuse or hypoplasia/agenesis of septal components is the presumed cause of most ventricular septal defects.

2. What is the anatomy of VSDs in small animals?

The interventricular septum is comprised of four components: the inlet septum, the outlet (or infundibular) septum, the trabecular septum, and the membranous septum. The latter is located in the subaortic region. The embryogenesis of the membranous septum involves the fusion of a number of separate components and the complexity of its formation probably explains the fact that most VSDs involve this region of the septum. Often, the defect extends into one of the other anatomic septal regions and the term peri- or paramembranous is used.

Most VSDs in small animals are perimembranous; the defect is typically subaortic and the right ventricular orifice of the VSD is immediately ventral to the septal tricuspid valve leaflet.

3. What is the prevalence of VSDs?

VSDs are among the most common cardiac anomalies in cats and are observed as isolated lesions or as components of more complex anomalies such as the endocardial cushion defect and tetralogy of Fallot. VSDs are somewhat less common in dogs; in a recent survey VSDs were the fourth most common congenital cardiac malformation observed in dogs.

4. What is a typical signalment for VSD in dogs? What about cats?

VSDs are most commonly identified in young dogs, but there is no known sex predisposition. A few purebred dogs, including the English bulldog and the English springer spaniel, are more likely to develop a congenital VSD than dogs in the general veterinary hospital population. Breed or sex predispositions are not recognized for VSDs in the cat.

5. What are the pathophysiologic consequences of a VSD? How does the presence of a VSD alter blood flow?

If the VSD is the only cardiac lesion and pulmonary vascular resistance is normal, then a portion of the left ventricular stroke volume enters the pulmonary circulation. The shunted blood augments the right ventricular output and is conveyed to the lungs. From the lungs, the enlarged pulmonary blood volume returns to the left atrium and left ventricle via the pulmonary veins. Thus, a *left-to-right* VSD results in a volume load on the *left atrium and left ventricle*.

6. What is the shunt fraction?

The shunt fraction, or Qp/Qs, expresses the relationship between pulmonary and systemic blood flow. This quantity can be measured indirectly through the determination of blood oxygen saturations in various parts of the circulation. Additionally, noninvasive estimates of the shunt fraction can be obtained echocardiographically. When obtained in a patient with a left-to-right VSD, the shunt fraction measures the relative extent to which pulmonary blood flow exceeds systemic blood flow.

7. What determines the shunt fraction or size of the shunt?

When a VSD is the only cardiac lesion, the size and direction of the shunt is determined by: (1) size of the defect; and (2) relationship between pulmonary and systemic resistance.

The size of the defect can be classified in relation to the size of the aorta. If the area of the VSD is less than 40% of that of the aortic orifice, the defect is said to be small. Large defects are as large or larger than the aortic orifice and moderately sized VSD are intermediate with regards to this characteristic. Small VSD are said to be restrictive, that is, the pressure difference between the left ventricle, which normally generates a high pressure, and the right ventricle, in which the systolic pressure is relatively low, is preserved. When the VSD is moderately sized, there is some "spillover" of pressure into the right ventricle. If the VSD is large, the pressures within the left and right ventricles equilibrate and the direction and size of the shunt depends entirely on the relationship between pulmonary and systemic vascular resistance.

Resistance is the hydraulic force that must be overcome in order to achieve or maintain flow through a vessel. Vascular resistance is related, in an approximate fashion, to flow and pressure by Ohm's law (BP = R × Q, where BP is blood pressure, R is vascular resistance, and Q is flow, or cardiac output). It is clear then that flow depends not only on pressure but also on resistance. When the pulmonary vessels are normal, systemic vascular resistance far exceeds pulmonary vascular resistance. Thus if a large and nonrestrictive VSD is present, a large left-to-right shunt is expected. In this case, the pressures within the ventricles are the same; however, it is much "easier" for blood to enter the low-resistance pulmonary circulation than it is for blood to enter the systemic vasculature.

8. A left-to-right VSD imposes a volume load on the left atrium and left ventricle; how is the right ventricle affected?

The extent to which the right ventricle is affected depends primarily on the size of the VSD. In the case of a VSD that is restrictive, the shunt volume is necessarily small and right ventricular pressures are normal. Thus, the right ventricle is "spared." In contrast, a moderate or large VSD results in right ventricular hypertension and this pressure overload results in varying degrees of right ventricular hypertrophy.

9. What is the effect of concurrent cardiac anomalies?

Concurrent cardiac anomalies may affect intraventricular pressures and volumes, which can alter the clinical importance of the VSD. In dogs, two specific associated lesions are important to consider: (1) **pulmonic stenosis**, which increases the resistance to right ventricular emptying and therefore raises right ventricular pressure; and (2) **aortic valve incompetence**, which can develop as a consequence of poor structural support of the aortic annulus related to the presence of a subaortic VSD.

Pulmonic stenosis, if severe, can result in a right-to-left shunt and, even if the VSD is small, this can result in hypoxemia and weakness. Aortic valve regurgitation imposes a volume load on the left ventricle. Aortic regurgitation tends to be poorly tolerated and the development of severe aortic regurgitation can have an impact on the prognosis in a patient with a small VSD that would be otherwise well tolerated.

10. What is the usual outcome of patients with VSD?

The clinical outcome depends upon the variables that affect shunt size and direction. If the VSD is large, left-sided, or even biventricular, congestive failure develops early in life. Most VSDs in small animals are small and are well tolerated; in this case, the prognosis depends largely on whether or not concurrent defects are present.

The development of pulmonary vascular disease as a sequel to chronic hyperperfusion of the lung is a recognized complication in people with left-to-right shunts. In this case, medial hypertrophy of the pulmonary arterioles increases pulmonary vascular resistance and, therefore, the pressure required to maintain flow through the pulmonary arterial system. In cases in which pulmonary vascular resistance becomes suprasystemic, the shunt reverses, resulting in a right-to-left shunt, venous admixture, and cyanosis. This is uncommon in small animals. Right-to-left shunting VSD will be addressed in Chapter 57.

11. What is an endocardial cushion defect?
An endocardial cushion defect or atrioventricular canal is an anomaly that consists of a primum atrial septal defect together with a VSD. The endocardial cushions are embryonic structures that contribute to the development of the interventricular septum, the atrial septum, and the atrioventricular valves. A failure of the cushions to fuse is thought to explain the development of this anomaly, hence the name. Abnormalities of the mitral and tricuspid valves are commonly observed together with the defects in atrial and ventricular septation.

12. How is a VSD detected?
VSDs are most often detected when a cardiac murmur is heard during the routine examination of puppies and kittens.

13. What findings are expected on cardiac auscultation?
A VSD results in a systolic, plateau-shaped murmur; the pressure difference between the ventricles during diastole is insufficient to generate audible blood flow. The intensity of the murmur is inversely proportional to the size of the defect; small, restrictive defects, which are common, result in loud systolic murmurs that are often accompanied by a precordial thrill. Larger defects result in softer murmurs; if the VSD is as large as the aorta, the shunt may not result in a murmur at all. The point of maximal intensity of the murmur is variable and depends on the anatomy of the defect. However, most VSDs in dogs and cats have a right ventricular orifice that is immediately ventral to the septal tricuspid valve leaflet; thus, the murmur is typically heard best over the right cardiac apex.
In addition to the murmur generated by the shunt through the VSD, an additional murmur of "functional" pulmonic stenosis is occasionally heard.

14. What is functional pulmonic stenosis?
This murmur results when the shunt volume is large enough to substantially increase pulmonary artery flow velocity. The pathogenesis of this murmur is as follows. When a left-to-right VSD is present, more blood than is normal passes through the pulmonary valve. Since the duration of systole remains about the same, the enlarged right ventricular stroke volume must be ejected at high velocity. If the velocity of blood flow is sufficiently high that flow becomes disturbed, a murmur may result. This murmur is usually of low intensity, systolic, has a crescendo-decrescendo configuration, and is heard best over the left cardiac base. This murmur can develop in the absence of pulmonic valve pathology; thus, it is known as a murmur of functional pulmonic stenosis. When the VSD is large, this flow murmur might be the only auscultatory evidence of the defect.

15. Describe the radiographic abnormalities associated with VSD.
The cardiac silhouette is enlarged to a degree commensurate with the size of the shunt. Many patients that have a small and restrictive VSD have either a normal or mildly enlarged cardiac silhouette. Generalized cardiomegaly is expected if the VSD is moderate or large. Shunting through the VSD and into the pulmonary artery can result in enlargement of the proximal main pulmonary artery and this structure may be prominent. The increase in pulmonary blood flow tends to make the pulmonary arteries and veins prominent, resulting in the radiographic appearance of pulmonary hyperperfusion.

16. What abnormalities are detected on echocardiographic examination?
Often, the VSD can be seen directly; usually, the defect is subaortic and directed towards the ventral aspect of the septal tricuspid valve leaflet. Caution must be exercised; the membranous part of the interventricular septal defect is very thin, and so the spurious appearance of a septal defect ("septal dropout") is quite common.

Doppler echocardiographic examination is required for a definitive noninvasive diagnosis of a VSD (see figure below). Shunting through the defect can be demonstrated through color-flow Doppler mapping. Spectral Doppler studies confirm the direction and velocity of the shunt. The velocity of the jet is related to the pressure difference between the two ventricles. When continuous-wave Doppler studies are performed using a right parasternal transducer position, a positive velocity signal with a peak velocity greater than 5 m/s is recorded when the beam is aligned with the VSD jet.

Additional and related findings might include aortic valve regurgitation and, on occasion, other congenital anomalies such as pulmonic stenosis, atrial septal defect, or AV valve incompetence.

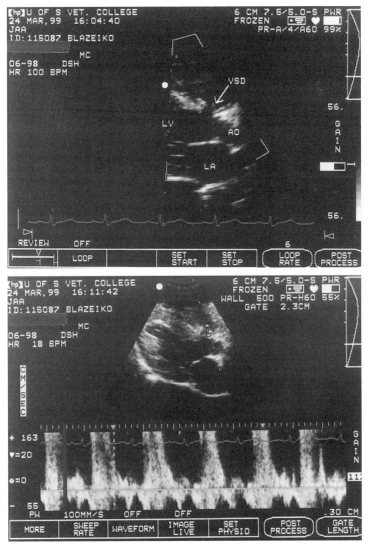

Top, Right parasternal long-axis echocardiographic image of the left ventricular outflow tract obtained from a 9-month-old male castrated domestic shorthair cat. The subaortic ventricular septal defect (VSD) is labeled. LV, left ventricle; LA, left atrium; AO, aorta. *Bottom*, Pulsed-wave Doppler study performed with the sample volume placed adjacent to the right ventricular orifice of the VSD. A systolic, high-velocity jet is evident; the spectral breadth of the signal is high, indicating disturbed flow.

17. Is echocardiography necessary for diagnosis of a VSD?

A presumptive diagnosis of a left-to-right VSD can be made based upon physical and radiographic findings. However, echocardiographic examination, including Doppler studies, is required for a definitive noninvasive diagnosis. The information that is obtained is essential for the formulation of an accurate prognosis and therapeutic plan. In fact, Doppler echocardiographic examination by an individual trained in the diagnosis and management of cardiovascular disease is recommended for all patients with congenital cardiovascular disease.

18. How else might one make a definitive antemortem diagnosis of a VSD?

Cardiac catheterization methods are well suited to the diagnosis of VSD. Selective angiographic studies performed following the injection of contrast material into the left ventricle will delineate the defect. Blood gas analyses performed on samples obtained from sites proximal and distal to the defect demonstrate an "oxygen step-up." Blood from the right atrium has a low oxygen saturation, as this blood represents the deoxygenated systemic venous return. The shunting of oxygenated blood from the left to the right ventricle through the VSD results in high oxygen saturations in the right ventricle and pulmonary artery. The magnitude of this oxygen step-up can be used in a modification of the Fick equation to obtain the shunt fraction or Qp/Qs.

Additionally, cardiac catheterization studies can provide useful hemodynamic information; the pressure within the cardiac chambers and great vessels can be measured directly and, if the cardiac output is measured, pulmonary vascular resistance can be calculated.

Cardiac catheterization provides a wealth of data that is probably most important when surgical repair of the defect is contemplated; however, when Doppler studies are performed by an experienced echocardiographer, catheterization is rarely necessary for diagnosis of the defect.

19. How is a VSD treated?

Small and restrictive VSDs are usually well tolerated and do not require treatment. When the shunt fraction (Qp/Qs) exceeds 2 or 2.5, or aortic valve regurgitation has contributed to substantial left ventricular enlargement, consideration can be given to surgical correction of the defect. Definitive repair of a VSD requires cardiopulmonary bypass, is relatively expensive, and is not without risk. Definitive surgical repair of VSDs is available at a few referral institutions and can be considered for appropriate candidates.

20. Are there medical alternatives to surgery for VSD?

The need for therapy in the absence of clinical signs can be debated; however, the use of an ACE inhibitor can be considered for patients that have echocardiographic evidence of a large left-to-right shunt or substantial aortic valve regurgitation. ACE inhibitors cause vasodilation, among other effects. The resultant decrease in systemic vascular resistance may limit shunting and is beneficial for patients with aortic valve regurgitation. Additionally, ACE inhibitors have neurohumoral effects that might preserve myocardial function. If CHF results from a VSD, standard medical therapy using a diuretic, ACE inhibitor, and digoxin is suggested. As for other congenital cardiac malformations that mechanically overload the heart, definitive therapy consists of surgical repair; medical therapy is only palliative.

21. What is the prognosis for patients with a VSD?

The prognosis for patients with an isolated, restricted VSD is very good; these patients are likely to live a normal lifespan without therapeutic intervention. Patients with clinically important aortic valve regurgitation may fare less well as this lesion tends to be poorly tolerated. The onset of congestive heart failure indicates that the defect is, without correction, terminal.

BIBLIOGRAPHY

1. Bonagura JD, Lehmkuhl LB: Congenital heart disease. In Fox PR, Sisson D, Moise NS (eds): Textbook of Canine and Feline Cardiology: Principles and Clinical Practice. Philadelphia, W.B. Saunders, 1999, pp 471–535.

2. Brown WA: Ventricular septal defects in the English springer spaniel. In Bonagura JD (ed): Current Veterinary Therapy XII: Small Animal Practice. Philadelphia, W.B. Saunders, 1995, pp 827–829.
3. Buchanan JW: Prevalence of cardiovascular disorders. In Fox PR, Sisson D, Moise NS (eds): Textbook of Canine and Feline Cardiology: Principles and Clinical Practice. Philadelphia, W.B. Saunders, 1999, pp 457–470.
4. Kittleson MD: Septal defects. In Kittleson MD, Kienle RD (eds): Small Animal Cardiovascular Medicine. St. Louis, Mosby, 1998, pp 231–239.
5. Patterson DF: Congenital defects of the cardiovascular system of dogs: Studies in comparative cardiology. Adv Vet Sci Comp Med 20:1–37, 1976.

52. ATRIAL SEPTAL DEFECTS

Donald P. Schrope, D.V.M.

1. Explain the normal embryologic development of the atrial septum.

The *septum primum* originates in the roof of a common atrium and grows ventrally, dividing the atrium into a left and right side (see figure below). An opening between the atria called the *ostium primum* is initially present ventrally, adjacent to the floor of the atria. Over time, as the septum primum extends ventrally to close the ostium primum, a portion of the septum primum degenerates, creating an opening called the *ostium secundum*. The ostium secundum develops in the caudodorsal aspect of the septum primum, maintaining an opening between the atria. In the fetus, it is important for there to be direct communication between the right and the left atria. This opening acts as a "pop-off valve" for the right fetal heart, where pressures are elevated due to the collapsed state of the lungs. As the septum primum completes its development, a second septum develops to the right of the septum primum, called the *septum secundum*. The septum secundum originates cranially and extends caudally adjacent to the septum primum. The septum stretches across the atria, leaving a small opening caudally called the *foramen ovale*. In the fetus, the space between the septum primum and the septum secundum is maintained. This allows blood to pass from the right atrium, through the foramen ovale, into the space between the atrial septa, and then out the ostium secundum into the left atrium. Soon after birth, the elevation in left atrial pressure forces the septum primum and septum secundum together, collapsing the space between the septa and therefore closing the opening between the left and the right atria. At this point, normally the septa will fuse and become the *interatrial septum*.

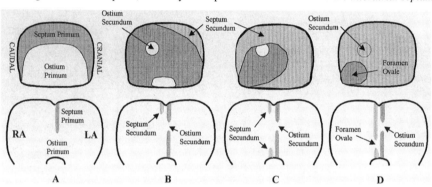

Diagram of normal embryonic development of the interatrial septum. The upper row of diagrams depicts the atria cut in the sagittal plane with the observer looking from the right atrium into the left atrium. The cranial aspect of the heart is to the right. The lower row of diagrams depicts the atria in a transverse plane with the right atrium on the left. *A,* The septum primum can be seen growing down from the roof of the common atrium. The septum primum forms the upper border of the ostium primum ventrally. *B,* As the septum primum closes the ostium primum and reaches the floor of the atrium, an opening in the caudodorsal aspect of the septum primum develops. This is called the ostium secundum. At the same time, the septum secundum begins to develop to the right of the septum primum, and in the craniodorsal aspect of the roof of the atria. *C,* The septum secundum continues to extend caudally across the ostium secundum. *D,* The septum secundum completes its development, leaving an opening caudoventrally, called the foramen ovale. A small space remains between the septum primum and the septum secundum in the fetus to allow right-to-left blood flow.

2. Explain the differences among an ostium primum atrial septal defect (ASD), an ostium secundum ASD, a sinus venosus ASD, and a patent foramen ovale.

Atrial septal defects (ASDs) are generally named based upon their presumed embryologic origin. An ostium primum ASD is found adjacent to the floor of the atria near the atrioventricular

(AV) valves where the embryonic ostium primum is found (see figure). This defect is often associated with defects of the endocardial cushions that are integral to the formation of the AV valves and a portion of the ventricular septum.

An ostium secundum ASD involves the persistence of an exceptionally large ostium secundum in the septum primum. This type of ASD is generally seen more dorsally and centrally in the atrial septum.

A patent foramen ovale results from lack of fusion of the septum primum and the septum secundum in the neonatal period. The structure of the patent foramen ovale allows only right-to-left flow across the interatrial communication. Therefore, a patent foramen ovale is often not recognized diagnostically unless pressures are higher in the right atrium than in the left atrium. The patent foramen ovale is not considered by some to be a true ASD because the resulting interatrial communication is secondary to elevations in right atrial pressure and is not the result of a true deficiency of the atrial septum. Patency of the foramen ovale can occur with tricuspid valve disease (congenital or acquired), pulmonary hypertension, and other diseases that abnormally elevate right atrial pressure.

A sinus venosus ASD is a defect in the atrial septum at the junction of the atrial septum and the cranial or caudal vena cava. Because the defect is present at the junction of the vena cava and the atrial septum, the cranial or caudal vena cava may straddle the atrial septum to some degree, emptying into both the right and the left atria. A sinus venosus ASD can also be associated with malposition and malformation of the pulmonary veins.

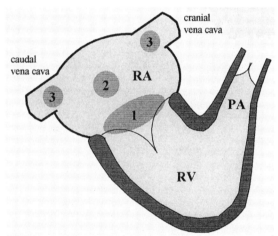

Types of atrial septal defects (ASD). This is a sagittal plane through the heart depicting the locations of the different types of atrial septal defects: *1*, ostium primum ASD; *2*, ostium secundum ASD; and *3*, sinus venosus ASD. RA, right atrium; RV, right ventricle; PA, pulmonary artery.

3. What is the typical signalment of a patient with an atrial septal defect?

Atrial septal defects appear to be fairly uncommon in the dog and the cat. It has been suggested that the boxer dog may be predisposed to atrial septal defects. There does not seem to be a sex predisposition in either dogs or cats, although the small number of reported cases makes this difficult to evaluate. Although defects in atrial septation are congenital, they are often detected only later in life for multiple reasons. First, a murmur, if present, may be very soft. Additionally, an ASD is often small and may not show signs of cardiac compromise until very late in life, if ever. Larger defects, especially a septum primum ASD, which may be seen in conjunction with ventricular septal abnormalities, may create signs of cyanosis, exertional dyspnea, and heart failure within the first year of life.

4. What are the expected findings on thoracic auscultation of a patient with a clinically important ASD? What are the origins of these abnormalities?

The production of a cardiac murmur is dependent upon the development of turbulence. Because of the low pressure gradient across the atrial septum, audible turbulence rarely develops at the site of an ASD. However, the excessive blood volume associated with the left-to-right shunt seen with an ASD can cause turbulence as it passes through the normal pulmonic valve, resulting in a murmur. Because the valve is anatomically normal, but is not large enough to handle the excess volume of blood, this is called a "relative pulmonic stenosis." This leads to a moderately loud systolic ejection murmur over the left heart base. Similar circumstances can occasionally lead to a soft diastolic murmur over the tricuspid valve. Therefore, a murmur associated with an ASD is related to the volume overload of the right heart, and does not result from the septal defect itself.

Normally, the second heart sound originates from the near-simultaneous closure of the aortic and pulmonic valves. The excessive volume of blood passing through the pulmonic valve associated with an ASD may delay the closure of the pulmonic valve relative to the closure of the aortic valve. If this delay is sufficiently great, the aortic and pulmonic components of the second heart sound can be distinguished by the examiner. This is known as splitting of the second heart sound.

5. Why do uncomplicated atrial septal defects cause right heart enlargement, while uncomplicated ventricular septal defects cause left heart enlargement?

Blood associated with an intracardiac shunt will always take the path of least resistance. In the instance of an uncomplicated ASD or ventricular septal defect (VSD) this causes a left-to-right shunt because normally pressure in the right heart is lower than that in the left throughout the majority of the cardiac cycle. When an isolated ASD is so large that the interatrial pressure difference is eliminated, blood continues to shunt from left to right because the right-sided chambers are more compliant than the left and also because the tricuspid orifice is somewhat larger than the orifice of the mitral valve.

The reason for the difference in cardiomegaly associated with an ASD or VSD is related to the anatomic site of the shunt. Because the filling pressure of the left ventricle exceeds that of the right, blood tends to shunt from left to right across the ASD during diastole, passing through the open tricuspid valve to enter the right ventricle. Dilation of the right ventricle is caused by this excess blood volume entering the right ventricle when the pulmonic valve is closed. During systole, the shunted blood enters the more compliant right atrium and is impeded by the closed tricuspid valve until the onset of diastole, at which time it contributes to right ventricular filling. This results in right atrial dilatation. Thus, an ASD results in dilation of both the right atrium and right ventricle.

In the presence of a VSD, shunting occurs at the level of the ventricles. The pressure difference between the left ventricle and the right ventricle is greatest during systole; therefore, the greatest shunting volume occurs during systole. The shunt volume passes from the left ventricle into the right ventricle and then immediately out the pulmonary artery into the lungs. This excess blood volume then empties into the left atrium and subsequently the left ventricle, resulting in left ventricular and left atrial dilation.

6. Explain what is meant by Eisenmenger's physiology in relation to an ASD.

Pulmonary artery pressures are related to pulmonary vascular resistance and pulmonary blood flow by Ohm's law such that PAP = Q × PVR (where PAP is mean pulmonary artery pressure, Q is pulmonary blood flow, and PVR is pulmonary vascular resistance). When pulmonary blood flow is increased, as is the case in a left-to-right shunting ASD, pulmonary vascular resistance (PVR) can decrease through distention and recruitment of pulmonary vessels in order to minimize increases in pulmonary artery pressures. However, the capacity for the pulmonary vascular system to accommodate excessive flow volumes is finite and large shunts necessarily result in elevations in pulmonary artery pressures, or *pulmonary hypertension*. If pulmonary hypertension is severe enough, significant damage to the pulmonary vasculature can occur. This can result in pulmonary vasoconstriction and narrowing of the pulmonary arteries through medial hypertrophy, which elevates PVR and therefore PAP.

With the development of elevated PVR, pressures in the right heart may exceed those in the left heart. This may lead to development of right-to-left shunting across a septal defect.

This reversal from a left-to-right to a right-to-left shunt secondary to elevated PVR is called Eisenmenger's physiology. It should be stated that the phenomenon of shunt reversal is a well-recognized complication of uncorrected left-to-right shunts in people. The incidence of Eisenmenger's physiology in small animals is unknown, although clinical experience with other, more common left-to-right shunts, such as ventricular septal defects or patent ductus arteriosus, would suggest that it is uncommon. It is likely that shunt reversal, when it does happen, occurs early in life and in association with large left-to-right shunts.

7. Describe the radiographic and electrocardiographic findings of a patient with an ASD.

The presence or absence of changes on radiographs or an electrocardiogram is dependent on the size of the ASD and whether right heart enlargement results. On an EKG, evidence of right ventricular enlargement such as a right axis shift, tall R-waves in right chest leads, and deep S-waves in left chest leads may be seen. Evidence of right atrial enlargement, such as P-pulmonale, may also be present.

With large defects, chest radiographs may show evidence of right ventricular and right atrial enlargement. The excessive volume of blood entering the pulmonary vasculature may be reflected as a bulging of the main pulmonary artery and evidence of overcirculation of the pulmonary vasculature. If an ostium primum ASD is associated with an endocardial cushion defect resulting in abnormalities of the mitral valve, left atrial and left ventricular enlargement may also be seen.

8. Describe the 2D echocardiographic findings in a patient with an ASD.

An ASD can generally be identified by an "echo-free" space in the atrial septum. An ostium primum ASD will show an echo-free space adjacent to the AV valves and membranous septum. In contrast, an ostium secundum ASD will be present more centrally and closer to the dorsal aspect of the atrial septum. A sinus venosus ASD will result in an echo-free space at the junction of the right atrium and the cranial or caudal vena cava. A patent foramen ovale will often appear as a bulging and thinning of the atrial septum centrally, and possibly as a small echo-free space.

The angle of interrogation of the atrial septum is important when evaluating for an ASD. The echo beam should be perpendicular to the long axis of the atrial septum, similar to the angle utilized to obtain a right parasternal long or short axis view. If the beam is parallel with the atrial septum, such as it is in an apical four-chamber view, the ultrasound beam may not reflect off the atrial septum. This can cause an artifactual echo-free space mimicking an ASD. Color-flow Doppler should be used when possible to confirm the presence of blood flow across a suspect ASD. Some small ASDs, such as a patent foramen ovale, may only be identifiable with Doppler evaluation. The right ventricle and right atrium may be dilated if the size of the ASD is moderate or large. The main pulmonary artery may also appear dilated.

The left heart is generally normal with an ASD. If the right heart enlargement and elevation in right heart pressures secondary to an ASD are severe, however, the LV may appear relatively small and abnormally shaped. This is due to flattening of the interventricular septum and paradoxical septal motion resulting from right ventricular volume overload.

9. Describe the Doppler echocardiographic findings in a patient with an ASD.

Color-flow Doppler should confirm the presence of a septal defect and help identify other secondary complications such as tricuspid regurgitation and mitral regurgitation. Spectral Doppler evaluation of an uncomplicated ASD will typically show predominantly left-to-right flow with two main peaks. The first peak begins in late systole and ends in middiastole, while the second peak is associated with atrial contraction in late diastole. Transient right-to-left shunting across an uncomplicated ASD, or "flow reversal," can be seen at the onset of systole. If pulmonary hypertension is present, the typical flow pattern may be altered and predominantly right-to-left flow may be seen across the defect throughout the cardiac cycle.

The right ventricular pressure may be estimated if a tricuspid regurgitation (TR) jet is identified with spectral or color-flow Doppler by using the modified Bernoulli equation as is discussed in Chapter 46.

10. Can echocardiography provide any other diagnostically useful information?

Microscopic air bubbles contained within agitated saline are highly reflective on ultrasound. Thus, the intravenous administration of agitated saline, or even saline mixed with the patient's blood, provides a form of echocardiographic contrast. The sonographically visible bubbles in saline are extracted during the passage through the patient's lungs. Thus, the use of "bubble contrast" studies is best suited to the diagnosis or right-to-left shunting cardiac defects; the visualization of even a small number of bubbles within the left atrium or left ventricle is certain evidence of a communication between the left and right heart. When shunting is from left-to-right, the negative contrast that results when "bubble-free" blood from the left atrium enters the opacified right atrium can suggest the presence of an ASD.

Additionally, even in cases of left-to-right ASD, momentary shunt reversal during the course of the cardiac cycle is common. Because of this and the diagnostic specificity of observing echocardiographic contrast within the left heart chambers, bubble contrast studies can provide supportive evidence whenever an ASD is suspected.

11. What is the pathophysiology of clinical signs associated with atrial septal defects?

As discussed, most patients with a small ASD will have few if any clinical signs related to this disease. Although uncommon, a significant volume overload secondary to a large ASD can result in heart failure due to multiple mechanisms. If right ventricular (RV) dilation is severe, systolic dysfunction associated with damage and fibrosis of the RV myocardium may develop resulting in elevated right atrial pressures and potentially, congestive heart failure. As mentioned above, a significant volume overload can elevate pulmonary artery pressures leading to pulmonary hypertension. Pulmonary hypertension may elevate RV diastolic pressures due to hypertrophy and through the development of systolic myocardial dysfunction. Again, the potential result is right-sided congestive heart failure (CHF). Patients with right heart failure may present with dyspnea due to pleural effusion, abdominal distension due to ascites, or exercise intolerance and weakness. Often, significant weight loss is seen associated with right-sided CHF.

In the event of shunt reversal, hypoxemia and potentially polycythemia develops secondary to the right-to-left shunt. Polycythemia can result in dyspnea, exercise intolerance, syncope/collapse, thromboembolism, or cerebral vascular accidents.

12. How is the severity of an ASD judged?

The following can be used to subjectively evaluate the severity of an ASD:
• Size of an ASD on echocardiography
• Severity of right heart enlargement as seen on echocardiogram
• Presence of congestive heart failure
• Evidence of abnormal right-to-left shunting (cyanosis and polycythemia)
• Presence of pulmonary hypertension

Objectively, the severity of an ASD can be evaluated by comparing the volume of blood passing out the pulmonary artery to the lungs, known as Qp or RV stroke volume, versus the volume of blood passing out of the aorta to the systemic circulation known as Qs or LV stroke volume. This is called the Qp/Qs ratio. Normally, the volume of blood leaving the RV through the PA is equal to the volume of blood leaving the LV through the aorta, resulting in a Qp/Qs ratio of 1.0. In the case of a left-to-right shunt, the Qs is decreased because a portion of the blood in the left heart passes through the shunt into the right heart. This results in an increased volume of blood in the right heart and thus an increased Qp. An increased Qp and a decreased Qs will cause an increase in the Qp/Qs ratio (> 1.0) typical of a left-to-right shunt. A decreased Qp and an increased Qs will cause a decrease in the Qp/Qs ratio (< 1.0) as occurs with a right-to-left shunt. The Qp/Qs ratio can be calculated by cardiac catheterization or by the use of Doppler echocardiography. If the Qp/Qs ratio is greater than 2.0, the left-to-right shunt is considered significant and the patient is a candidate for surgical correction. A ratio of 1.0 to 2.0 is generally considered a minor shunt.

13. What are the therapeutic options for a clinically important ASD?

In veterinary medicine, therapeutic options for an ASD are limited. A significant left-to-right shunt in a human patient would lead to surgical correction, or occlusion of the defect with one of a variety of catheter-delivered occlusion devices that are being evaluated. Although often cost prohibitive, the availability of these therapies is increasing in veterinary medicine. Fortunately, it is common for dogs and cats with small to moderate-sized defects to live a near normal life span before clinical signs develop.

Several approaches to medical therapy are recommended. Clinical signs of right heart failure should be treated with furosemide. The use of digoxin could also be considered in the face of persistent right heart failure. Enalapril and other ACE inhibitors may also be used to treat right heart failure due to an ASD. By inhibiting the renin-angiotensin system, they may help to alleviate vascular congestion. However, it is theoretically possible that the use of ACE inhibitors could lead to a decrease in left atrial pressure, predisposing to right-to-left shunting, and, therefore, caution is justified.

If right-to-left shunting develops, the treatment options are even more limited. If concurrent CHF is present, it should be treated as discussed above. If polycythemia develops, phlebotomy may be necessary based on the presence and progression of clinical signs. Medical management with hydroxyurea or pentoxifylline could be considered at this time. The efficacy and safety of these medications in the face of an ASD and pulmonary hypertension are unknown.

BIBLIOGRAPHY

1. Bonagura JD, Darke PGG: Congenital heart disease. In Ettinger SJ, Feldman EC (eds): Textbook of Veterinary Internal Medicine. Philadelphia, W.B. Saunders, 1995, pp 892–943.
2. Bonagura JD, Lehnkuhl LB: Congenital heart disease. In Fox PR, Sisson D, Moise NS (eds): Textbook of Canine and Feline Radiology. Philadelphia, W.B. Saunders, 1999, pp 471–535.
3. Eyster GE: Atrial septal defect and ventricular septal defect. Semin Vet Med Surg (Small Anim) 9:227–233, 1994.
4. Hamlin RL, Smith CR, Smetzer DL: Ostium secundum type interatrial septal defects in the dog. J Am Vet Med Assoc 143:149–157, 1963.
5. Jeraji K, Ogburn PN, Johnston GR, et al: Atrial septal defect (sinus venosus type) in a dog. J Am Vet Med Assoc 177:342–346, 1980.
6. Noden DM, de Lehunta A: Cardiovascular system II: Heart. In Noden DM, De Lahunta A (eds): The Embryology of Domestic Animals. Baltimore, Williams & Wilkins, 1985, pp 231–256.
7. Olivier NB: Congenital heart disease in dogs. In Fox PR (ed): Canine and Feline Cardiology. New York, Churchill Livingstone, 1988, pp 357–389.

53. TRICUSPID VALVE DYSPLASIA

William A. Brown, D.V.M.

1. What is tricuspid valve dysplasia?

Tricuspid valve dysplasia (TVD) is a congenital malformation of the right atrioventricular valve. Generally, this anomaly results in incompetence of the tricuspid valve and subsequent tricuspid regurgitation. However, in rare cases malformation of the tricuspid valve may result in stenosis and physical impairment of right ventricular filling. TVD may occur in combination with other congenital cardiac defects such as mitral valve dysplasia, atrial septal defect, and ventricular septal defects, but it most frequently occurs as an isolated defect.

2. What is Ebstein's anomaly?

Ebstein's anomaly is a malformation of the tricuspid valve apparatus that is observed in children. It is characterized by a downward or apical displacement of the point of tricuspid leaflet apposition so that part of the right ventricle is effectively incorporated into the right atrium. Some cases of TVD in dogs have features of Ebstein's anomaly and the term does appear in the veterinary literature; however, there is a great deal of variability in the gross appearance of canine tricuspid malformations, and TVD, as the more general term, is probably preferable when referring to congenital tricuspid valve abnormalities in dogs.

3. Describe the gross pathologic changes associated with TVD.

TVD is characterized by variable thickening of the tricuspid valve leaflets, elongation of the leaflets, fibrous thickening and shortening of the chordae tendineae, abnormal insertion of the chordae tendineae onto the valve leaflets, and underdevelopment of the papillary muscles. In severely affected individuals, the tricuspid valve leaflets may be fused directly to the right ventricular wall.

4. What is the pathophysiology of TVD?

Mild tricuspid valve dysplasia may result in only mild tricuspid regurgitation. In this instance, the corresponding volume overload is relatively small and the right atrium and right ventricle undergo only minimal eccentric hypertrophy (dilation). However, in more severe cases, massive tricuspid regurgitation leads to severe volume overload and marked dilation of the right atrium and right ventricle. This decrease in right heart pumping efficiency (stroke volume) leads to a compensatory activation of the renin-angiotensin-aldosterone system (RAAS) and ultimately right heart failure as characterized by hepatomegaly, splenomegaly, ascites, and pleural effusion. In the rare case of tricuspid stenosis, the right atrium may become disproportionately dilated when compared to the right ventricle due to physical obstruction of venous return into the right ventricle and corresponding increases in the mean right atrial pressure.

5. Are there any breeds that are at increased risk for developing TVD?

Recent studies of the prevalence of congenital heart disease in dogs revealed that TVD is most commonly seen in Labrador retrievers, German shepherds, and great Pyrenees. The majority of dogs with TVD are male (71%). The finding of several affected puppies within certain families of Labrador retrievers is strongly suggestive of a genetic component to this disease. Thus far, no specific feline breeds have been demonstrated to be at increased risk for developing TVD. However, a 6:1 male predominance was also noted in cats with TVD.

6. What are the typical clinical signs of an animal with TVD?

TVD is usually first identified when a cardiac murmur is detected during routine examination of an apparently healthy puppy. Other affected dogs with soft murmurs may not be diagnosed until later in life or the onset of right heart failure. Puppies that are severely affected may demonstrate reduced exercise tolerance and signs of right heart failure (ascites, pleural effusion) within the first year of life. In addition to signs of congestive heart failure, dogs with a stenotic tricuspid valve may show signs of reduced cardiac output during periods of exercise or excitement when high heart rates further limit ventricular filling. This may manifest itself as exercise intolerance or syncope. Because of their leisurely lifestyle and subsequent lack of clinical signs, cats with TVD are frequently not diagnosed until middle age.

7. What abnormalities might be present on the physical examination of an animal with TVD?

Animals with TVD typically have a holosystolic murmur heard best on the right hemithorax over the tricuspid valve area. A palpable precordial thrill may also accompany the murmur. Rarely, a systolic valve click or soft diastolic rumble is ausculted, suggesting concurrent tricuspid valve stenosis or severe tricuspid regurgitation. The intensity of the murmur does not always correlate with the severity of the lesion. In some animals with massive tricuspid regurgitation the murmur will be very soft or absent. The femoral arterial pulse quality is typically normal. Occasionally, jugular pulses, hepatomegaly, and ascites may be present in animals with severe TVD and right heart failure.

8. Describe the typical radiographic findings of TVD.

The cardiac silhouette generally has a normal appearance in animals with mild TVD. However, animals with more severe TVD typically have severe cardiomegaly. In the lateral radiographic view, there is loss of the cranial waist corresponding to severe right atrial enlargement. In addition, the right ventricle is markedly enlarged with evidence of increased sternal contact and elevation of the left ventricular apex off the sternum. The cardiac silhouette in the dorsoventral view shows enlargement of the right atrium and right ventricle, giving the heart a "reverse D" appearance, and the left ventricular apex is often markedly shifted into left hemithorax. The pulmonary vasculature is normal or occasionally diminished, reflecting reduced right ventricular output and decreased pulmonary blood flow. The caudal vena cava may be dilated and tortuous in severe cases of TVD.

9. What abnormalities might be noted in the electrocardiogram (ECG) of an animal with TVD?

Despite the severe right heart enlargement caused by TVD, the resting electrocardiogram frequently does not have the classic criteria of right heart enlargement (a right axis shift with deep S waves in leads I, II, III, and aVF). However, evidence of right heart enlargement (deep S waves) is generally present in the left precordial (chest) leads. In addition, the P waves are typically wide and may be increased in voltage, which is supportive of right atrial enlargement. Some dogs with TVD may display a unique "splintering" of the QRS complex in leads II, III, and aVF. The reason for this pattern is not known, but an intraventricular conduction disturbance is suspected. Atrial arrhythmias such as atrial premature beats, atrial fibrillation, and supraventricular tachycardia are common due to severe right atrial dilation. Ventricular arrhythmias are rare in animals with TVD.

10. What echocardiographic findings are recognized in TVD?

Echocardiography is the diagnostic test of choice for evaluating animals with TVD (see figure). Abnormal location, shape, motion, or attachment of the tricuspid valve apparatus is generally observed on 2-D echocardiography. The tricuspid valve leaflets typically appear thickened. The septal leaflet may appear to be tethered or adhered to the interventricular septum. The chordae tendineae are often shortened, thickened, and abnormally inserted onto the valve leaflets. In addition, the papillary muscles may be fused. Generally, there is massive dilation of the right atrium and right ventricle. In rare cases of tricuspid valve stenosis, diastolic doming of the valve may be evident with a normal to small right ventricle. The left ventricle in animals with TVD may be reduced in size due to decreased pulmonary venous return or may appear small relative to the severely dilated right ventricle. M-mode echocardiography usually demonstrates right ventricular dilation and paradoxical motion of the interventricular septum due to right ventricular volume overload. Evaluation using color-flow or spectral Doppler typically reveals a jet of tricuspid regurgitation or less frequently tricuspid stenosis.

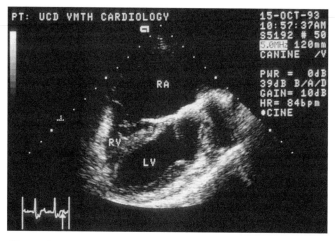

Right parasternal long-axis echocardiographic image obtained from a Labrador retriever with tricuspid stenosis due to valvular dysplasia. The right atrium is extremely large while the right ventricle is relatively small. LV, Left ventricle; RV, right ventricle; RA, right atrium. (From Brown WA, Thomas WP: Balloon valvuloplasty of tricuspid stenosis in a Labrador retriever. J Vet Intern Med 9:419–424, 1995, with permission.)

11. What is the prognosis for an animal with TVD?

The prognosis varies based on the degree of tricuspid regurgitation and associated cardiac enlargement. Animals with mild TVD and mild cardiomegaly often remain asymptomatic and may have a normal life span. However, more severely affected animals often experience clinical signs, atrial arrhythmias, and right-sided congestive heart failure within the first few months or years of life. In some cases, cats with moderate to severe TVD may live with the disease for several years before the onset of clinical signs.

12. How are right-sided congestive heart failure (CHF) and atrial arrhythmias best managed in an animal with TVD?

There are two main goals in treating an animal with TVD and subsequent congestive heart failure. First, the preload must be manipulated to control clinical signs of congestion. This is typically achieved with judicious use of diuretics (furosemide), ACE inhibitors (enalapril), and a low-salt diet to reduce excessive salt intake and water retention. In animals with large volumes of ascites that are causing respiratory difficulty or inability to rest comfortably, abdominocentesis should be performed to stabilize their clinical condition. In addition, nitrate venodilators (nitroglycerine) and thiazide diuretics (hydrochlorothiazide) may be beneficial in severe cases that are refractory to initial treatment with furosemide and enalapril. Second, heart rate control must be established for good long-term results. Animals with TVD are at increased risk for developing atrial arrhythmias. These are often responsive to concurrent treatment with digoxin and calcium channel blockers (diltiazem). In some cases, beta-blockers (atenolol) may be used in addition to or instead of calcium channel blockers. The author uses a target heart rate of 120–150 bpm for dogs with TVD and 150–180 bpm for cats. Of course the kidney function should periodically be monitored in all animals with TVD that are concurrently receiving diuretics and ACE inhibitors. In addition, monitoring of the serum digoxin level is suggested for those animals receiving digoxin.

BIBLIOGRAPHY

1. Bonagura JD, Lehmkuhl LB: Congenital heart disease. In Fox PR (ed): Textbook of Canine and Feline Cardiology. Philadelphia, W.B. Saunders, 1999, pp 471–535.
2. Brown WA, Thomas WP: Balloon valvuloplasty of tricuspid stenosis in a Labrador retriever. J Vet Intern Med 9:419–424, 1995.
3. Buchanan JW: Prevalence of cardiovascular disorders. In Fox PR (ed): Textbook of Canine and Feline Cardiology. Philadelphia, W.B. Saunders, 1999, pp 457–470.
4. DeMadron E, Kadish A, Spear JF, et al: Incessant atrial tachycardias in a dog with tricuspid dysplasia. J Vet Intern Med 1:163–169, 1987.
5. Liu SK, Tilley LP: Dysplasia of the tricuspid valve in the dog and cat. J Am Vet Med Assoc 169:623–630, 1976.
6. Moise NS: Tricuspid valve dysplasia in the dog. In Bonagura JD (ed): Current Veterinary Therapy XII: Small Animal Practice. Philadelphia, W.B. Saunders, 1995, pp 813–816.
7. Weirich WE, Blevins WE, Conrad CR, et al: Congenital tricuspid insufficiency in a dog. J Am Vet Med Assoc 164:1025–1028, 1974.

54. MITRAL VALVE DYSPLASIA

Mark E. Stamoulis, D.V.M.

1. What is mitral dysplasia?

Mitral valve dysplasia is a congenital malformation of the mitral apparatus that is observed in both dogs and cats. Any part of the mitral apparatus may be affected. The leaflets may be deformed, adherent to adjacent structures, or cleft (as noted with endocardial cushion defects). Chordae tendinae may be excessively long, short, or absent altogether (i.e., valve leaflet inserts directly into the papillary muscles). The papillary muscles may be abnormal in number, position, or shape. The valve annulus can be abnormal in shape or location. Less commonly, a fibrous ring or membrane may be located above the valve (see figure below).

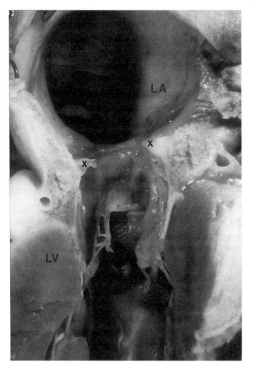

Post-mortem specimen from a young cat. A fibrous ring is located just above the mitral valve (x). This is a rare example of supravalvular mitral stenosis. Left atrial enlargement and hypertrophy are also evident. This disease differs from cor triatriatum because the left atrial appendage communicates with the proximal part of the atrium. LA, left atrium; LV, left ventricle.

2. How common is mitral valve dysplasia?

Mitral dysplasia is thought to be one of the most common congenital heart diseases of cats. However, due to the variable course of the disease, diagnosis is often delayed until later in life. Mitral dysplasia is less common in dogs. Studies performed in the U.S. and Europe indicate that mitral dysplasia occurs in about 8% of dogs with congenital heart disease.

3. What is the cause of mitral valve dysplasia? Is there any breed or sex predilection?

There is no known cause of mitral dysplasia. However, it is believed that a genetic predisposition exists in certain breeds, although detailed studies to support this are lacking. The Great Dane, German shepherd, golden retriever, Newfoundland, mastiff, and bull terrier (both standard and miniature) are predisposed to dysplasia of the mitral valve. While no apparent breed predilection is found in cats, there is an increased incidence of atrioventricular (either mitral, tricuspid, or both) malformations in males of this species.

4. What is the pathophysiology of mitral valve dysplasia?

Abnormal coaptation of dysplastic valve leaflets results in mitral regurgitation. Occasionally mitral stenosis is present as well. Two factors influence the severity of mitral regurgitation: the size of the regurgitant orifice and aortic impedance to blood flow during systole. Left atrial compliance and left ventricular function dictate how long the lesion is tolerated before signs of congestive heart failure occur.

Mitral regurgitation results in a volume overload to the left side of the heart. Compensatory dilation with hypertrophy (i.e., eccentric hypertrophy) of the left atrium and ventricle occurs in an attempt to reduce wall stress and preserve cardiac output. Left ventricular systolic performance is initially hyperdynamic as the regurgitant volume is ejected into the low-pressure atrium. Over time, increased left atrial pressure is transmitted to the pulmonary veins and pulmonary capillaries, resulting in pulmonary edema. Cardiac output is eventually diminished as myocardial fibrosis limits both systolic and diastolic function.

Mitral stenosis limits blood flow into the left ventricle during diastole. Left atrial pressure rises in proportion to the severity of the obstruction. This atrial hypertension is transmitted to the pulmonary veins and pulmonary capillaries, resulting in pulmonary edema. Furthermore, elevated pulmonary venous pressure causes reflex pulmonary arteriolar vasoconstriction and pulmonary hypertension.

Cardiac arrhythmias may occur and are most likely secondary to left atrial enlargement. Atrial and ventricular arrhythmias may be detected. Atrial fibrillation may be particularly damaging, as loss of atrial contraction may lead to significant hemodynamic compromise and clinical deterioration.

5. How does an animal with mitral valve dysplasia present?

Clinical signs are variable in dogs and cats with mitral dysplasia. While some animals may present with signs suggestive of congestive heart failure, others may have no signs other than a murmur or arrhythmia detected during physical examination.

6. Describe the expected findings of cardiac auscultation.

The most common finding is a holosystolic regurgitant murmur of variable intensity heard best at the left fifth intercostal space at the costochondral junction in dogs, and along the left sternal border in cats. If mitral stenosis is present or mitral valve regurgitation is very severe, a soft diastolic rumble may be heard. A gallop rhythm associated with atrial contraction (S_4), rapid ventricular filling (S_3), or both also may be detected.

7. What electrocardiographic abnormalities are seen?

Atrial arrhythmias, particularly atrial fibrillation, are seen most commonly. Sinus tachycardia and premature ventricular complexes also may be observed, especially if congestive heart failure is present. Patterns consistent with left atrial and left ventricular enlargement also may be noted. It should be remembered that the electrocardiogram is an insensitive predictor of chamber enlargement.

8. Why are chest radiographs so important?

While radiographic findings vary greatly depending on the duration and severity of the lesion, much is learned with respect to clinical signs, pulmonary hemodynamics, and response to therapy. Left atrial enlargement is usually detected as the first radiographic change, causing the typical bulge at the 2 to 3 o'clock position in the ventrodorsal view and dorsal displacement of the mainstem bronchus in the lateral view. Left ventricular enlargement occurs next as the caudal cardiac border becomes convex in the lateral view. In cases of mitral stenosis the left atrium may enlarge without noted changes in the left ventricle.

Detection of pulmonary venous congestion with left atrial enlargement suggests elevated pulmonary venous pressure, usually coinciding with early clinical signs of congestive heart failure. These changes are followed by interstitial and alveolar pulmonary edema. While these changes are most often seen in the hilar region in dogs, a much more variable distribution is observed in cats. Pleural effusion, typically a result of right-sided heart failure in dogs, may be detected in cats with left-sided heart failure.

9. How does one definitively diagnose mitral dysplasia?

Echocardiography enables noninvasive assessment of the mitral valve apparatus. Careful inspection may reveal abnormal anatomy or function of the papillary muscles, chordae tendinae, or valve leaflets. In rare instances a supravalvular fibrous ring or membrane may be detected. M-mode echocardiography allows measurement of cardiac dimensions and contractile indices. Doppler studies are used to document and quantitate the presence of mitral regurgitation, mitral stenosis, or both. Cardiac catheterization and angiocardiography may also be used to establish a diagnosis, although much less frequently.

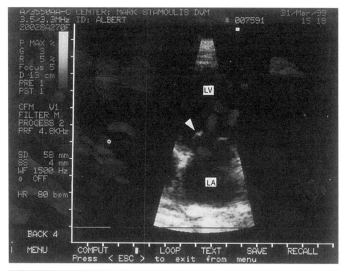

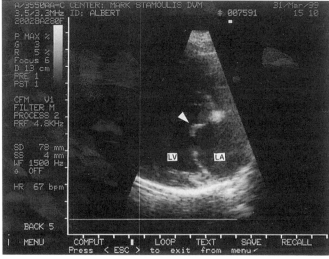

Apical *(top)* and parasternal *(bottom)* views of a two-dimensional echocardiogram from a bull terrier with mitral valve dysplasia. The mitral valve is stenotic and characteristic doming of the septal leaflet during diastole is seen *(arrow)*. LA, left atrium; LV, left ventricle.

10. What are the specific echocardiographic features of mitral stenosis?

Two-dimensional echocardiography reveals doming of the anterior mitral leaflet in diastole (see figure above). M-mode studies demonstrate two diastolic events: abnormally prolonged closure of the mitral valve leaflets (i.e., E to F slope), and upward or anterior motion of the posterior leaflet. Doppler findings of the transmitral gradient are an increased filling velocity (both E and A waves) with a characteristic prolongation in decline of the inflow velocity (see figure below). Color-flow Doppler imaging demonstrates turbulence within the valve orifice that extends into the left ventricle.

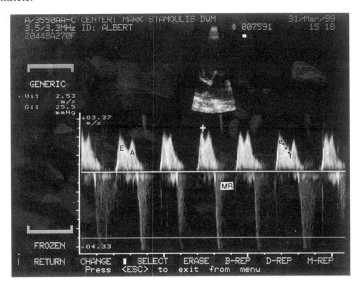

Continuous-wave Doppler examination of the same bull terrier. An increased transmitral velocity of greater than 2.0 m/s is noted for both early filling (E) and atrial contraction (A). The abnormally prolonged E to F slope (e…f) indicates delayed emptying of the left atrium. These changes are consistent with mitral stenosis. Mitral regurgitation is also present (MR).

11. What factors influence the prognosis?

Concomitant congenital defects, such as aortic stenosis (Newfoundland, golden retriever, bull terrier), tricuspid valve dysplasia, or endocardial cushion defects may hasten the onset of clinical signs. Cats appear to be able to tolerate isolated mitral valve dyplasia for years; however, when significant cardiomegaly is detected, the prognosis is generally poor for both species.

12. What type of medical therapy is indicated?

Asymptomatic animals without evidence of atrial or ventricular enlargement are examined every 6 months. Recent studies suggest that early modulation of the sympathetic nervous system and renin-angiotensin-aldosterone system in animals with chronic valvular disease might be beneficial. It seems appropriate that asymptomatic animals with moderate or progressive left atrial and left ventricular enlargement should be treated with angiotensin-converting enzyme inhibitors (e.g., enalapril or benazepril). Diuretics should be added when signs of congestion occur. Digitalis is indicated to control atrial arrhythmias and to support systolic dysfunction.

13. What other treatment options are available?

Interventional procedures such as balloon valvuloplasty are being performed with increasing frequency by veterinary cardiologists. Although difficult, a catheter could be introduced across the interatrial septum to dilate a stenotic mitral valve. Surgical procedures to replace, repair, or dilate abnormal valves are not performed routinely.

BIBLIOGRAPHY

1. Bonagura JD, Darke PG: Congenital heart disease. In Ettinger SJ, Feldman EC (eds): Textbook of Veterinary Internal Medicine, 4th ed. Philadelphia, W.B. Saunders, 1995, pp 892–943.
2. Bonagura JD, Miller MW, Darke PG: Doppler echocardiography I: Pulsed-wave and continuous-wave examinations. Vet Clin North Am 28:1325–1360, 1998.
3. Bonagura JD, Miller MW: Doppler echocardiography II: Color Doppler imaging. Vet Clin North Am 28:1360–1390, 1998.
4. Fyler DC: Mitral valve and left atrial lesions. In Fyler DC (ed): Nadas' Pediatric Cardiology. Philadelphia, Hanley & Belfus, 1992, pp 611–617.
5. Lemkuhl LB, Ware WA, Bonagura JD: Mitral stenosis in 15 dogs. J Vet Intern Med 8:2–17, 1994.
6. Ryan T: Congenital heart disease. In Feigenbaum H (ed): Echocardiography, 5th ed. Baltimore, Williams & Wilkins, 1994, pp 358–361.
7. Stamoulis ME, Fox PR: Mitral valve stenosis in three cats. J Small Animal Pract 34:452–456, 1993.
8. Tidholm A: Retrospective study of congenital heart defects in 151 dogs. J Small Animal Pract 38:94–98, 1997.

55. CYANOTIC CONGENITAL HEART DISEASE

Davin J. Borde, D.V.M, and John-Karl Goodwin, D.V.M.

1. What is cyanosis?

Cyanosis is a physical sign manifested by bluish discoloration of the skin or mucous membranes. It occurs when there is an increased delivery of reduced hemoglobin or abnormal hemoglobin pigment (e.g., methemoglobinemia) to the affected area. Cyanosis can be classified as central or peripheral. Peripheral cyanosis is typically a consequence of cutaneous vasoconstriction (e.g., secondary to low cardiac output or exposure to cold). Central cyanosis primarily occurs as a result of reduced arterial oxygen saturation and can be seen secondary to right-to-left shunting congenital heart disease or impaired pulmonary function. Cyanosis is typically noted in dogs and cats when arterial oxygen saturation is less than 70% and arterial oxygen tension less than 40 mmHg.

2. What are examples of congenital cardiac diseases in dogs and cats that can result in cyanosis and which breeds are predisposed to these defects?

Congenital cardiac defects that can be associated with cyanosis include tetralogy of Fallot, right-to-left shunting patent ductus arteriosus (PDA), pulmonic stenosis with an atrial-level shunt, and Eisenmenger's complex or syndrome. Other less common examples of cyanotic congenital heart disease include double-outlet right ventricle with pulmonic stenosis, tricuspid atresia, pulmonary atresia (with intact ventricular septum), truncus arteriosus, and pseudotruncus arteriosus. Keeshonds and English bulldogs are predisposed to tetralogy of Fallot. This congenital defect has also been reported in the cat. Patent ductus arteriosus is commonly observed in German shepherd dogs, collies, Pomeranians, toy and miniature poodles, Shetland sheepdogs, Maltese, English springer spaniels, keeshonds, Chihuahuas, cocker spaniels, Kerry blue terriers, Newfoundlands, and Yorkshire terriers.

3. Describe the characteristic cardiac defects that define tetralogy of Fallot.

Tetralogy of Fallot is a congenital cardiac defect that is characterized by a ventricular septal defect, an overriding aorta, right ventricular hypertrophy, and pulmonic stenosis. In the keeshond, the defect has been shown to be a polygenic trait that results in abnormal formation of the conotruncal septum. Abnormal positioning and alignment of the components of the cranial ventricular septum result in the development of a ventricular septal defect (VSD), narrowing of the right ventricular outflow tract, and dextroposition of the aorta. Right ventricular hypertrophy (RVH), the fourth element of the tetralogy, is a consequence of the abnormal hemodynamics that results from septal malalignment. Typically, the VSD in tetralogy is large or "nonrestrictive"; when this is the case, the two ventricles behave as a single chamber and pressures within the right ventricle are necessarily systemic. This abnormally high pressure within the ventricle is the stimulus for RVH. Alternatively, if the VSD is restrictive and prevents equilibration of right and left ventricular pressures, RVH results from the increased afterload associated with the presence of pulmonic stenosis.

4. Through what pathophysiologic mechanism does cyanosis occur in tetralogy of Fallot?

In patients with an isolated ventricular septal defect, left ventricular pressures typically exceed right ventricular pressures and blood consequently shunts from left to right. In patients with tetralogy of Fallot, however, resistance to right ventricular outflow is increased due to pulmonic stenosis. If the resistance to right ventricular ejection exceeds systemic vascular resistance, right-to-left shunting through the ventricular septal defect results. This allows poorly oxygenated blood (reduced hemoglobin) to enter the systemic circulation and cyanosis is the result.

5. Besides cyanosis, what other physical findings and clinical signs could be expected in a patient with tetralogy of Fallot?

Besides cyanosis, patients with tetralogy of Fallot typically present with clinical signs of exercise intolerance. Cyanosis may be induced or worsened by exercise. Weakness, syncope, shortness of breath or seizures may also be noted. The patient is often underweight and may show a failure to thrive. A cardiac murmur consistent with pulmonic stenosis can be found on physical examination (systolic, possibly high-intensity murmur heard best at the left cardiac base), although flow through the ventricular septal defect may also result in a murmur. Occasionally, the combination of a nonrestrictive ventricular septal defect, increased blood viscosity due to polycythemia, and very severe pulmonic stenosis fails to produce a cardiac murmur.

6. What are the diagnostic findings in a patient with tetralogy of Fallot?

Radiographs will typically demonstrate right ventricular enlargement and diminished pulmonary circulation. There is usually no main pulmonary artery dilation as there is with uncomplicated pulmonic stenosis. Electrocardiography commonly demonstrates a right axis deviation in the frontal plane; however, a left axis shift can be seen in some cats. The hypoxemia induced by right-to-left shunting of blood can produce polycythemia in many patients with tetralogy of Fallot. Arterial blood gas analysis can demonstrate severity of disease and arterial oxygen tension is usually less than 35 mmHg.

Echocardiography will demonstrate the large ventricular septal defect and overriding aorta. Hypertrophy of the right ventricular free wall and stenosis of the right ventricular outflow tract are also noted. The pulmonic stenosis present can be valvular, subvalvular, or both. Color Doppler interrogation of the pulmonic valve demonstrates turbulent flow, and interrogation of the subaortic region can usually delineate the ventricular septal defect. Contrast echocardiography will document right-to-left shunting with contrast being visualized from the right ventricle through the ventricular septal defect to the aorta and occasionally being seen in the left ventricle.

Cardiac catheterization will typically demonstrate equilibration of the right and left ventricular pressures. Angiocardiography will reveal pulmonic stenosis, a dextropositioned aorta, a subaortic ventricular septal defect, and right-to-left shunting of blood. Bidirectional shunting can also be noted.

7. What treatment options are available for a patient with tetralogy of Fallot?

Definitive surgical correction with use of cardiopulmonary bypass is commonly performed in human medicine and involves relieving or bypassing the pulmonic stenosis and patching the ventricular septal defect. This procedure has been reported once in the dog. Attempting to relieve the pulmonic stenosis without closure of the ventricular septal defect will result in severe left-to-right shunting and left ventricular failure. The more typical surgery performed in canine patients is palliative and involves creation of a systemic to pulmonary shunt. The most common surgery performed in dogs involves anastomosis of the left subclavian artery and pulmonary artery (Blalock-Taussig shunt), but anastomosis of the ascending aorta to pulmonary artery (Potts shunt) and aorta to right pulmonary artery (Waterston-Cooley shunt) have also been reported. The modified Blalock-Taussig shunt involves use of a synthetic graft to anastomose the subclavian artery or aorta and the pulmonary artery.

Medical management of tetralogy of Fallot involves use of phlebotomy to reduce polycythemia when clinical signs can be attributed to increased blood viscosity. Polycythemia in patients with cyanotic heart disease is a compensatory measure and overly aggressive reduction in hematocrit is to be avoided. The optimal hematocrit for patients with cyanotic heart disease is not known. However, increases in hematocrit beyond 65% result in an exponential rise in blood viscosity; therefore, phlebotomy performed to attain a hematocrit of 60–68% is probably reasonable. Intravenous fluid replacement of 1–2 times the blood volume removed is recommended. The volume of blood to be removed is calculated from the following formula, where BW stands for body weight, AH for actual hematocrit, and DH for desired hematocrit.

$$\text{Volume (ml)} = [\text{BW (kg)} \times 0.08] \times 1000 \text{ ml/kg} \times [\text{AH} - \text{DH/AH}]$$

Use of hydroxyurea as a myelosuppressive agent in cases that require frequent phlebotomies may also be tried, but is often associated with severe side effects. Propranolol can also be administered in attempt to reduce hypoxemic episodes. Propranolol is a negative inotrope that may act to decrease the severity of dynamic right ventricular outflow tract obstruction. Additionally, because propranolol is a nonselective beta blocker, it may prevent the decrease in systemic vascular resistance that accompanies exercise and thus limit right-to-left shunting and cyanosis.

8. What is a patent ductus arteriosus?

The ductus arteriosus is a vessel normally patent in the fetus connecting the pulmonary trunk and descending aorta. It allows most of the right ventricular output to bypass the unexpanded lungs of the fetus, an organ of high resistance, and enter the descending aorta where it will eventually travel to the placenta (the fetal organ of oxygenation). Shortly after birth, initial closure of the ductus occurs through a sudden increase in the partial pressure of oxygen initiated by ventilation and resultant changes in the metabolism of vasoactive eicosanoids. Intimal proliferation and fibrosis gradually follow to produce complete anatomic closure. Patent ductus arteriosus (PDA) is a congenital cardiac defect whereby the ductus remains open after birth.

9. Why would cyanosis occur in patients with a patent ductus arteriosus?

A PDA typically results in shunting of blood from the systemic circulation (with higher vascular resistance) to the pulmonary circulation, thus flow is left to right. Cyanosis can be seen in patients with a PDA when clinically significant right-to-left shunting occurs. This is also called a "reversed PDA" and most commonly arises consequent to the development of high pulmonary vascular resistance. Elevated pulmonary vascular resistance is thought to occur secondary to a failure of the normal maturation of the pulmonary vasculature toward a low-resistance vascular bed. Additionally, increased pulmonary flow results in changes to the pulmonary arteries over time, which increases pulmonary resistance to the point of exceeding systemic vascular resistance. Right-to-left shunting is the end result.

10. What are the physical findings and clinical signs in a patient with right-to-left shunting PDA? How might they differ from those found in other congenital cardiac defects resulting in cyanosis?

Typically, rear limb weakness or collapse is the presenting complaint in patients with right-to-left shunting PDA. Lethargy, seizures, shortness of breath, syncope, or pain may also be noted. Physical examination usually demonstrates no murmur; however, a split-second heart sound is commonly noted.

In contrast to other congenital cardiac defects, like tetralogy of Fallot, that cause generalized cyanosis, a right-to-left shunting PDA commonly produces differential cyanosis, which affects the prepucial, penile, and vulvar mucous membranes while normal oral mucous membrane color is noted. The differential cyanosis is usually exacerbated by exercise. It occurs because the deoxygenated blood delivered by the right-to-left shunting PDA to the aorta occurs downstream of the brachiocephalic trunk and left subclavian arteries. As a result, normally oxygenated blood is supplied to the head, neck, and forelimbs, while poorly oxygenated blood is supplied to the caudal portion of the body.

11. What are the typical diagnostic findings in a patient with right-to-left shunting PDA?

The CBC will usually demonstrate polycythemia with a hematocrit greater than 55%. This occurs as a result of poorly oxygenated blood being delivered to the kidneys and a consequent increase in erythropoietin production. Femoral arterial blood gas analysis will commonly reveal an oxygen tension less than 40 mmHg in symptomatic dogs. Thoracic radiographs may demonstrate right ventricular enlargement, aneurysmal dilation of the descending aorta, and hypoperfusion of the peripheral pulmonary vasculature. Dilation of the main pulmonary artery may be noted. Electrocardiography will usually show evidence of right ventricular enlargement, such as a right axis deviation.

Echocardiography demonstrates right ventricular concentric hypertrophy. The left chambers are normal or reduced in diameter. The ductus may be visualized as a large, completely open vessel in contrast to the funnel-shaped appearance of the ductus in most left-to-right shunting PDA. Contrast echocardiography (microbubble-laden saline injected into a cephalic vein) will demonstrate the appearance of contrast in the right atrium, right ventricle, main pulmonary artery, and, via the right-to-left shunting ductus, in the descending abdominal aorta. Tricuspid regurgitation and pulmonic insufficiency may be noted with color Doppler echocardiography. Cardiac catheterization is rarely required to make the diagnosis. It reveals severe pulmonary hypertension, with similar systolic pressures in the left and right ventricles, aorta, and pulmonary artery. Angiography reveals right-to-left shunting and, occasionally, bidirectional shunting. Right ventricular hypertrophy is also noted.

12. How is a right-to-left shunting PDA treated?

Treatment of a right-to-left shunting PDA is aimed at reducing the polycythemia. Increased erythropoiesis and polycythemia eventually result in increased blood viscosity, which increases resistance to blood flow, decreases tissue oxygen delivery, and increases workload on the heart. Phlebotomy is typically performed and the volume of blood to be removed is calculated by the formula described for tetralogy of Fallot (see question 7). As described previously, hydroxyurea (a myelosuppressive agent) may also be tried. Surgical ligation of a right-to-left shunting PDA is contraindicated because it worsens pulmonary hypertension and frequently results in death.

13. Why would cyanosis occur in a patient with pulmonic stenosis?

Pulmonic stenosis occurring concurrently with a congenital cardiac defect such as an atrial septal defect, patent foramen ovale, or ventricular septal defect can result in right-to-left shunting of blood and cyanosis. If pulmonic stenosis is severe enough, it can result in significantly increased right ventricular and right atrial pressure. Once right chamber pressures exceed left chamber pressures, right-to-left shunting can occur through a communication between the chambers, such as an atrial septal defect or ventricular septal defect.

14. Suggest physical findings and clinical signs that would be expected in a patient with severe pulmonic stenosis and an atrial septal defect or patent foramen ovale.

As with congenital cardiac defects previously mentioned, exercise intolerance or cyanosis may be the presenting complaint. Cyanosis may increase with exercise. Similar to other cyanotic congenital cardiac defects, polycythemia can be noted. Auscultatory findings typical of severe pulmonic stenosis are also evident.

15. What options are available for treatment of severe pulmonic stenosis and a right-to-left shunting septal defect?

Balloon valvuloplasty may benefit patients with pulmonic stenosis and a right-to-left shunting atrial or ventricular septal defect. This may reduce resistance to right ventricular ejection and subsequently decrease right-to-left shunting. However, caution must be exercised because there is a risk that effective valvuloplasty may lead to the development of a clinically important left-to-right shunt in patients with moderate or large septal defects.

16. What is Eisenmenger's complex and Eisenmenger's syndrome?

Eisenmenger's complex is a term used to describe the combination of a ventricular septal defect and pulmonary vascular disease resulting in right-to-left shunting of blood and cyanosis. Eisenmenger's syndrome is a broader term used to describe other systemic to pulmonary communications, pulmonary vascular disease, and cyanosis.

17. How does cyanosis develop in patients with Eisenmenger's complex?

In a young puppy or kitten with a large ventricular septal defect and no other complicating abnormalities, left-to-right shunting typically occurs. Because pulmonary vascular resistance is normally less than systemic vascular resistance, pulmonary circulation and venous return to the left heart are significantly increased and left heart failure through massive left-to-right shunting of blood is the end result. Eisenmenger's complex can arise in those patients with a large ventricular septal defect where pulmonary vascular resistance remains elevated in the postnatal period. In these patients, left-to-right shunting is reduced, and left heart failure may not occur. In time, chronic pulmonary overcirculation through the left-to-right shunting of blood may result in pathologic changes to the pulmonary vasculature, with resultant increasing pulmonary hypertension. Eventually, pulmonary vascular resistance can exceed systemic vascular resistance, with consequent right-to-left shunting through the ventricular septal defect and cyanosis.

BIBLIOGRAPHY

1. Bonagura JD, Lehmkuhl LB: Congenital heart disease. In Fox PR, Sisson D, Moise NS (eds): Textbook of Canine and Feline Cardiology: Principles and Clinical Practice, 2nd ed. Philadelphia, W.B. Saunders, 1999, p 471.
2. Buchanan JW: Patent ductus arteriosus, ductal aneurysm, and pulmonary hypertension. Proc Annu Vet Med Forum, 1994, p 307.
3. Cote E, Ettinger SJ, Sisson DD: Long-term management of reversed patent ductus arteriosus (RPDA) in four dogs using phlebotomy alone. J Vet Intern Med 11:139, 1997 (abstract).
4. Eyster GE, Anderson LK, Sawyer DC, et al: Beta-adrenergic blockade for management of tetralogy of Fallot in a dog. J Am Vet Med Assoc 169:637, 1976.
5. Feldman EC, Nimmo-Wilkie JS, Pharr JW: Eisenmenger's syndrome in the dog: Case reports. J Am Anim Hosp Assoc 17:477, 1981.
6. Friedman WF: Congenital heart disease in infancy and childhood. In Braunwald E (ed): Heart Disease: A Textbook of Cardiovascular Medicine, 5th ed. Philadelphia, W.B. Saunders, 1997, p 877.
7. Herrtage ME, Hall LW, English TAH: Surgical correction of the tetralogy of Fallot in a dog. J Small Anim Pract 24:51, 1983.
8. Kittleson MD: Patent ductus arteriosus. In Kittleson MD, Kienle RD (eds): Small Animal Cardiovascular Medicine. St. Louis, Mosby, 1998, p 219.
9. Kittleson MD: Tetralogy of Fallot. In Kittleson MD, Kienle RD (eds): Small Animal Cardiovascular Medicine. St. Louis, Mosby, 1998, p 240.
10. Patterson DF, Pyle RL, Van Mierop L, et al: Hereditary defects of the conotruncal septum in keeshond dogs: Pathology and genetic studies. Am J Cardiol 34:187, 1974.
11. Pyle RL, Park RD, Alexander AF, et al: Patent ductus arteriosus with pulmonary hypertension in the dog. J Am Vet Med Assoc 178:565, 1981.
12. Ringwald RJ, Bonagura JD: Tetralogy of Fallot in the dog: Clinical findings in 13 cases. J Am Anim Hosp Assoc 24:33, 1988.
13. Turk JR, Miller JB, Sande RD: Plexogenic pulmonary arteriopathy in a dog with ventricular septal defect and pulmonary hypertension. J Am Anim Hosp Assoc 18:608, 1982.

58. FELINE AORTIC THROMBOEMBOLISM

Nancy J. Laste, D.V.M.

1. Define the syndrome of feline aortic thromboembolism (FATE).

FATE refers to the clinical syndromes associated with the occlusion of an artery by an infectious (septic) embolus, a neoplastic (tumor) embolus, or, most commonly, a sterile embolus. This chapter will discuss only sterile emboli.

2. Where do the peripherally located emboli originate?

Although not commonly identified antemortem, emboli are presumed to originate from thrombi formed in the heart. The most typical sites for thrombus formation are the left atrium, particularly in the left auricular appendage. Thrombi have also been identified associated with the left ventricular endocardium, the valves, and the right heart.

3. List the most common sites for thromboembolism.
- Saddle embolus: distal aortic trifurcation
- Forelimb embolus: brachial artery embolization
- Visceral arteries (including mesenteric artery, renal arteries)
- Cerebral artery

4. What are the clinical signs associated with a saddle embolus?

The "six Ps" are a mnemonic used to remember the signs of peripheral embolism: pain, pallor, paresthesia, paralysis, pulselessness, and poikilothermy. Patients often also display firm hindlimb musculature. Coexistent congestive heart failure is frequently present, manifesting as dyspnea and tachypnea.

5. What are the clinical signs associated with a forelimb embolus?

The signs can be mild (intermittent limping) or more severe (knuckling, disuse of a forelimb). With complete obstruction there is absence of the brachial pulse. The footpad is typically cool and pale when compared to the contralateral limb.

6. Are there any known underlying predispositions for aortic thromboembolism?

The major predisposing factor is the presence of cardiac disease. More specifically, increase in left atrial size seems to be associated with increased risk for FATE. The presence of spontaneous contrast effect in the left atrium on the echocardiogram has been suggested to be positively correlated with thromboembolic complications. Increases in platelet responsiveness to adenosine diphosphate (ADP) in cardiomyopathic cats suggests that platelet hyperaggregability also plays a role in this disease syndrome.

7. What diagnostic tests can confirm the presence of a limb embolus in a case in which clinical signs may be equivocal?

The absence of bleeding after clipping a toenail short enough to transect the arterial nail bed would confirm obstruction to arterial flow. This can be determined less invasively using a Doppler ultrasound probe (or other indirect blood pressure system) to confirm the absence of arterial flow to the limb. Two-dimensional and Doppler ultrasound imaging can also help visualize emboli. The gold standard test for documenting an embolus would be a nonselective angiogram.

8. List the most common hematologic abnormalities commonly noted with aortic thromboembolism.

Hyperglycemia, leukocytosis, increases in alanine aminotransferase (ALT), aspartate aminotransferase (AST), and creatinine phosphokinase (CPK), and hypocalcemia.

9. **Which types of cardiac disease are most commonly associated with cases of FATE?**
Hypertrophic cardiomyopathy (present in 57% of cases of saddle embolus) and intermediate-form or restrictive cardiomyopathy (present in 17% of cases). These are the most frequent forms of cardiac disease overall and are frequently associated with left atrial enlargement. However, any type of cardiac disease can presumably lead to FATE.

10. **Are there any age or sex predilections for FATE?**
The typical FATE patient, a middle-aged male cat, likely reflects the age and sex predilection for hypertrophic cardiomyopathy. Mean age has been described as 7.7 years with 67% of cases occurring in male cats.

11. **What are the therapeutic options for treating FATE?**
Supportive care
  • Fluid therapy
  • Oxygen
  • Pain control
  • Providing warmth to the hind legs
Vasodilator therapy
  • Acetylpromazine
  • Hydralazine
Therapy for the cardiac disease
  • As determined by echocardiography
Anticoagulants
  • Heparin
  • Warfarin
Thrombolytic agents
  • Streptokinase (SK)
  • Recombinant tissue plasminogen activator (rt-PA)
Surgery

12. **What are the potential risks and benefits of vasodilator therapy in FATE?**
The potential benefit of vasodilator therapy is to encourage collateral circulation to the limbs, allowing oxygen and nutrient delivery and removal of the by-products of impaired circulation. Impaired circulation helps prevent permanent nerve damage and muscle necrosis. Unfortunately, FATE patients, with their accompanying cardiac disease, are very susceptible to hypotension, which may result in shock. In addition, the hypotension may promote poor renal perfusion, a risk factor for the development of oliguric or anuric renal failure. Renal infarction, which is a common finding in FATE patients, puts these patients at risk for renal decompensation. Vasodilator therapy should be used carefully and guided by measurement of blood pressure to guide appropriate use. The additive effects of other hypotensive medications should be considered.

13. **Briefly discuss the most common thrombolytic agents.**
  • **Streptokinase (SK)**. This is a bacterial enzyme produced by streptococci and it is thus antigenic. SK is a relatively inexpensive agent given intravenously or locally at the site of a thrombus. The administration of SK results in a systemic thrombolysis: it binds to plasminogen to form plasmin, which lyses fibrin. This results in depletion of prothrombin, clotting factors V and VIII, fibrinogen, plasminogen, and fibrinogen degradation products (FDPs).
  • **Recombinant tissue plasminogen activator (rt-PA)**. This is produced by recombinant DNA technology and is thus expensive. rt-PA is given intravenously and achieves a local thrombolysis due to its high affinity for plasminogen in the presence of fibrin bound to the surface of a thrombus.

14. What are the advantages of thrombolytic therapy for FATE?

Successful thrombolysis results in earlier reestablishment of circulation to the tissues, resulting in less tissue damage and an earlier return to function.

15. What are the disadvantages of thrombolytic therapy for FATE?

The major disadvantage of thrombolytic therapy is the need for very close monitoring and frequent hematologic testing. Frequent phlebotomies and repeat coagulation tests can deplete the blood volume in the smaller feline patient. Venous access may be limited due to hematoma formation or venous thrombosis.

The major complication associated with thrombolytic agents would be reperfusion injury and bleeding complications. Reperfusion injury occurs as a result of the release of toxins, potassium, free radicals, and acidemic blood into the general circulation. Bleeding complications are more likely to arise with the use of streptokinase, due to the systemic thrombolysis that occurs.

16. It is often unclear when an embolic event has occurred. Does the timing of the event impact on the decision of how to treat cats with FATE?

It is widely believed that thrombolysis is more successful and safer in patients with an embolus less than 8 hours old. However, this widely held concept needs to be reevaluated to establish more clear-cut guidelines. In human patients, thrombolytic therapy is no longer thought to be just an acute intervention but the risks would differ in treating myocardial infarctions as opposed to aortic occlusion with the larger volume of infarcted tissue. Many would argue that the risk of reperfusion injury is too high for cats with more chronic aortic occulsion.

17. There are several potential surgical interventions for FATE. Briefly discuss these interventions.

Open aortic embolectomy via laparotomy allows for easy removal of the saddle embolus. This approach has the advantage of predicting the degree of abdominal organ involvement. Reperfusion injury may also result, but the reestablishment of circulation is predictable and thus bicarbonate and free-radical scavengers can be administered prior to reestablishing circulation. The second major type of surgical intervention would be embolectomy by way of a peripheral approach (via the femoral artery). The use of the Fogarty catheter system is very difficult in the cat due to the small size of the femoral artery. The development of sophisticated embolectomy devices for people will likely lead to devices that will also make this more feasible in the feline patient.

18. What is the major advantage of surgical therapy?

The major advantage to surgery is the early reestablishment of circulation.

19. What is the major disadvantage of surgical therapy?

The need for general anesthesia in an unstable cardiac patient has generally resulted in an unacceptably high mortality rate. Surgical wounds create a challenge in anticoagulation to prevent recurrent episodes of thromboembolism in the postsurgical patient.

20. What is currently thought to be the best therapy for cats affected with a saddle embolus?

This is currently open for debate. Streptokinase is a promising drug for clot thrombolysis in cats. Whether there is a correlation among the return of femoral pulses and earlier return to function and improved overall survival has yet to be established. More study needs to be done to decide if SK therapy is the optimal therapeutic approach and if so to develop a dose schedule to maximize favorable outcome while minimizing complications.

More conservative therapy consisting of analgesic therapy, heparin, and supportive care can be considered as an alternative. Heparin is dosed at 200 IU/kg subcutaneously every 8 hours and the APTT monitored daily with a goal of prolongation to 1.5 to 2.0 times the normal value. Patients need to be monitored for signs of external or internal hemorrhage associated with the heparin therapy. To date, data has not been generated to support the success of any of the described strategies for treating FATE.

21. Discuss the prognosis for cats with saddle embolus.
The overall prognosis is guarded to poor. Overall survival rate in one study was 37%. Individual prognosis depends on the degree of paralysis, the degree of ischemic damage, the degree of collateral circulation to the limbs, the severity of the underlying heart disease, the severity of coexistent congestive heart failure, and the extent of visceral organ involvement.

22. What is the prognosis for a cat presenting with forelimb embolus?
Cats presenting with a forelimb embolus almost uniformly recover completely and in less than 24 hours. However, the development of a forelimb embolus is an important harbinger of future major thromboembolic events.

CONTROVERSY

23. What is the best therapy for preventing recurrent thromboembolic episodes in the cat?
Aspirin, considered a platelet-modifying drug, has traditionally been prescribed at 81 mg every 48 to 72 hours to try to prevent embolic complications. Experimentally, aspirin has been shown to decrease platelet responsiveness, but clinical results with aspirin have been disappointing; aspirin appears to be relatively ineffective in preventing thromboembolism.

Warfarin sodium is the anticoagulant most routinely prescribed in both human and animal patients who have suffered an embolic event. Recent pharmokinetic studies in the cat indicate that the tablets should be compounded into a suspension as the drug is unevenly distributed in the tablets. Cats are generally started at a dosage of 0.25 to 0.5 mg once daily and the dose adjusted weekly to maintain the prothrombin time (PT) at 1.5–2.0 times baseline, but less than 30 seconds. Difficulties with warfarin therapy are many: erratic fluctuations of the PT, bleeding complications (sometimes not predicted by the PT), and repeat thromboembolic episodes, even when the patient appears to be adequately anticoagulated. The international normalization ratio (INR) is a better way to monitor anticoagulant therapy, as it corrects for variations in thromboplastin reagent and laboratory technique.

Although randomized studies for FATE survivors comparing aspirin, placebo, and warfarin therapy are desperately needed, randomization of such cases is extremely complicated due to numerous clinical and prognostic variables.

BIBLIOGRAPHY

1. Allen DG, Johnstone IB, Crane S: Effects of aspirin and propranolol alone and in combination on hemostatic determinants in the healthy cat. Am J Vet Res 46:1820–1823, 1985.
2. Baty CJ: Warfarin prophylaxis in feline aortic thromboembolism. Proc Am Coll Vet Intern Med 11:519–520, 1993.
3. Baty CJ, Harpster NK: Warfarin therapy of the cat at risk of thromboembolism. In Bonagura J (ed): Current Veterinary Therapy XII. Philadelphia, W.B. Saunders, 1995, pp 473–480.
4. Greene CE: Effects of aspirin and propranolol on feline platelet aggregation. Am J Vet Res 43:1647–1650, 1982.
5. Handin R, Loscalzo J: Hemostasis, thrombosis, fibrinolysis, and cardiovascular disease. In Braunwald E (ed): Heart Disease: A Textbook of Cardiovascular Medicine. 4th ed. Philadelphia, W.B. Saunders, 1996, pp 1767–1789.
6. Helenski MS, Ross JN: Platelet aggregation in feline cardiomyopathy. J Vet Int Med 1:24–28, 1987.
7. Kellerman DL: Heparin therapy: What we do and don't know. Proc Am Coll Vet Intern Med 16:438–439, 1998.
8. Laste NJ, Harpster NK: A retrospective study of 100 cases of feline distal aortic thromboembolism: 1977–1993. J Am Animal Hosp Assoc 31:492–500, 1995.
9. Smith SA: Warfarin therapy in small animal patients: What we do know, what we don't know. Proc Am Coll Vet Intern Med 16:440–442, 1998.

57. CARDIAC PACING

Dana A. Buoscio, D.V.M.

1. When is cardiac pacing indicated?

Cardiac pacemaker implantation is the treatment of choice for symptomatic bradyarrhythmias. Dogs and cats with bradyarrhythmias may exhibit clinical signs, including weakness, exercise intolerance, and syncope, as well as signs of overt congestive heart failure.

2. What are the most common arrhythmias that require pacing?

The most common bradyarrhythmia requiring pacing in dogs and cats is high-grade second-degree or third-degree atrioventricular block (two-thirds of cases). Sick sinus syndrome, including sinus bradycardia, sinus arrest, sinoatrial block, and bradycardia-tachycardia syndrome is also a common finding, accounting for 25% of cases. Less common is persistent atrial standstill (less than 10% of cases).

3. Do clinical signs resolve after pacing?

Dogs with advanced atrioventricular block often develop signs of congestive heart failure as a result of the chronic bradycardia. Sick sinus syndrome may precipitate the development of congestive heart failure, particularly in animals with pre-existing mitral valve endocardiosis. Many animals with chronic and severe bradycardia develop heart murmurs of atrioventricular incompetence related to stretch of the mitral or tricuspid valve annulus. Additionally, a flow murmur that is associated with a large stroke volume is sometimes heard in dogs with atrioventricular block and slow ventricular rates. The presence of a cardiac murmur in association with chronic and profound bradycardia does not necessarily imply the presence of serious underlying myocardial or valvular dysfunction; however, careful, preoperative echocardiographic evaluation is certainly warranted. When the heart rate is returned to normal the signs usually resolve, since the congestive heart failure is a result of the chronic bradycardia. The presence of underlying systemic or cardiac diseases should be ruled out as this might alter the prognosis and result in persistent clinical signs despite adequate rhythm control.

Animals with persistent atrial standstill are in a different situation. They often have progressive myocardial failure, which is evident at the time of presentation or develops despite appropriate management of the arrhythmia with pacing. These cases are given a guarded prognosis as a result of their progressive disease.

4. What are the components of a pacemaker?

A pacemaker is a device that senses electrical activity and delivers an electrical stimulus. The electrical stimulus is supplied by a battery and conducted over a lead that contains electrodes in direct contact with the heart. The first component of a pacemaker is the pulse generator. The pulse generator contains the power source in the form of a lithium battery, which is required to generate the electrical impulse. The lithium battery has a high energy density, long shelf-life, and predictable characteristics that allow early detection of battery depletion. In most models, the pacing rate declines gradually as the battery becomes depleted, indicating that the pulse generator should be replaced; this and other features ensure that depletion of the battery does not lead to a sudden and unexpected pacing failure. The life of a lithium battery is between 7 and 12 years for most types of pulse generators that are used in dogs and cats.

The second component is the lead. The lead is an insulated wire with an electrode on one end that conducts the electrical impulse from the pulse generator to the heart and senses spontaneous electrical activity within the heart. Leads are either epicardial or endocardial. Epicardial leads are implanted into the myocardium from the outer surface of the heart, either by screwing or suturing the lead to the heart. Endocardial leads are implanted transvenously so that the electrode contacts the inner surface of the heart. Leads are also classified based upon the nature of the electrical circuit that they complete. Unipolar leads have one electrode in the heart (cathode) and a second electrode outside of the heart within the pulse generator casing (anode). Bipolar leads have both electrodes within the heart. Unipolar leads have better sensing characteristics, but bipolar leads have greater resistance to electromagnetic and myopotential interference.

5. Discuss the pacemaker identification code.

All pacemaker pulse generators are categorized with a basic three-letter identification code. The first letter denotes the chamber that is paced, the second letter the chamber that is sensed, and the third letter the response to sensing.

1ST LETTER CHAMBER(S) PACED	2ND LETTER CHAMBER(S) SENSED	3RD LETTER RESPONSE TO SENSING
	0 (none)	0 (none)
A (atrium)	A (atrium)	T (triggered)
V (ventricle)	V (ventricle)	I (inhibited)
D (dual; A+V)	D (dual; A+V)	D (dual; T+I)

Inhibited response means that the pacemaker discharge is suppressed by a sensed signal, while triggered response means that the pacemaker is triggered to discharge when it senses a signal.

A fourth and fifth letter can also be used to describe other qualities of a pulse generator. The fourth letter indicates its ability to be programmed (P or M) or modulate its rate (R). The fifth letter indicates whether it can perform antitachycardia pacing (P).

6. Which type of pacemaker is most often used?

The most common type of pulse generator used in veterinary medicine is the VVI, which is a single-chamber, ventricular-demand pacemaker. Most of these are also rate- and output-programmable (VVIPO or VVIMO). The VVI pulse generator senses and paces only the ventricle, and is inhibited or will not deliver an impulse if a spontaneous beat is sensed. This type of pulse generator prevents the heart rate from falling below a predetermined level, which usually is set between 80 and 100 bpm in most dogs. Ventricular pacing at this rate usually obtains a good clinical result in dogs with otherwise normal cardiac function. When this type of pulse generator is used in a cat, the rate is usually set at 120 bpm.

Occasionally other types of pulse generators are used, such as the DDD or VAT. These are dual-chamber pacemakers that require implantation of an atrial lead as well as a ventricular lead. Dual-chamber pacemakers offer the advantage of having the atria contract in synchrony with the ventricles, which can improve cardiac output. These types of pacemakers are more expensive and are harder to obtain for use in veterinary patients. These potentially would offer a better clinical result in active dogs or dogs with underlying valvular or myocardial disease who may not show a good response to a ventricular pacemaker.

7. Outline the typical work-up for a veterinary patient in need of a pacemaker.

Prior to implanting a pacemaker, animals are assessed in a thorough manner to exclude any underlying cause for the bradyarrhythmia, such as neurologic, metabolic, or endocrine disease. A routine physical examination is performed, and a complete blood count, serum chemistry analysis, heartworm test, and urinalysis is obtained. In order to document the arrhythmia an electrocardiogram is recorded, and if the arrhythmia is not evident, a 24-hour Holter electrocardiogram or event recording is obtained. Thoracic radiographs and an echocardiogram are then performed to evaluate for congestive heart failure and underlying cardiac disease. If signs of congestive heart failure are present, medical therapy is begun to stabilize the patient prior to pacemaker implantation.

8. How is the pacemaker implanted?

The permanent pacemaker is implanted under general anesthesia in most cases. Since these animals are at a high risk for developing life-threatening arrhythmias, a temporary pacemaker should be used prior to induction of anesthesia if possible. Controlling the rate with a temporary endocardial pacemaker prevents the development of high-degree atrioventricular block, severe sinus node dysfunction, or asystole, which is often seen when these animals are placed under anesthesia. Many dogs are cooperative enough to place the temporary lead while awake. This is done by placing a bipolar lead through a large-bore venous catheter into the jugular vein and then passing the lead into the right ventricle either blindly or with fluoroscopic guidance. The lead is connected to an external pulse generator which is adjusted to maintain the heart rate at a safe level while anesthesia is induced.

Permanent pacemaker implantation is then performed using either the endocardial or epicardial approach. The endocardial transvenous implantation is the preferred method since it is less invasive and offers less morbidity and mortality related to the implantation process. Successful use of this method requires meticulous attention to technique in order to reduce the incidence of complications occurring after implantation. Using fluoroscopic guidance, the unipolar or bipolar lead is introduced into the jugular vein and directed into the apex of the right ventricle, where it is placed or secured. The best type of endocardial lead used for this method is either a tined lead or an active fixation lead. A tined lead has small projections at its tip that are entangled in the trabeculae, and an active fixation lead has a small retractable screw that is extruded to penetrate the myocardium once the lead is properly positioned. The lead is then ligated within the jugular vein and connected to the pulse generator, which is placed in a subcutaneous pocket through a separate incision in the dorsolateral aspect of the neck. The pulse generator is secured in its position by suturing it to the underlying muscle and fascia.

The epicardial method requires surgical implantation via either a lateral thoracotomy, caudal median sternotomy, or a ventral abdominal transdiaphragmatic approach. These methods are more invasive and have more complications associated with the surgical procedure. The epicardial lead is implanted into an avascular site on the left ventricular apex. The pulse generator is placed either in the flank or within the abdomen. When placed within the abdomen the pulse generator may be too deep to be reached by an external noninvasive reprogramming unit.

9. What postoperative care is required? How often are rechecks necessary?

Immediately following implantation, thoracic radiographs (lateral and dorsoventral) and an electrocardiogram are obtained to document lead placement and pacemaker function. The pulse generator pocket site is bandaged for several days, and the animal's activity is restricted for 10–14 days. Broad-spectrum antibiotics are used prophylactically for 1–2 weeks after implantation. The electrocardiogram and pulse rate is monitored intermittently for 48 hours to detect arrhythmias and to ensure proper pacemaker function (see figure at top of next page). The patient is released to the owner's care in 3–5 days if no serious complications are evident. For dogs with transvenously implanted pacemakers, the owners are instructed to use a shoulder harness instead of a collar. Additionally, the jugular vein should not be used for venipuncture, and prophylactic antibiotics should be used for routine surgeries and dental cleanings.

The patient is rechecked at the time of suture removal (10–14 days), at which time a physical examination and electrocardiogram are performed. Further rechecks are scheduled at 3 and 6 months postimplantation, and every 6–12 months thereafter.

10. Discuss the most common complications associated with pacemaker implantation.

• **Arrhythmias** can occur during or after pacemaker implantation. The most common postimplantation arrhythmia is ventricular tachycardia or ventricular premature beats. Some of these require treatment, but infrequent premature beats are closely monitored and often resolve without treatment. More serious arrhythmias are seen with the epicardial implantation procedure, including ventricular fibrillation and asystole.

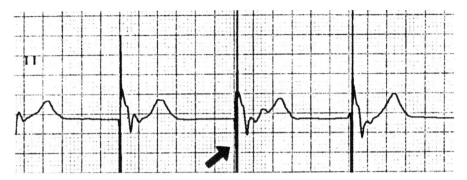

Normal electrocardiogram of a dog after permanent pacemaker implantation for complete heart block. The pacemaker impulse (arrow) occurs regularly at a rate of 100 bpm and is followed by a wide, bizarre QRS complex. Paper speed 50 mm/sec; 1 cm = 1 mV.

- **Lead dislodgement** can occur with both endocardial and epicardial leads. Endocardial lead dislodgement is more common, usually occurring within 48 hours, but occasionally may occur later. Endocardial lead dislodgement was more common prior to the availability of tined or active fixation leads. Strict cage confinement in the early postoperative period minimizes the incidence of this complication. Dislodgement of leads also can occur if there is repeated rotation of the pulse generator within the subcutaneous pocket (twiddler's syndrome). Repositioning or replacement of the lead is required since intermittent or complete loss of pacing occurs as a result of dislodgement.

- **Infection** of the pulse generator can also occur, requiring antibiotic therapy and usually removal of the infected pacemaker and reimplantation of a new pacemaker. This complication is seen more often in animals not receiving prophylactic antibiotics perioperatively.

- **Seroma or hematoma formation** at the pulse generator site can be a complication, sometimes resulting in migration of the pulse generator and erosion of the overlying skin, or pacemaker twiddler's syndrome. This can be minimized by careful operative technique, application of a bandage over the pulse generator site, and restriction of activity.

- **Synchronous muscle twitching** of cervical or shoulder skeletal musculature can be seen in the early postimplantation period, and often disappears within a few days. Occasionally a normally functioning unipolar pulse generator without an insulation leak can cause a persistent muscle twitch by flipping over within its pocket, which can be remedied by flipping the pulse generator back into its original position.

- **Pacemaker malfunction** also can occur, including loss of capture, loss of pacing stimulus, undersensing, or oversensing.

11. What causes pacemaker malfunction?

Many different problems can cause pacemaker malfunction. **Loss of capture** is seen when the pulse generator produces a stimulus but fails to "capture" or produce a myocardial contraction. This can be corrected by reprogramming the pulse generator, but may require replacement of the lead if it is a result of damage to the lead, dislodgement, or exit block. Exit block occurs when the impulse from the lead electrode is blocked from traveling into the surrounding myocardium. This is seen after implantation as a result of development of nonexcitable fibrous tissue around the electrode. **Loss of pacing stimulus** can occur as a result of lead fracture, loose connection to the pulse generator, or failure of the pulse generator battery. This requires replacement of the pulse generator and/or the lead. Impending battery failure can be detected by a reduction in the pacing rate. When this occurs, the patient is monitored more frequently until a new pulse generator is required.

Undersensing occurs when the pacemaker fails to recognize spontaneous electrical activity and delivers its impulse when it should be inhibited. **Oversensing** occurs when the pacemaker is inappropriately inhibited from delivering an impulse according to its programmed automatic interval. These complications may occur due to poor lead placement, dislodgement, or interference with skeletal muscle potentials. Reprogramming or reimplantation may be required to correct these complications.

BIBLIOGRAPHY

1. Barold SS, Zipes DP: Cardiac pacemakers and antiarrhythmic devices. In Braunwald E (ed): Heart Disease: A Textbook of Cardiovascular Medicine, 5th ed. Philadelphia, W.B. Saunders, 1997, pp 705–741.
2. Bonagura JD, Helphrey ML, Muir WW: Complications associated with permanent pacemaker implantation in the dog. J Am Vet Med Assoc 182:149–155, 1983.
3. Darke PGG: Update: Transvenous pacing. In Kirk RW, Bonagura JD (eds): Current Veterinary Therapy XI: Small Animal Practice. Philadelphia, W.B. Saunders, 1992, pp 708–713.
4. Darke PGG, McAreavey D, Been M: Transvenous cardiac pacing in 19 dogs and one cat. J Small Anim Pract 30:491–499, 1989.
5. Klement P, Del-Nido PJ, Wilson GJ: The use of cardiac pacemakers in veterinary practice. Comp Contin Educ 6:893–902, 1984.
6. Lombard CW, Tilley LP, Yoshioka M: Pacemaker implantation in the dog: Survey and literature review. J Am Anim Hosp Assoc 17:751–758, 1981.
7. Schollmeyer M: Pacemaker therapy. In Fox PR (ed): Canine and Feline Cardiology. New York, Churchill Livingstone, 1988, pp 625–634.
8. Sisson, DD: Bradyarrhythmias and cardiac pacing. In Kirk RW (ed): Current Veterinary Therapy X: Small Animal Practice. Philadelphia, W.B. Saunders, 1989, pp 286–295.
9. Sisson DD, Thomas WP, Woodfield J, et al: Permanent transvenous pacemaker implantation in forty dogs. J Vet Intern Med 5:322–331, 1991.

58. CANINE HEARTWORM DISEASE

Clay A. Calvert, D.V.M.

1. What is heartworm disease?

Heartworm (HW) disease, or dirofilariasis, is the consequence of parasitic infection by a filarid nematode, *Dirofilaria immitis*. The dog is the primary host although other carnivores may harbor the parasite. Adult heartworms reside primarily within the pulmonary arteries but are occasionally found in the right atrium, right ventricle, or venae cavae. The adult female worms release a larval form directly into the bloodstream; transmission of the infection is by mosquitoes, which are an obligatory intermediate host for the parasite.

2. Other than the U.S., in which countries has *D. immitis* infection of dogs been detected?

Canada, Mexico, Japan, South America, southern and southeastern Asian countries, Australia, Italy, and southern European countries all are known to have an incidence.

3. Are there any areas of the U.S. and Canada where the HW infection has not been detected?

HW infection is generally uncommon in Canada but is reported in southern regions adjacent to Washington, Minnesota, New York, and lakes Huron, Ontario, and Erie. HW infection is rare in mountainous regions of the U.S., Alaska (one case reported), Idaho, Montana, Wyoming, Nevada, Utah, Arizona, and the western parts of the Dakotas.

However, a mobile public guarantees that infected dogs will be transported to nonendemic regions and, if the climate is suitable, infections can be established. Feral dogs and wild *Canidae* (principally coyotes and foxes) can become reservoirs, making the problem difficult to eradicate.

4. What species other than dogs and cats are susceptible to *D. immitis* infections?

Other *Canidae*, sea lions, and ferrets have been reported with HW infection.

5. What does the term "occult" HW infection mean?

Occult HW infection is a term often applied to infections in which microfilariae are absent or inconsistently retrieved at low numbers by serial venipuncture samples.

There are several potential causes, including:

- Immune-mediated entrapment and destruction of microfilariae in the pulmonary microcirculation.
- Unisex infections: more likely to occur in nonendemic regions when the adult HW burden is low.
- Drug-induced: several drugs, most importantly the macrolide preventative drugs milbemycin oxime, ivermectin, and moxadectin, will reduce microfilarial production and kill microfilariae over a variable time span. Thus, patent infections in dogs receiving these preventatives will become "occult" over a period of months.

6. Are all mosquitos capable of transmitting infective *D. immitis* larvae?

Many (at least 60) species can transmit the infection. *Culex* and *Aedes* spp. are the primary culprits, most preferring to feed on dogs, but *Culex pipiens*, and perhaps others, prefer to feed on cats.

7. What are the microfilariae?

Microfilariae are first-stage larvae (L1) that are produced by a gravid female *D. immitis*. It is believed that microfilariae produce little or no pathology and are a "dead end" for the parasite unless they are taken up by a mosquito feeding on the infected host. If that mosquito is capable of being a transport host, the L1 may develop to the infective stage (L3) within the mosquito. Otherwise, the primary significance of microfilariae is their diagnostic value relative to infection.

8. How long does it take for the L1 to develop to the infective (L3) stage within the mosquito?
This varies linearly with the ambient temperature. For example, maturation time is 130 days at 15°C, 65 days at 16°C, 32–33 days at 17°C, and 16 days at 18°C.

9. How long after a dog is infected by L3 does it take for microfilariae to appear in the peripheral blood of the host?
The patency period is approximately 6 months.

10. Which stages of development are found in the pulmonary arteries?
The fifth-stage larvae develop via the molt from L4 50–70 days after L3 inoculation. They reach the pulmonary arteries 70–110 days after L3 inoculation. Most are found in the caudal lobar pulmonary arteries, with more in the right artery, simply because these vessels have the highest blood flow. The L5 grow and mature in the pulmonary arteries and are sexually mature 190–285 days after L3 inoculation. Thus the L5 (young adults) and adults are found in the pulmonary arteries.

11. If microfilariae of *D. immitis* are detected, are the adult HW always present?
Usually, unless adulticide treatment has been administered. It is very uncommon for microfilariae to be present without adult worms in an untreated dog because the adult HW life span is thought to be longer. The true life span of adult HW is poorly documented, but microfilariae can live for 2–4 years.

12. Microfilariae are occasionally detected in puppies. What is the significance of this finding?
Microfilariae (L1) can be transmitted via the placenta to the fetus. The microfilariae probably do little or no harm but the puppy serves as a reservoir host. Also, confusion could arise if these microfilariae were not detected until the dog was more than 6–7 months old. However, a negative antigen test at that time, suggesting no or very few adult HW, would help clarify the situation.

13. Is there any significance to the concentration of microfilariae in the peripheral blood?
The concentration of microfilariae detected by small blood samples varies throughout the day. Sometimes there are midday peaks but often the periodicity is unpredictable. In general, the concentration of microfilariae does not correlate with the adult HW burden. The incidence of acute adverse reactions following the administration of microfilaricide treatment (milbemycin or ivermectin, 50 µg/kg) is greater when the microfilarial counts are highest. However, microfilarial counts are not routinely done.

14. Is there a distinction between HW infection or infestation and HW disease?
It is true that HW infection does not always produce clinical, radiographic, ECG, or echocardiographic abnormalities and thus the term HW disease is not always applied to infected dogs. On the other hand, it is doubtful that any HW infection will fail to produce at least mild histologic changes of the pulmonary arterial endothelium.

15. What actually causes the pulmonary artery disease associated with HW infection?
Sloughing of strips of endothelium occurs quickly after HW contact. Some antigenic substance from the worm is probably the inciting factor. Platelets and leukocytes adhere to the damaged endothelium and growth factors are thought to be released from these cells, stimulating multiplication and migration of smooth muscle cells. This leads to villus hypertrophy of the arteries characterized by protuberances consisting of smooth muscle covered by a healed or subsequently redamaged endothelium. Thickening of artery and arteriole walls leads to decreased blood flow, thromboembolism, and decreased compliance.

16. Do all dogs with HW infection have pulmonary hypertension?

No, or at least it is mild in most cases. Two-thirds of the pulmonary circulation must be obstructed before severe hypertension develops. However, some degree of pulmonary hypertension exists in most dogs with radiographic evidence of HW infection, although radiograph artery size does not necessarily correlate with the degree of hypertension.

Since the vasculature cannot dilate when it is severely diseased and recruitment of collateral vessels does not occur (because the vessels are already in use or obstructed), hypertension is exacerbated by exercise; hence, there may be exercise-induced symptoms including right-sided heart failure and syncope.

17. What causes right heart enlargement in some dogs with HW disease?

The exact mechanism is not completely understood. One would expect hypertrophy in response to a pressure overload (pulmonary hypertension). However, the geometry of the right ventricle is ill-suited to the generation of high pressures and this probably contributes to the development of tricuspid valve regurgitation and systolic myocardial failure. Thus, the right ventricular response to chronic pulmonary hypertension is characterized by both dilation and hypertrophy. Right heart failure is often, but not always, associated with moderate to severe pulmonary hypertension.

18. Why is the pathology worse in some dogs compared to others?

High adult HW burden (increased contact with endothelium) and especially immune-mediated responses cause more severe damage. Presumably, the duration of infection and exercise level are also important contributing factors.

In any case, severe lobar arterial dilation, tortuosity, and obstruction tend to be more severe in highly endemic regions (higher worm burden) and in occult infections.

Loss of pulmonary arterial compliance secondary to thickening of the walls and more importantly, embolism and obstruction leads to pulmonary hypertension. It is the latter that leads to right ventricular dilation and hypertrophy.

19. When should dogs be tested for HW infection?

In general, there are several specific recommendations:
- All dogs should be tested when they reach 6 months of age.
- Whenever an adult dog is presented that is not or may not have been on an adequate HW preventative program, it should be tested.
- A microfilarial test is mandatory prior to initiating diethylcarbamazine prophylaxis.
- Dogs already receiving prophylaxis should be tested annually.

20. Is it really necessary to test annually?

It is well documented that client compliance is often poor. However, if a macrolide is given every 2 months, the likelihood of infection is small. Clinical judgment is required.

21. Has serology supplanted microfilarial detection as the preferred method of diagnosis?

Yes, the incidence of false-negative test results using HW antigen tests is lower than the incidence of occult or amicrofilaremic infections.

22. What is the best antigen test for the detection of HW infection?

There are numerous tests available, mostly utilizing ELISA technology, and all are very sensitive and specific and are continually being refined. No doubt advances in serologic diagnosis will continue.

The two basic types are the so-called "stat" tests, which provide a quick answer while the client is at the clinic, and those more suitable for batching numerous samples to be run later in the day. Antigen tests are used for:
- Screening
- Diagnosis of occult infections

- As part of the clinical database for a dog with signs, radiographs, and laboratory findings consistent with HW infection
- Monitoring adulticide efficacy

23. Do we need to worry about a weakly positive HW antigen test?

A weakly positive antigen test indicates a low antigen burden. The risk of symptomatic HW disease developing in such a patient is relatively low.

24. Then what is recommended when one encounters this situation?

Usually an antigen test is repeated, preferably using a different methodology. Also, a microfilarial test can be useful, but a negative result is more likely when the worm burden is low. Thoracic radiographs will probably be normal or equivocal.

25. Should these dogs be treated?

The risk of serious adverse reactions in such dogs treated with melarsomine is low; therefore, many clinicians recommend treatment. On the other hand, since the severity and rate of progression of pathology is usually limited, another choice is to initiate ivermectin prophylaxis since this will kill the adult worms slowly over a period of months. Some worms may survive as long as 18 months.

26. False-positive test results are not supposed to happen, but they do. Why?

Theoretically, heartworm antigen tests have absolute specificity. The primary causes for false positive results are cross-contamination and improper methodology.

In addition, the interpretation of some test results is made difficult due to subtle reactions that indicate either low-level antigenemia or a truly negative result; there is a learning curve involved. HW antigen test kit manufacturers provide a confirmatory service; thus, appropriate samples can be submitted.

27. Can false-negative test results occur?

Yes. There are several situations that can lead to a false-negative result. It is only the female worm that contributes to a positive result. Thus, a unisex male infection will test negative. Furthermore, currently none of these tests will detect early (up to 5–6 months after L3 inoculation) infections. When three or more female worms 8 months or more of age are present, most tests are 100% sensitive. If only one or two females are present, and especially if they are less than 8 months old, negative results are possible.

Dogs with very few worms are unlikely to develop clinical signs and thus the false-negative test result is not really a problem as long as prophylaxis is underway, thus preventing further infection. Ivermectin will eventually kill adult worms.

28. What tests are used to detect circulating microfilaria; which of these are the best?

Microfilaria can be detected through examination of a direct blood smear. However, tests that concentrate the microfilariae are more sensitive. The modified Knott test utilizes centrifugation to concentrate microfilariae; the sediment is stained and examined microscopically. Commercially available filter tests rely on a small-pore filter in order to concentrate the heartworm larvae.

Both the concentrating filter tests and modified Knott test are equally sensitive. The direct blood smear, while quick and facilitating the identification of microfilariae (D. immitis versus D. reconditum), is at least 25% less sensitive than the concentration tests, which are approximately 75% sensitive when microfilariae are present.

29. How often will microfilarial tests miss microfilariae in dogs with live adult HW?

This varies by geographic region, but in general 15–50% of all HW infections are not associated with circulating microfilariae. The higher incidences of occult infections occur in highly endemic regions. It is estimated that in the southeastern United States 20–30% of all infections are occult, while in Hawaii the incidence may be as high as 50%. Fewer than 10% of dogs with *D. immitis* microfilariae do not have live adult worms.

30. Are *Dipetalonema reconditum* infections of any significance?

Dipetalonema reconditum is a benign subcutaneous parasite commonly found in *D. immitis* endemic regions. The microfilariae of *D. reconditum* tend to be of lower concentration than those of *D. immitis*, can cause profound eosinophilia, and closely resemble those of *D. immitis*. Thus, confusion can arise. On a direct smear, the microfilariae of *D. reconditum* progress across the microscopic field while those of *D. immitis* tend to undulate in place without steady progression. The former have a more rounded or blunt "nose" and a hooked tail. However, differentiation is best accomplished by measuring their length and width (see table).

In addition, if a HW antigen test is positive, then it is known that adult worms are present and adulticide treatment is probably indicated. Milbemycin and ivermectin at the microfilaricidal dose (50 mg/kg) will kill both types of microfilariae.

Differentiation of the Microfilariae of D. immitis from D. reconditum

	D. immitis	*D. reconditum*
Filter test		
Length (μm)	235–285	215–240
Width (μm)	> 6	< 6
Knott test		
Length (μm)	> 290	< 275
Width (μm)	> 6	< 6

31. Can HW serology be of value in determining the severity of infection?

Yes. All HW antigen tests are a semiquantitation of the HW burden. It is generally assumed that a relatively high worm burden will be associated with:

• More severe signs
• The emergence of signs in an asymptomatic HW-infected dog
• Increased likelihood of thromboembolic complications following administration of an adulticide

Some tests provide a negative, low-burden positive, and high-burden positive result. Semiquantitation of other tests can be done by serial dilution (phosphate buffered saline) of the serum and determining to which titer (dilution) a positive result persists. A titer of more than 1:32 may be associated with greater risk of thromboembolic disease. Armed with this information, and the history, physical examination, and thoracic radiographs, the appropriate choice of therapy can be selected.

32. Are there any new tests that can detect early infections?

Yes. A highly sensitive ELISA test that can detect infections as young as 3 months after L3 inoculation may become available.

33. What are the most common signs of HW disease?

Coughing, exercise intolerance, and dyspnea are most frequent.

34. What is the protocol for classifying the severity of HW disease?

Patients with class I infections are asymptomatic or have only occasional coughing. Patients with class II infections have clinical signs such as cough or mild exercise intolerance. Class III is comprised of severely affected dogs, such as those with overt congestive heart failure, syncope, and severe exercise intolerance (see table at top of next page).

Classification of Heartworm Disease by Severity

CLASS	SIGNS	RADIOGRAPHS
I	Absent-mild	Normal to slightly abnormal
II	Cough Mild exercise intolerance Mild weight loss	Slightly to moderately abnormal
III	Severe cough Exercise intolerance Poor condition Anemia Ascites Syncope Dyspnea Weight loss	Severely abnormal

35. Are there clinical signs that are associated with severe HW disease?

Syncope, dyspnea, hemoptysis, ascites, anemia, weight loss, and a general unhealthy appearance, if caused by HW disease, all are associated with class III infections.

36. Which classification of HW severity is most common?

In one study, approximately two-thirds of the dogs had class II disease. These dogs are typically about 5 years of age compared to an average of 3–4 years of age for dogs with class I infection and approximately 7–8 years of age for dogs in class III.

37. What determines why some dogs are more severely affected than others?

Worm burden, duration of infection, and the host immune response are the factors that determine severity. Dogs with class I disease tend to be younger and have a lower serum antigen concentration than most dogs in class II. Dogs with class III infections are typically a little older but frequently their serum antigen concentration is lower. Presumably their worm burden was higher but some of the worms have died (dead worms produce a severe reaction in the lungs). Necropsy of dogs with class III disease sometimes reveals relatively few live worms. Worm death may be the cause of or the result of a strong immune reaction.

38. What clinical findings indicate that pulmonary thromboembolism is occurring?

Coughing, dyspnea, hemoptysis, fever, pulmonary crackles, an inflammatory leukogram, thrombocytopenia, hemoglobinuria, and patchy interstitial-alveolar pulmonary infiltrates (especially in the caudal lobes) are all associated with thromboembolism.

39. What clinical findings are associated with congestive heart failure due to HW disease?

These dogs with class III disease exhibit ascites; jugular vein distention/pulsation, hepatomegaly, coughing, dyspnea, exercise intolerance, and syncope are variably present. Invariably thoracic radiographs contain severely enlarged and tortuous lobar arteries (best viewed on the dorsoventral projection). The ECG often reflects right ventricular hypertrophy (large S waves in leads I, V_2 and V_4).

40. What is the appropriate minimum clinical database that should be obtained prior to HW treatment?

Although this question has been debated for many years, with the advent of rapid cost-effective laboratory services, all infected dogs should be evaluated by a CBC, serum chemistry profile, and urinalysis.

41. Are thoracic radiographs necessary?

The single most useful test for determining the severity of HW infection is thoracic radiography, and radiographs should be obtained if the infection is occult, symptomatic, of unknown or long-standing duration, and in older dogs. Unfortunately, this component of the database is the one most often omitted. Unexpected complications following adulticide adminstration could often have been anticipated if thoracic radiographs had been obtained.

42. Not all the radiographic abnormalities associated with HW disease consist of arterial enlargement and tortuosity. What causes the interstitial and alveolar changes commonly seen?

Small pulmonary arterioles are also damaged by HW infection and these can leak fluid and inflammatory cells. This produces interstitial and alveolar infiltrates that are most concentrated in the caudal lung lobes adjacent to the lobar arteries. Extensive infiltrates sometimes develop. These changes are most common and severe after adulticide therapy (3–30 days, mostly 10–21 days) but can occur earlier, especially following exertion.

Another cause is associated with immune-mediated occult infections in which an unusually severe allergic reaction occurs. Heavy concentrations of eosinophils are found in the lungs and the radiographic pattern can resemble left-sided congestive heart failure (pulmonary edema), blastomycosis, and allergic pneumonitis unrelated to HW.

43. Aren't liver enzyme elevations not only common, but also indicative of adulticide intolerance?

Markedly increased SAP and ALT activities are not common nor are they predictive of adulticide toxicity, efficacy, or prognosis, if the increases are less than tenfold.

44. Is proteinuria an important abnormailty?

Proteinuria is common with class III disease, but if mild (urine protein/creatine ratio < 3) with a normal serum albumin, the best course of action is to eliminate the possible cause—heartworms.

Severe proteinuria, particularly with a mildly low or low normal albumin is cause for concern. An irreversible, progressive glomerulopathy may exist. Nonetheless, if the patient is otherwise a good candidate for treatment, then treat. The nephrotic syndrome (ascites or edema together with hypoalbuminemia and proteinuria) is indicative of a grave prognosis and HW treatment is ill advised.

45. Is the ECG an important component of the clinical database?

Not in most instances since it is usually normal. Evidence of right ventricular hypertrophy is always associated with class III (severe) HW infection. However, a thorough history and physical examination coupled with thoracic radiographs will identify such patients and radiographs provide more information. Heart rhythm disturbances due to HW infection are uncommon and seldom severe. Atrial fibrillation can occur with class III infections with overt or impending congestive heart failure.

46. How valuable is echocardiography for HW detection or assessment of severity?

Most dogs with mild HW disease have normal "echo" results. Right ventricular dilation may be seen with moderate and will be seen with severe disease.

HW echos (two parallel, short, linear densities separated by a narrow lucent linear region) can be seen in the right heart, main pulmonary artery, and proximal lobar arteries when the burden is relatively high.

Pulmonary hypertension can be detected and quantitated if spectral Doppler echocardiography detects tricuspid or pulmonic reguritation with a high flow velocity.

47. Should all HW-infected dogs be treated with the same protocol?

No. The standard melarsomine protocol is highly effective for class I and class II HW disease; however, the alternative protocol is recommended for class III disease because of the increased risk of severe thromboembolic complications following adulticide therapy if many worms are initially killed.

48. When is corticosteroid treatment appropriate for HW disease?

Anti-inflammatory dosages of corticosteroids (1.0 mg/kg once or twice daily of prednisolone or prednisone, for example) are sometimes administered empirically for thromboembolism. Some clinicians routinely prescribe these agents following adulticide administration, believing that the incidence of fever, coughing, and anorexia during the first few weeks is reduced.

Anti-inflammatory dosages of corticosteroids are highly effective for allergic pneumonitis associated with occult heartworm disease. The duration of treatment for this purpose is 3–5 days and adulticide therapy is then initiated quickly.

In general, protracted corticosteroid administration promotes thromboembolism and causes reduced pulmonary arterial blood flow.

49. When is heparin indicated for HW disease?

Heparin (75 U/kg subcutaneously, 3 times/day) can be used for class III infections in an attempt to reduce pulmonary thromboembolism. It is administered for several days prior to, during, and for several weeks following adulticide treatment. It is coupled with severe exercise restriction.

Heparin is also useful for complications of thromboembolism associated with hemoglobinuria and/or plummeting platelet counts. Again, strict cage confinement is a part of the treatment.

50. When is aspirin indicated for HW infection?

This controversial treatment is only indicated for class III infections. Aspirin in doses of 5–7 mg/kg once daily may help ameliorate the severity of pulmonary endothelial damage and reduce the severity of thromboembolism. It takes 1 week or longer to produce significant benefits and is therefore used prophylactically prior to, during, and following adulticide treatment rather than as an acute treatment for thromboembolism.

Aspirin can cause gastric bleeding and thus the hematocrit must be monitored and the patient should be observed for vomiting and anorexia.

51. Some veterinarians do not believe that it is necessary to treat asymptomatic HW infections. Is this position tenable?

It is true that if there are no signs, and if radiographs reveal no or only equivocal abnormalities, there is no urgency for treatment. Some argue that such dogs can be monitored for clinical signs and by radiographs, with treatment withheld until progressive disease is detected. Arguments against this approach are:

• Client compliance is often poor and some dogs will be lost to followup.
• The risks associated with melarsomine treatment in such dogs are small.

Alternatively, if a wait-and-see approach is chosen, prophylaxis should logically be prescribed. Ivermectin is the best choice since it will eradicate the adult worms in less than 18–24 months.

52. What about the "ancient" dog?

Old dogs, especially those with concomitant disorders, are not always treated. Considerable clinical judgment is required and decisions are made on an individual patient basis.

Ivermectin treatment may be an option since this will kill adult heartworms slowly over many months (up to 18–24 months) and adverse effects appear to be minimal.

53. Then why not use ivermectin more often as an adulticide?

Since the success rate of melarsomine for patients with class I and II infections is very high and adverse results are not usually severe when the proper protocol and posttreatment confinement are enforced, there is little reason to deviate from the recommendations of the American Heartworm Society. Furthermore, the slow rate of kill produced by ivermectin might allow progressive pulmonary arterial pathology and complications to develop before improvement begins.

54. Are there some dogs that should not be treated for adult HW infection?

Clearly, treatment is of no value in some cases. The most obvious instances are in dogs with:
- The nephrotic syndrome
- Overt right-sided congestive heart failure together with hepatic failure
- Severe renal failure
- Life-limiting comorbid disease not related to HW infection.

Congestive heart failure or class III HW disease alone are not necessarily contraindications for treatment, although treatment complication risk is greater and survival time may be less than that for patients in class I and II.

55. Is there any advantage of thiacetarsemide over melarsomine?

Other than lower cost, there is little or no justification for the continued use of thiacetarsemide.

56. What then are the advantages of melarsomine over thiacetarsemide?

The most important advantages of melarsomine are:
- Melarsomine produces fewer acute arsenical reactions due to the lower dose of arsenic/dog as compared to that of thiacetarsemide.
- The intramuscular administration of melarsomine is preferable.
- Melarsomine results in as high or higher percentages of *D. immitis* larvae and adults of both genders killed versus thiacetarsemide. (Melarsomine does not kill L1, microfilariae.)
- Melarsomine has a dose-related kill rate. By administering 50% of the standard dosage (one dose rather than two), approximately 50% fewer worms are killed, thus reducing pulmonary thromboembolic complications.

57. What is the difference between the standard and alternative melarsomine treatment protocols?

The standard protocol is one intramuscular (epaxial) injection, followed by a second injection on the opposite side 24 hours later. If an antigen test is positive 4 months later, the treatment is repeated.

The alternative protocol (for class III disease) consists of an initial injection followed in one month by two injections given 24 hours apart. If an antigen test is positive 4 months later, two more injections are administered 24 hours apart (see table).

Standard and Alternative Melarsomine Treatment Protocols

	STANDARD	ALTERNATIVE
Indication	Class I–II*	Class III
Dosage	2.5 mg/kg (0.1 ml/kg)	2.5 mg/kg
Route	IM, deep	IM, deep
Location	Epaxial, L_3–L_5	Epaxial, L_3–L_5
Needle	22-gauge	22-gauge
≤ 15 kg	¾ inch	¾ inch
> 15 kg	1 inch	1 inch
Repeat	24 hours (opposite side)	1 month (2 doses at 24 hours apart)
Follow-up		
Antigen test	4 months	4 months
Positive test	Repeat 2 doses as above	Repeat 2 doses at 24 hours apart

* If high antigen burden (> 1.7 µg/ml) class II, use alternative protocol.

58. How effective is the standard protocol?

Approximately 75% of dogs will be antigen-negative 4 months later. If the second set of injections is required, over 95% of dogs will be antigen-negative 4 months later.

59. If an antigen test is weakly positive 4 months after the first two injections, is it appropriate to wait 1–2 additional months and then repeat the test?

Yes.

60. Should all dogs with persistent low-grade antigenemia be retreated.

Clinical judgment is required. The decision is based on initial severity, degree of improvement, age, concomitant problems, whether or not physical exertion is required of the dog, and how many doses were administered. After three or four doses, very few worms will survive and the pathology usually improves dramatically over a 3–6 month period. Also, ivermectin (prophylactic) administration will gradually kill the remaining worms.

61. How effective is the melarsomine alternative dosing regimen?

The first injection kills approximately 90% of the male worms and 15–20% of the females. Overall, 50–60% of the worms are killed by the first injection. Four months after the second set of injections, an antigen test will be negative in 90% of the dogs.

62. Is it appropriate to use the alternative dosing regimen for all HW infected dogs?

It is not inappropriate, but it is not necessary for patients with class I disease.

63. Isn't it true that some clinicians routinely use the alternative melarsomine protocol for all HW infections?

Yes, the logic is that since melarsomine kills more adult worms, pulmonary thromboembolic complications following its administration should be more severe. This has not been reported to be the case in experimental studies. However, anecdotal accounts relating the impression of more severe thromboembolic complications with the use of melarsomine compared to retrospective experience persist.

64. Isn't it true that dogs become tolerant to organic arsenicals so that retreatment is not likely to cause problems?

Yes. Furthermore, since the worm burden is no doubt reduced, the risk of thromboembolism is reduced and is unlikely if no such problems were encountered with the first treatment.

65. Since young female worms are most resistant, isn't it a waste of time to retreat within a few months of the first treatment?

That might be true with thiactersemide, but female worm resistance is less of a problem with melarsomine.

66. Are there any indications for surgical removal of heartworms?

Forceps removal of worms is the treatment of choice for the vena cava syndrome. Affected dogs have hundreds of worms in the venae cavae and right heart. The procedure requires considerable expertise but is highly effective and can be lifesaving.

Dogs with class III disease and echocardiographically confirmed high worm burden in the right heart and main pulmonary artery can be saved by the Ishihara technique. Under anesthesia and fluoroscopic guidance, a long, flexible Ishihara alligator forceps is introduced via a jugular vein and repeatedly passed into the heart and pulmonary arteries with multiple retrievals of none to many worms. In experienced hands, 80% or more of adult worms can be retrieved.

67. How much of the pulmonary pathology of HW disease is reversible?

Most dogs will experience significant improvement, even if a few worms persist. Even dogs with class III disease can be saved, although the risk of mortality is high during the first month after administration of adulticide therapy. These dogs may never improve enough to allow vigorous exertion, but many return to adequate functional status. Unfortunately, some of the most severely affected never experience enough pulmonary pathology improvement to survive. In addition, some dogs whose treatment appears to be complete develop severe pulmonary hypertension months later.

Presumably some "point-of-no-return" had been reached and the disease progressed after adulticide. The exact factors responsible for such progression are unknown.

68. What steps can be taken to minimize the risk of severe thromboembolic lung disease after treatment?

The first step is a good pretreatment evaluation so that high-risk patients (with class III disease) can be identified. The alternative protocol is recommended for class III. Severe restriction of activity for 4–6 weeks after treatment is imperative. Although controversial, aspirin (5–7 mg/kg once daily) or heparin (75 U/kg 3 times/day subcutaneously) can be administered prior to (1–3 weeks), during, and for 3–7 weeks after adulticide. Such treatment is naturally combined with strict confinement. This approach is recommended only for the most severely affected dogs.

Some veterinarians administer corticosteroids for 1–2 weeks after treatment. This may reduce the severity of inflammation, fever, and coughing. Corticosteroids do promote coagulation and decreased pulmonary blood flow so that their use should be not longer than 1–2 weeks.

69. How much toxicity is one likely to see after melarsomine treatment?

The therapeutic index is relatively low and the lungs are the most susceptible to overdosage. At 2.5 mg/kg, adverse effects are common but mild and include lethargy, anorexia, fever, and vomiting. Tenderness at the injection site is common but of short duration and is probably due to drug leakage out of the needle tract. Therefore, digital pressure should be applied during needle withdrawal and for 1–2 minutes thereafter.

70. Should dogs with congestive heart failure (ascites) be treated?

All dogs with class III disease should be evaluated carefully. Many can be treated successfully but mortality is greater than with dogs in class I and II. If the mucous membranes are gray or cyanotic, dyspnea is severe and constant, or if the dog is anorexic, obviously unhappy, and in distress, death is the likely outcome. However, if the dog is eating, has at least pale pink mucous membranes, does not require oxygen supplementation, and looks reasonably happy, there is at least a 75% chance of survival. Among the patients, in class III, the subset with ascites does not necessarily have a worse prognosis.

71. What about diuretics and cardiac drugs for dogs with congestive heart failure?

Furosemide 1–2 mg/kg 2 times/day and a low-salt diet are recommended. Angiotensin-converting enzyme inhibitors such as enalapril seem to help, but should be initiated at a low dosage (0.25 mg/kg, once daily). The dosage is based on the estimated lean weight. The dosage is gradually increased every several days (0.25 mg/kg 2 times/day) to a maximum of 0.5 mg/kg 2 times/day. Hypotension is a potential complication of vasodilator use in dogs with right-sided congestive heart failure and fixed pulmonary arterial resistance. Digoxin is notoriously ineffective for cor pulmonale. Hydralazine and diltiazem should not be administered since they usually cause systemic hypotension in patients with class III disease.

72. Do corticosteroids reduce the efficacy of adulticide treatment?

This is controversial and based on observations in one study of thiacetarsamide. A major impact of corticosteroids on melarsomine kill-rates is unlikely.

73. What is the treatment recommendation if hemoglobinuria occurs with HW disease?

Immediate, strict cage confinement and heparin (200 U/kg IV, followed by 75 U/kg subcutaneously 3 times/day). Oxygen therapy is advisable since hemoglobinuria is usually associated with class III disease and thromboembolism; oxygen is the only practical and effective way to dilate the pulmonary arteries. Short-term corticosteroid treatment (1.0 mg/kg once or twice daily) may be of value. Treatment is continued until there is clinical, radiographic, and laboratory evidence of marked improvement.

74. Is it necessary to treat microfilariae?

The American Heartworm Society recommends that microfilariae be treated. Because microfilariae produce little pathology, some veterinarians have chosen not to treat them in collies and related breeds. Furthermore, because of a low incidence of adverse reactions in all breeds, some veterinarians have elected to skip microfilarial treatment and prescribe prophylaxis.

75. Is there a good reason to treat microfilariae?

The primary reason is that a dog with persisting microfilariae serves as a reservoir for spreading HW infection.

76. When should microfilaricide treatment be administered?

Usually such treatment is given 3–4 weeks after adulticide in microfilaremic dogs.

77. Is ivermectin or milbemycin the preferred microfilaricide drug?

Both drugs are highly effective but neither are FDA approved for this use. Nonetheless, either drug can be used for this purpose.

Milbemycin is easier to use than ivermectin since the preventative dosage (500–999 µg/kg) is acutely microfilaricidal. The microfilaricidal dosage of ivermectin is 50 µg/kg (10 times the prophylactic dosage). Although the large dosage formulation (272 µg) can be used for a 5-kg dog, most HW infected dogs are medium to large-sized and this approach would thus be expensive. More often the cattle product, Ivomec (10,000 µg/ml) is diluted 1:10 with propylene glycol (suitable for storage) or water (for immediate use) yielding a concentration of 1000 µg/ml to be given at a dosage of 1 ml/20 kg. Most dogs object to the taste of propylene glycol. The parenteral route is not recommended for ivermectin.

78. How effective is the treatment?

Most (> 90%) microfilariae are killed by one dose of ivermectin (50 µg/kg) or milbemycin. A microfilaria detection test is performed 3–4 weeks later, and if positive, the treatment can be repeated.

79. Is it necessary to repeat the treatment?

Since most microfilariae are killed by the first dose, the rest can be killed over a period of 5–7 months simply by initiating macrolide prophylaxis. A low level of microfilaremia is not likely to serve as a good reservoir source.

80. Are adverse effects likely?

This depends on the microfilarial concentration. These drugs kill most of the microfilariae in less than 24 hours. If the count is very high, acute vomiting, diarrhea, and a degree of circulatory collapse can occur. The overall incidence of adverse reactions is less than 10% and is usually restricted to vomiting, diarrhea, lethargy, and anorexia. However, microfilarial counts are not routinely performed. Prednisone (1 mg/kg) given with milbemycin reduces the risk of reaction to almost zero.

81. When do reactions occur?

Most reactions begin within a few hours. Therefore, it is recommended that the treatment be given in the morning and the dog discharged in the late afternoon. Occasionally, mild lethargy and anorexia develop the following day and persist for 1–2 days.

82. Is death possible?

At recommended dosages, even more severe reactions, if detected quickly, are treatable with IV fluids and soluble corticosteroid (IV) administration. Therefore, each dog should be observed closely.

83. Is there any advantage to one or another HW preventative drug?

In general, the monthly prophylactic drugs have supplanted daily prophylaxis for the reason of convenience. All are highly effective and safe.

84. How long does it take for microfilariae to disappear from the blood in dogs given ivermectin prophylaxis?

Approximately 5–8 months.

85. Which prophylactic is safest to administer to a dog with circulating microfilaria?

The prophylactic dosage of ivermectin does not kill microfilariae quickly and therefore an acute reaction is rare. Milbemycin is acutely microfilaricidal and therefore some dogs will experience an adverse reaction during the first 48 hours.

86. Should year-round prophylaxis be maintained?

In the southeastern US, year-round prevention is maintained even though transmission is not likely during December and January in states such as Georgia. Prophylaxis should not be interrupted in Florida or the coastlines of the southeastern U.S., the Carribean region, and Hawaii.

In the midwest and further north wherever heartworm infection is known to occur, macrolide prophylaxis should be started by May or June and continued until October to December. The average daily temperature must be above 57°F for larval maturation to occur in time for transmission to a host.

87. Can ivermectin or milbemycin be given bimonthly?

Alternate month administration is effective, but not recommended.

88. Do the macrolide prophylactic drugs kill heartworms?

Both ivermectin and milbemycin, if given on a monthly basis starting 4 months or less post-inoculation with infective larvae (L3) and continued for 1 year or longer, will prevent the development of persistent adult infection. Ivermectin is approximately 98% effective.

89. Does a monthly dose of ivermectin kill preexisting adult HW infections?

Recent studies have demonstrated that adult infections can be terminated over a period of 18–24 months of administration.

90. Are ivermectin and milbemycin safe in collies?

High-dose ivermectin ($\geq$ 100 µg/kg) can cause serious toxicity in a subset (one-third) of collies wherein the drug can cross the blood-brain barrier. Both the preventative dose and recommended ivermectin microfilaricidal dose (50 µg/kg) are not more dangerous for this type of dog than others. Toxic dosages produce varying (dose-related) severities of hypersalivation, mydriasis, blindness, ataxia, bradycardia, decreased respiration, coma, and death.

91. Is milbemycin safer for collies than ivermectin?

No, the same collies that react to a 4 or more times ($\geq$ 200 µg/kg) dose of ivermectin will also react to a proportionately high dose of milbemycin.

92. Is diethylcarbamazine (DEC) still an acceptable prophylactic drug?

Yes. This drug has stood the test of time. At 5.5 mg/kg once daily, DEC is safe and highly effective. Extended parasite control is provided by the addition of oxybendazole, with a slight risk of reversible hepatotoxicity.

A microfilarial concentration test must be negative before DEC is initiated. The drug should be started at least 2 weeks before the mean daily temperature is above 57°F, and for 2 months after either the temperature drops below this level or the first frost. Year-round treatment is recommended if the mean daily temperature is less than 60°F for no more than 3 months.

The uncommon periportal hepatitis associated with DEC-oxybendazole is potentially lethal, reversible, and can be potentiated by concomitant phenobarbitol administration.

BIBLIOGRAPHY

1. Calvert CA, Rawlings CA, McCall JW: Canine heartworm. In Fox PR, Sisson D, Moise NS (eds): Textbook of Canine and Feline Cardiology: Principles and Clinical Practice, 2nd ed. Philadelphia, W.B. Saunders, 1999.
2. Case JL, Tanner PA, Keister DM, et al: A clinical field study of melarsomine dihydrochloride (RM340) in dogs with severe (class 3) heartworm disease. In Soll MD, Knight DH (eds): Proceedings of the Heartworm Symposium. Batavia, IL, American Heartworm Society, 1995.
3. DiSacco B, Vezzoni A: Clinical classification of heartworm disease for the purpose of adding objectively to the assessment of therapeutic efficacy of adulticidal drugs in the field. In Soll MD (ed): Proceedings of the Heartworm Symposium. Batavia, IL, American Heartworm Society, 1992.
4. Ishihara K, Sasaki Y, Kitagawa H: Development of a flexible alligator forceps: A new instrument for removal of heartworms in the pulmonary arteries of dogs. Jpn J Vet Sci 48:989–995, 1986.
5. Jackson RE: Surgical treatment of heartworm disease. J Am Vet Med Assoc 154:383–388, 1969.
6. Keith JC, Schaub RG, Rawlings C: Early arterial injury-induced myointimal proliferation in canine pulmonary arteries. Am J Vet Res 44:181–188, 1983.
7. McCall JW, McTeir TL, Supakorndej N, et al: Clinical prophylactic activity of macrolides on young adult heartworms, In Soll MD, Knight FH (eds): Proceedings of the Heartworm Symposium. Batavia, IL, American Heartworm Society, 1995.
8. Miller MW, Keister MD, Tanner PA, et al: Clinical efficacy of melarsomine dihydrochloride (RM340) and thiacetarsemide in dogs with moderate (class 2) heartworm disease. In Soll MD, Knight DH (eds): Proceedings of the Heartworm Symposium. Batavia, IL, American Heartworm Society, 1995.
9. Rawlings CA, Dawe DL, McCall JW, et al: Four types of occult *Dirofiolaria immitis* infections in dogs. J Am Vet Med Assoc 180:1323–1330, 1982.
10. Rawlings CA, Keith JCJ, Losonsky JM, et al: An aspirin-prednisone combination to modify postadulticide lung disease in heartworm infected dogs. Am J Vet Res 45:2371–2375, 1984.
11. Rawlings CA, Losonsky JM, Schaub RG, et al: Postadulticide changes in *Dirofilaria immitis*-infected beagles. Am J Vet Res 44:8–14, 1983.
12. Rawlings CA, Raynaud JP, Lewis R, et al: Pulmonary thromboembolism and hypertension after thiacetarsemide vs. melarsomine dihydrochloride treatment of *Dirofilaria immitis* infection in dogs. Am J Vet Res 54:920–929, 1992.
13. Schaub RG, Keith JCJ, Rawlings CA: Effect of acetylsalicylic acid vascular damage and myointimal proliferation in canine pulmonary arteries subjected to chronic injury by *Dirofilaria immitis*. Am J Vet Res 44:449–455, 1983.
14. Vezzoni A, Genchi C: Reduction of post-adulticide thromboembolism complications with low dose heparin therapy. In Otto GF (ed): Proceedings of the Heartworm Symposium. Washington, DC, American Heartworm Society, 1989.

59. FELINE HEARTWORM DISEASE

Jonathan A. Abbott, D.V.M.

1. What is feline heartworm disease? Is it caused by the same organism that is responsible for heartworm disease in the dog?

Heartworm disease is a consequence of infestation by parasite *Dirofilaria immitis*, a filarial nematode. Adult worms reside in the pulmonary arteries, and occasionally in the right atrium, ventricle, and cavae of carnivores. Embryonic larval forms of the worm, the microfilariae, are released by the gravid female into the bloodstream of the host. Mosquitoes that consume microfilariae during a blood meal are the obligate vectors for heartworm transmission.

2. Is heartworm infestation different from heartworm disease?

Because the presence of a small number of worms can result in histologic pulmonary artery abnormalities, the distinction between infestation, the presence of heartworms, and heartworm disease as the clinical syndrome that results from the presence of the worms is somewhat arbitrary. However, since heartworm infection does not necessarily result in clinical signs, many authors distinguish between heartworm disease and heartworm infestation.

3. How does feline heartworm disease differ from canine heartworm disease?

The cat is susceptible to heartworm infestation, but it is a more resistant host compared to the dog. In general, the worm burden of infected cats is low and patent infections are uncommon; as a result, the cat is not an important host for the heartworm since microfilariae generally must be obtained from a dog with a patent infection for spread of the parasite. Heartworm longevity is less in the cat than in the dog. In the feline host the life span is usually less than 2 years. In contrast, heartworms in the canine host may live 5–7 years. Heartworms tend to grow to a larger size in the dog than in the cat. Worm burdens in cats are usually smaller than in the dog; most cats have five or fewer worms, while a heavily infected dog might harbor more than 100 organisms. In part this is likely due to the fact that, relative to the dog, few infective larvae mature to adulthood in the cat. However, it is important to recognize that relatively low worm-burdens can have devastating clinical consequences in the cat.

4. Describe the pathogenesis of feline heartworm disease.

The final larval stage of *D. immitis* penetrates a systemic vein and is carried to the pulmonary arteries where maturation is completed. Sloughing of arterial endothelium occurs shortly after contact with adult heartworms; this damage to the arterial intima initiates an inflammatory cascade. Growth factors are released from platelets and leukocytes, which results in smooth muscle hyperplasia. A villous endarteritis characterized by myointimal proliferation results. Protuberances from the tunica muscularis extend into the vessel lumen, reducing the cross-sectional area of the pulmonary vascular lumen; potentially, there is an increase in pulmonary vascular resistance, which results in the development of pulmonary hypertension. Embolism of dead and dying adult worms contributes to increases in pulmonary vascular resistance.

However, clinical signs such as right-sided congestive failure are relatively uncommon in the cat; more often, the disease is manifest clinically when lung injury results in cough and dyspnea. The inflammatory response to the presence of heartworms increases pulmonary vascular permeability, which can cause local, noncardiogenic edema and the perivascular accumulation of inflammatory cells. These abnormalities likely explain some of the radiographic abnormalities and respiratory clinical signs associated with FHD. Additionally, the arrival of late-stage larvae in the pulmonary arteries induces the development of diffuse pulmonary infiltrates and, potentially, an eosinophilic pneumonitis.

5. What is occult heartworm disease?

Heartworm infection is said to be occult when microfilariae are not detected in the peripheral blood. Occult heartworm disease may develop in untreated patients under the following circumstances: (1) when there is immune mediated destruction of microfilariae; (2) the infection is pre-patent; (3) the adult heartworms are of the same sex; or (4) the worm burden is low and the sexes are physically separate.

Additionally, while generally not of great importance in the cat, the monthly administration of macrolide heartworm-preventive drugs such as ivermectin suppresses microfilaria production and can result in the development of occult infection. Most cats are infected with relatively few worms and the immunologic response to heartworms tends to be vigorous. As a result, occult heartworm infection is common and, from a diagnostic point of view, is of great clinical importance in the cat.

6. What is aberrant heartworm migration? What is its clinical importance?

While the cat is susceptible to heartworm infestation, it is not the preferred host for the organism; possibly because of this, the incidence of clinical signs related to the presence of heartworms in aberrant locations is higher than it is in the dog. Heartworms have been detected in the aorta, pleural space, and central nervous system of infected cats; clinical signs may result from the local effects of the parasite.

7. What is the prevalence of heartworm disease in the cat?

Based on surveys of veterinary practitioners in the U.S., FHD has been diagnosed in 38 states. Feline heartworm disease is less common than heartworm disease in the dog; the prevalence of feline heartworm infestation in any given geographical area is generally 5–20% of the comparable figure for dogs.

8. What signalment is typical for cats with heartworm infection?

Heartworm infection is most commonly confirmed in middle-aged male cats, although FHD has been reported in cats as young as 1 year and as old as 17. Breed predispositions for the development of feline heartworm infection are not recognized. Cats that spend part or all of their time out of doors are more prone to heartworm infestation, although FHD is also observed in cats that reside entirely indoors.

9. What are the typical historical findings?

Heartworm infestation in cats does not necessarily result in clinical signs. When clinical signs are observed, they may develop acutely as a result of pulmonary embolism of dead worms or aberrant migration of late-stage larvae. In such cases, clinical signs may include dyspnea, hemoptysis, circulatory collapse, head tilt, and blindness. Alternatively, clinical signs may be of a more chronic nature. Cough, dyspnea, vomiting, lethargy, and weight loss may be observed in affected cats. Sudden death is a relatively common manifestation of FHD. Signs of cor pulmonale, such as ascites, are uncommon in the cat.

10. What abnormalities are detected during physical examination of feline patients with heartworm disease?

Physical findings in FHD are generally nonspecific; dyspnea or poor body condition may be evident on inspection. Auscultation may reveal a cardiac murmur, gallop rhythm, diminished lung sounds, or adventitious pulmonary sounds. Right-sided congestive heart failure is an uncommon sequel of FHD; however, when present, jugular distention and ascites may be evident.

11. Is routine hematology helpful in the diagnosis of FHD?

Eosinophilia or basophilia may be associated with the development of FHD. However, these findings are transient and detected only in a relatively small subpopulation of cats with FHD. Further, in a prospective study the prevalence of eosinophilia or basophilia was not significantly greater than the prevalence of these abnormalities in cats with cardiorespiratory signs that did not have FHD. Thus, the presence of eosinophilia or basophilia might heighten diagnostic suspicion of FHD, but otherwise it has limited diagnostic utility.

12. What factors complicate the diagnosis of FHD?

FHD exhibits a number of features that make the diagnosis difficult. The clinical signs are varied and poorly localized, few infections are patent (i.e., most cats with FHD have occult disease), and the prevalence of FHD is, or at least is perceived to be, low and diagnostic efforts may be limited as a consequence.

13. How is a diagnosis of FHD made?

Potentially, a diagnosis of FHD can be made by any of the following methods:
* Examination of whole blood for the presence of microfilariae
* Serologic tests: (1) immunofluorescent antibody (IFA) test for antibodies directed against microfilarial antigens; (2) enzyme-linked immunosorbent assay (ELISA) for antibodies directed against adult antigens; and (3) ELISA for adult antigens
* Echocardiographic examination

14. Which of these diagnostic methods is superior?

If microfilaremia develops in cats with FHD, it is generally transient and associated with low numbers of microfilariae. Because of this and because occult FHD is common, tests that document the presence of microfilariae have low sensitivity and distinct limitations. IFA tests for the presence of antibodies against microfilarial antigens have been used to elucidate the biology of FHD, but do not generally have a clinical application. ELISA for adult antigens has a great utility in the diagnosis of canine heartworm disease. In the cat, low worm burdens reduce the sensitivity of the test; however, a positive test is virtually certain evidence that adult heartworms are present in the circulation.

Commercially available ELISA kits that test for antibodies against heartworms may have the greatest utility in the diagnosis of FHD. A negative result means, with near certainty, that the patient does not have FHD; however, a positive result has less clinical utility. The presence of antibodies indicates exposure to larval forms of the parasite and potentially could mean one of the following: (1) adult heartworms are present in the circulation; (2) past, now resolved infection; (3) larval forms (L4 or immature L5) are present; or (4) ectopic infection.

15. What is the role of radiography in the diagnosis and management of FHD?

Radiographic abnormalities in patients with FHD may include enlargement of the caudal pulmonary arteries and the presence of interstitial, bronchointerstitial, or alveolar pulmonary densities. Enlargement of the cardiac silhouette and pleural effusion may also be evident. However, radiographic abnormalities in FHD are inconsistent and may have similarities with other cardiorespiratory diseases that limit the utility of radiography as a screening test for FHD. When other diagnostic tests indicate the presence of heartworm, radiography may provide useful prognostic information.

16. What is the role of echocardiography in the diagnosis and management of FHD?

Heartworms may be visible as linear echogenicities in infected cats; the worms may be detected in the main pulmonary artery, the right ventricle, or occasionally the right atrium. Echocardiographic visualization of heartworms is confirmation of infection. However, the ability to detect heartworms depends on the index of suspicion and technical skill of the operator.

17. What therapy is recommended for patients with confirmed feline heartworm disease?

Therapy for FHD is controversial. The adverse effects of arsenical heartworm adulticides may be greater in cats than in dogs; noncardiogenic edema has been observed in healthy cats following the administration of thiacetarsemide. Additionally, clinical deterioration associated with pulmonary thromboembolism following worm death can be catastrophic and appears to be common in cats. Because the life span of heartworms in cats is generally less than 2 years, some advocate conservative therapy of respiratory signs using anti-inflammatory doses of corticosteroids as an alternative to adulticide administration. However, peracute presentations associated with spontaneous worm death can have devastating consequences and because it is difficult to predict such an occurrence, adulticide administration can be justified in some cases. Patients in whom a diagnosis of FHD is confirmed should receive heartworm prophylaxis in order to prevent reinfection.

18. How is thromboembolism associated with FHD treated?

Pulmonary thromboembolism associated with spontaneous worm death or the administration of heartworm adulticide can result in marked clinical deterioration. Clinical signs may include dyspnea, circulatory collapse, cough, and hemoptysis. The administration of injectable corticosteroids is indicated as are supportive measures that may include supplemental oxygen administration, cage rest, and the administration of intravenous fluids.

19. Is aspirin indicated in the management of FHD?

The administration of standard doses of aspirin does not alter the development of pulmonary artery lesions in experimentally infected cats and the use of aspirin is not recommended.

20. What is the prognosis in FHD?

The prognosis associated with feline heartworm infection is variable. In some cases, feline heartworm infection does not result in clinical signs, while in others severe morbidity or death is the result.

21. Is FHD preventable? Is heartworm prophylaxis for cats necessary?

Feline heartworm infestation can be prevented by the monthly administration of macrolide endectocides; both ivermectin and milbemycin are approved by the FDA for this purpose. The need for heartworm prophylaxis depends on the geographic region in which the cat resides. The diagnostic difficulties and risks associated with feline heartworm infection justify the use of prophylaxis in highly endemic regions.

BIBLIOGRAPHY

1. Atkins CE, Ryan WG: CVT Update: Diagnosis and prevention of heartworm disease in cats. In Bonagura JD: Current Veterinary Therapy XIII-Small Animal Practice. Philadelphia, W.B. Saunders, 2000, pp 782–787.
2. Atkins CE, DeFrancesco TD, Miller M, et al: Prevalence of heartworm infection in cats with signs of cardiorespiratory abnormalities. J Am Vet Med Assoc 212:571–520, 1997.
3. DeFrancesco TD, Atkins CE, Miller MW, et al: Diagnostic utility of echocardiography in feline heartworm disease. In Soll MD, Knight DH (eds): Proceedings of the American Heartworm Symposium '98. Batavia, IL, American Heartworm Society, 1998.
4. Dillon R: Feline heartworm disease. In Fox PR, Sisson D, Moise NS (eds): Textbook of Canine and Feline Cardiology: Principles and Clinical Practice. Philadelphia, W.B. Saunders, 2000, pp 727–735.
5. Kittleson MD: Heartworm infestation and disease (dirofilariasis). In Kittleson MD, Kienle RD: Small Animal Cardiovascular Medicine. St Louis, Mosby, 1998, pp 370–401.
6. Rawlings CA, Farrell RL, Mahood RM: Morphologic changes in the lungs of cats experimentally infected with *Dirofilaria immitis*-response to aspirin. J Vet Intern Med 4:292–300, 1990.

INDEX

Page numbers in **boldface type** indicate complete chapters.